# Hair Transplantation

## Procedures in Cosmetic Dermatology

**Series Editor: Jeffrey S. Dover MD FRCPC**
**Associate Editor: Murad Alam MD**

**Botulinum Toxin**
*Alastair Carruthers MABM BCh FRCPC FRCP(Lon) and Jean Carruthers MD FRCS(C) FRC(OPHTH)*
*ISBN 1 4160 2470 0*

**Soft Tissue Augmentation**
*Jean Carruthers MD FRCS(C) FRC(OPHTH) and Alastair Carruthers MABM BCh FRCPC FRCP(Lon)*
*ISBN 1 4160 2469 7*

**Cosmeceuticals**
*Zoe Diana Draelos MD*
*ISBN 1 4160 0244 8*

**Laser and Lights: Volume 1**
Vascular • Pigmentation • Scars • Medical Applications
*David J. Goldberg MD JD*
*ISBN 1 4160 2386 0*

**Laser and Lights: Volume 2**
Rejuvenation • Resurfacing • Hair Removal • Treatment of Ethnic Skin
*David J. Goldberg MD JD*
*ISBN 1 4160 2387 9*

**Photodynamic Therapy**
*Mitchel P. Goldman MD*
*ISBN 1 4160 2360 7*

**Liposuction**
*C. William Hanke MD MPH FACP and Gerhard Sattler MD*
*ISBN 1 4160 22082*

**Scar Revision**
*Kenneth A. Arndt MD*
*ISBN 1 4160 31316*

**Chemical Peels**
*Mark G. Rubin MD*
*ISBN 1 4160 30719*

**Hair Transplantation**
*Robert S. Haber MD and Dowling B. Stough MD*
*ISBN 1 4160 31049*

**Treatment of Leg Veins**
*Murad Alam MD and Tri H. Nguyen MD*
*ISBN 1 4160 31596*

**Blepharoplasty**
*Ronald L. Moy MD and Edgar F. Fincher MD PhD*
*ISBN 1 4160 29966*

**Advanced Face Lifting**
*Ronald L. Moy MD and Edgar F. Fincher MD PhD*
*ISBN 1 4160 29974*

PROCEDURES IN COSMETIC DERMATOLOGY

Series Editor: Jeffrey S. Dover MD FRCPC

Associate Editor: Murad Alam MD

# Hair Transplantation

**Edited by**

**Robert S. Haber** MD FAAD FAAP

Assistant Professor, Dermatology and Pediatrics, Case Western Reserve University School of Medicine; Director, University Hair Transplant Center, Cleveland, OH, USA

**Dowling B. Stough** MD

Medical Director, The Dermatology Clinic, Hot Springs, AR; Clinical Assistant Professor, Department of Dermatology, University of Arkansas for Medical Sciences, Little Rock, AR, USA

**Series Editor**

**Jeffrey S. Dover** MD FRCPC

Associate Professor of Clinical Dermatology, Yale University School of Medicine, Adjunct Professor of Medicine (Dermatology), Dartmouth Medical School, Director, SkinCare Physicians of Chestnut Hill, Chestnut Hill, MA, USA

**Associate Editor**

**Murad Alam** MD

Chief, Section of Cutaneous and Aesthetic Surgery, Department of Dermatology, Northwestern University, Chicago, IL, USA

ELSEVIER
SAUNDERS

ELSEVIER
SAUNDERS

An imprint of Elsevier Inc.

First published 2006



ISBN-10 1 4160 31049
ISBN-13 9781416031048

British Library Cataloguing in Publication Data
A catalogue record for this book is available from the British Library

Library of Congress Cataloging in Publication Data
A catalog record for this book is available from the Library of Congress

**Notice**

Medical knowledge is constantly changing. Standard safety precautions must be followed, but as new research and clinical experience broaden our knowledge, changes in treatment and drug therapy may become necessary or appropriate. Readers are advised to check the most current product information provided by the manufacturer of each drug to be administered to verify the recommended dose, the method and duration of administration, and contraindications. It is the responsibility of the practitioner, relying on experience and knowledge of the patient, to determine dosages and the best treatment for each individual patient. Neither the Publisher nor the editor assumes any liability for any injury and/or damage to persons or property arising from this publication.

**The Publisher**

Printed in China
Last digit is the print number: 9 8 7 6 5 4 3 2 1



Commissioning Editor: **Karen Bowler**
Development Editors: **Martin Mellor Publishing Services Ltd, Seán Duggan, Louise Cook**
Project Managers: **Naughton Project Management, Cheryl Brant**
Illustration Manager: **Gillian Murray**
Design Manager: **Andy Chapman**
Illustrators: **Richard Prime, Tim Loughhead**

# Contents

# Series Foreword
## Procedures in Cosmetic Dermatology

While dermatologists have been procedurally inclined since the beginning of the specialty, particularly rapid change has occurred in the past quarter century. The advent of frozen section technique and the golden age of Mohs skin cancer surgery has led to the formal incorporation of surgery within the dermatology curriculum. More recently technological breakthroughs in minimally invasive procedural dermatology have offered an aging population new options for improving the appearance of damaged skin.

Procedures for rejuvenating the skin and adjacent regions are actively sought by our patients. Significantly, dermatologists have pioneered devices, technologies and medications, which have continued to evolve at a startling pace. Numerous major advances, including virtually all cutaneous lasers and light-source based procedures, botulinum exotoxin, soft-tissue augmentation, dilute anesthesia liposuction, leg vein treatments, chemical peels, and hair transplants, have been invented, or developed and enhanced by dermatologists. Dermatologists understand procedures, and we have special insight into the structure, function, and working of skin. Cosmetic dermatologists have made rejuvenation accessible to risk-averse patients by emphasizing safety and reducing operative trauma. No specialty is better positioned than dermatology to lead the field of cutaneous surgery while meeting patient needs.

As dermatology grows as a specialty, an ever-increasing proportion of dermatologists will become proficient in the delivery of different procedures. Not all dermatologists will perform all procedures, and some will perform very few, but even the less procedurally directed amongst us must be well-versed in the details to be able to guide and educate our patients. Whether you are a skilled dermatologic surgeon interested in further expanding your surgical repertoire, a complete surgical novice wishing to learn a few simple procedures, or somewhere in between, this book and this series is for you.

The volume you are holding is one of a series entitled "Procedures in Cosmetic Dermatology." The purpose of each book is to serve as a practical primer on a major topic area in procedural dermatology.

If you want to make sure you find the right book for your needs, you may wish to know what this book is and what it is not. It is not a comprehensive text grounded in theoretical underpinnings. It is not exhaustively referenced. It is not designed to be a completely unbiased review of the world's literature on the subject. At the same time, it is not an overview of cosmetic procedures that describes these in generalities without providing enough specific information to actually permit someone to perform the procedures. And importantly, it is not so heavy that it can serve as a doorstop or a shelf filler.

What this book and this series offer is a step-by-step, practical guide to performing cutaneous surgical procedures. Each volume in the series has been edited by a known authority in that subfield. Each editor has recruited other equally practical-minded, technically skilled, hands-on clinicians to write the constituent chapters. Most chapters have two authors to ensure that different approaches and a broad range of opinions are incorporated. On the other hand, the two authors and the editors also collectively provide a consistency of tone. A uniform template has been used within each chapter so that the reader will be easily able to navigate all the books in the series. Within every chapter, the authors succinctly tell it like they do it. The emphasis is on therapeutic technique; treatment methods are discussed with an eye to appropriate indications, adverse events, and unusual cases. Finally, this book is short and can be read in its entirety on a long plane ride. We believe that brevity paradoxically results in greater information transfer because cover-to-cover mastery is practicable.

Most of the books in the series are accompanied by a high-quality DVD, demonstrating the procedures discussed in that text. Some of you will turn immediately to the DVD and use the text as a backup to clarify complex points, while others will prefer to read first and then view the DVD to see the steps in action. Choose what suits you best.

We hope you enjoy this book and the rest of the books in the series and that you benefit from the many hours of clinical wisdom that have been distilled to produce it. Please keep it nearby, where you can reach for it when you need it.

*Jeffrey S. Dover MD, FRCPC and*
*Murad Alam MD*

To the women in my life

My grandmothers, Bertha and Lillian
My mother, Nina
My daughters, Sophie and Isabel
And especially to my wife, Tania

For their never-ending encouragement, patience, support, love, and friendship

To my father, Mark
A great teacher and role model

To my mentor, Kenneth A. Arndt for his generosity, kindness, sense of humor, joie de vivre, and above all else curiosity and enthusiasm

At Elsevier, Sue Hodgson who conceptualized the series and brought it to reality

and

Martin Mellor for polite, persistent, and dogged determination

*Jeffrey S. Dover*

The professionalism of the dedicated editorial staff at Elsevier has made this ambitious project possible. Guided by the creative vision of Sue Hodgson, Seán Duggan and Martin Mellor have attended to the myriad tasks required to produce a state-of-the-art resource. In this, they have been ably supported by the graphics team, which has maintained production quality while ensuring portability. We are also deeply grateful to the volume editors, who have generously found time in their schedules, cheerfully accepted our guidelines, and recruited the most knowledgeable chapter authors. Finally, we thank the chapter contributors, without whose work there would be no books at all. Whatever successes are herein are due to the efforts of the above, and of my teachers, Kenneth Arndt, Jeffrey Dover, Michael Kaminer, Leonard Goldberg, and David Bickers, and of my parents, Rahat and Rehana Alam.

*Murad Alam*

# Preface

The purpose of this volume in the Dover series is to cover the tenets of hair transplantation by considering the philosophy, basic science, and techniques in a practical clinical text. The result is a practical text that covers a wealth of knowledge compressed into a digested form. The book has been an international endeavor, with professionals and true experts from around the world contributing on their area of expertise. We hope that you find it both compact and readable, with each chapter reflecting the author's style yet supporting the overall content. The concepts and philosophy are supported by videos of techniques and surgical procedures, which we believe will enhance the utility of the book.

We considered this a very important book because surgeons use their experience and knowledge daily to make sound judgments and recommendations for their patients. As in all areas of medicine, techniques and approaches evolve with advancing knowledge, and we intend this volume to provide a fund of background information of current thinking for those working in hair restoration, which will support surgeons in choosing the most effective paths to follow.

After the many, many hours that have gone into producing this volume, the editors have only a few small paragraphs to express their gratitude to all those who have contributed so much of their expertise and time. We must also acknowledge the large debt owed to the dedicated individuals who built the foundation of hair restoration surgery. We have been lucky in that we have been able to combine close friendship with the opportunity to write, compose, and edit this volume. We are indebted to each other as co-editors of this volume. Dow Stough has appreciated Robert Haber's organizational skills, wisdom, common sense and large breadth of knowledge, which are evident in every chapter. Robert Haber has been honored to work with one of the world's most respected hair surgeons, and collaborating with him on this textbook has demonstrated how much that respect is deserved. We are most grateful to Dr. Jeffrey Dover, senior editor of the Dover series, for the opportunity to write this book and must thank Martin Mellor and the team at Elsevier Publishing for their professionalism and the ability to organize, provide encouragement, and keep the process on course. We also would like to thank our secretaries, Deborah Barrett and Darla Kelsay, for the extra work that the book has entailed and for enduring with grace our occasionally frazzled attitudes. We also regret the precious time stolen from our families, whose support has enabled us to complete this volume. Thank you to the Stoughs: Shannon, Burke, Bradley, and Sara. And thanks also to the Habers: Maxwell and Isabel.

*Robert S. Haber MD and Dowling B. Stough MD*

# List of Contributors

**Marc R. Avram** MD
Clinical Associate Professer in Dermatology, Weill Cornell Medical School; Private Practice, New York, NY, USA

**Michael Beehner** MD
Medical Director, Saratoga Hair Transplant Center, Saratoga Springs, NY, USA

**Robert M. Bernstein** MD FAAD
Associate Clinical Professor, Department of Dermatology, College of Physicians and Surgeons, Columbia University; Director, Private Practice, Bernstein Medical Center for Hair Restoration, New York, NY, USA

**Bernard Cohen** MD
Voluntary Professor, University of Miami School of Medicine, Department of Dermatology and Cutaneous, Miami, FL, USA

**Jerry E. Cooley** MD
Director, Private Practice, The Hair Center, Charlotte, NC, USA

**Robert S. Haber** MD FAAD FAAP
Assistant Professor, Dermatology and Pediatrics, Case Western Reserve University School of Medicine; Director, University Hair Transplant Center, Cleveland, OH, USA

**James A. Harris** MD, FACS
Clinical Instructor, University of Colorado School of Medicine, Denver; Medical Director, Hair Sciences Center of Colorado, Greenwood Village, CO, USA

**Victor Hasson** MD
Cosmetic Surgeon, Private Practice, Hasson & Wong Aesthetic Surgery, Vancouver, BC, Canada

**Francisco Jiménez** MD
Dermatologist, Private Practice, Clinic Dr. Jimenenz Acosta, Las Palmas, Spain

**Sajjad H. Khan** MD
Medical Director for ILHT Overseas Operations, Private Practice, International Laser Hair Transplant, Lahore, Pakistan; Formerly Professor, University of California, Los Angeles, CA, USA

**Shagufta Khan** MD, FAACS
Medical Director, Private Practice, International Laser Hair Transplant, San Diego, CA; Lecturer, Facial Plastic Department, University of California, San Diego, CA, USA

**Russell Knudsen** MB, BS
Private Practice, Melbourne & Sydney, Australia

**Matt L. Leavitt** MD
Medical Director, Medical Hair Restoration, Orlando, FL, USA

**Bradley Limmer** MD
Assistant Clinical Professor, Department of Internal Medicine, Division of Dermatology; Associate Clinical Professor, Department of Plastic and Reconstructive Surgery; Surgeon, Private Practice, Limmer Clinic, San Antonio, TX, USA

**Bobby L. Limmer** MD
Professor of Dermatology, University of Texas Health Sciences Center; Surgeon, Private Practice, Limmer Clinic, San Antonio, TX, USA

**Mario Marzola** MBBS
Private Practice, Norwood, SA, Australia

**William M. Parsley** MD
Associate Clinical Professor, Department of Dermatology, University of Louisville Medical Center, Louisville, KY, USA

**Damkerng Pathomvanich** MD, FACS
Consultion Staff, Bumrungrad Hospital and Vichaiyuth Hospital, Bangkok, Thailand

**Enrique Poblet** MD
Associate Professor of Pathology, Universidad de Castilla, La Mancha; Staff Pathologist, Anatomia Patologica, Hospital General Universitario, Albacete, Spain

**Carlos J. Puig** DO
Medical Hair Restoration, Houston, TX, USA

**William R. Rassman** MD
Director, Private Practice, New Hair Institute, Los Angeles, CA, USA

**Paul T. Rose** MD
Medical Director, Private Practice, Rose Hair Restoration, Tampa, FL, USA

**David Seager** MD
Private Practice, Toronto, ON, Canada

**Richard Shiell** MD
Private Practice, Melbourne, VIC, Australia

**Dowling B. Stough** MD Medical Director, The Dermatology Clinic, Hot Springs, AR; Clinical Assistant Professor, Department of Dermatology, University of Arkansas for Medical Sciences, Little Rock, AR, USA

**James E. Vogel** MD, FACS Associate Professor of Plastic Surgery, The Johns Hopkins School of Medicine, Division of Plastic Surgery, Baltimore, MA, USA

# 1 Pathogenesis and Medical Therapy of Male and Female Pattern Hair Loss

*Robert S. Haber*

## Introduction

Male and female pattern hair loss represents the clinical endpoints of two processes that may share some pathways, but which are clearly different entities. The current state of knowledge about the pathogenesis of these conditions can at best be considered incomplete, as there are no current theories that can adequately explain the variation in presentation of these conditions, nor the lack of consistent clinical response of many patients to the available therapeutic modalities.

It is difficult to understand the hair loss process if the normal state of hair growth is also poorly understood. The specific factors that determine the rate of hair growth, the timing of anagen, telogen and catagen as well as the unique programming of specialized hairs, including eyebrows and eyelashes, are in the earliest stages of identification. A better understanding of the receptors or processes that govern these functions will not only clarify the mechanisms of the disease processes, but will give rise to novel and perhaps more effective therapies.

The development of new pharmacologic remedies for hair loss has been made possible through advances in the understanding of pattern hair loss on a pathophysiologic level. It is important for practitioners of diverse specialties to understand the causes and treatments of hair loss and subsequently educate the affected population regarding how to best decide on an appropriate treatment plan. Conventional reporting methods significantly underestimate the true incidence of pattern hair loss, which is problematic in that medical management should emphasize prevention of further loss at the earliest stages. Underestimating the prevalence can negatively impact the allocation of resources devoted to the diagnosis and management of the condition.

The terminology used to describe pattern hair loss in men and women has been inconsistent. Although **androgenic alopecia** (AGA) is an appropriate term for use in men, in whom sufficient data exist to identify the combined elements of androgens and genetic susceptibility to produce predictable patterns of hair loss, this term is no longer appropriate for women, in whom other pathways are likely to predominate. In this chapter the terms **male pattern hair loss** (MPHL) and **female pattern hair loss** (FPHL) will be used to represent the respective patterns of hair loss that occur in each sex that are not related to other causes of hair loss.

## Male Pattern Hair Loss

As implied in the term androgenetic alopecia, both androgens and genetic factors work together to produce this recognized clinical hair loss pattern, and in fact the androgen receptor gene has been positively associated with MPHL. The widely held belief that a man's hair loss pattern will mirror the pattern seen in his maternal grandfather is clearly incorrect. Current evidence implicates both maternal and paternal ancestry, and can involve either an autosomal dominant and/or a polygenic inheritance pattern.

Furthermore, there may be variable penetrance, all of which makes accurately predicting future hair loss for a given individual based on his genetic family pedigree all but impossible. It is clear though, that without a built-in genetic susceptibility, pattern hair loss will not occur, regardless of the presence or levels of various hormones. It may be that future identification of subsets of balding men based on specific receptors or other factors will permit genetic classification that is more accurate.

Topical minoxidil, a potassium channel opener and a vasodilator, has been shown to effectively treat MPHL, yet no specific role for potassium channels or vasoactivity in hair loss has been determined.

## Role of Androgens in Pattern Hair Loss

The role of androgens was first identified through observations of eunuchs, who did not develop MPHL unless androgen replacement therapy was administered. The androgen most closely implicated in the expression of MPHL is dihydrotestosterone (DHT). This was determined through the study of a kindred of individuals from the Dominican Republic, in which certain males were lacking Type II 5α-reductase (5AR), and were therefore deficient in DHT. In addition to major phenotypic abnormalities, these males did not develop MPHL. Finasteride, a competitive inhibitor of Type II 5AR, was developed and found to decrease levels of DHT and effectively treat MPHL, further confirming the importance of DHT in the hair loss process.

Androgens exert their influence on hair by way of an involved pathway that begins with circulating testosterone derived from the adrenal gland or testes (Fig. 1.1). More than 97% is bound by plasma-binding proteins such as albumin and specific testosterone and corticosteroid-binding globulins, and is therefore inactive (Fig. 1.1, Step 1). The remaining free testosterone diffuses passively into skin cells (Fig. 1.1, Step 2) and is converted to DHT, a more potent metabolite, by 5AR (Fig. 1.1, Step 3). Two isoenzymes of 5AR exist, with Type I being located in the pilosebaceous unit and sebaceous gland, while Type II 5AR is found in the outer root sheath of scalp hair follicles, prostate, and dermal papillae. A protein cytosol androgen receptor then forms a complex with DHT (Fig. 1.1, Step 4), permitting transport into the cell nucleus (Fig. 1.1, Step 5). DHT induces a conformational change in the receptor, permitting binding to DNA, production of cell-specific messenger RNA (Fig. 1.1, Step 6), and synthesis of specific proteins that lead to inactivation of hair follicles (Fig. 1.1, Step 7). Alternate pathways exist for most of these steps. Testosterone can be converted to DHT in the circulation and then enter the cell, bypassing the cellular 5AR step. Testosterone might bind to a different cytosol receptor (Fig. 1.1, Step 8), enter the nucleus as a testosterone–protein complex, and induce mRNA production (Fig. 1.1, Step 9). In addition, other androgens such as dehydroepiandrosterone might enter the cell directly and then be converted to DHT. These alternate pathways might

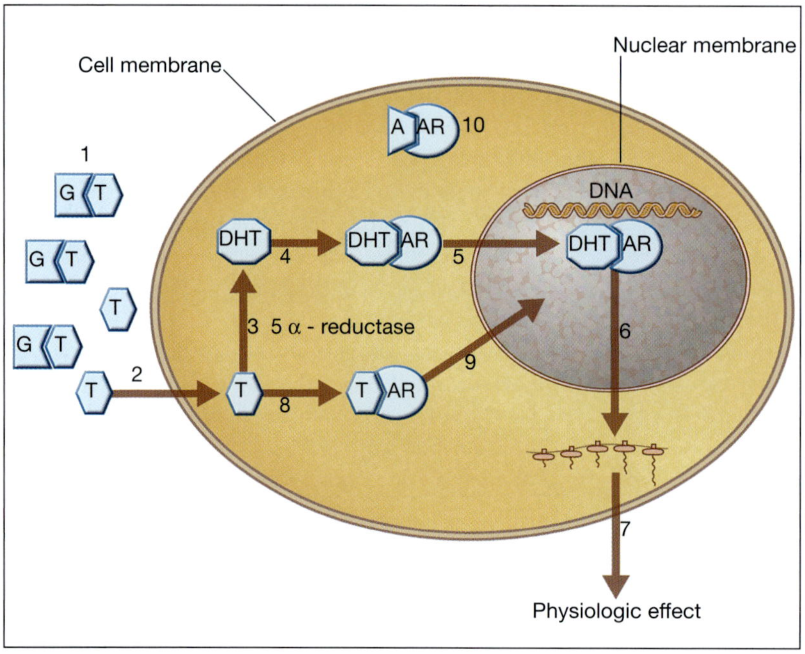


**Fig. 1.1** Key steps in androgen pathway. 1. Testosterone (T) bound to circulating binding globulins (G). 2. T enters target cell. 3. Conversion of T to dihydrotestosterone (DHT) by 5α-reductase. 4. DHT binds to cytosol androgen receptor (AR). 5. DHT-AR complex enters cell nucleus. 6. DHT-AR complex binds to DNA, producing cell-specific mRNA. 7. Protein synthesis produces physiologic effect. 8. Direct binding of T to alternate cytosol AR. 9. T-AR complex enters cell nucleus. 10. Antiandrogen (A) binds to cytosol AR

explain why some patients do not experience the expected benefits of available therapies. Many therapeutic interventions for MPHL will target one or more steps in the androgen pathway. Certain androgens, such as dihydrotestosterone, have no known beneficial role after puberty and can therefore be targeted specifically without significant concern.

There may be important roles for aromatase and adenylate cyclase in this process as well, as diminished levels of these enzymes and cyclic-AMP in association with elevated levels of DHT and 5AR are possibly associated with diminished hair growth. Unfortunately, the details of this process are not known, and no specific role has been elucidated for these enzymes. This may explain why not all men benefit from finasteride-induced DHT reduction.

The clinical effects of DHT consist of the progressive miniaturization of the terminal hair. With each successive anagen cycle, the hair grows in somewhat thinner and lighter, and the anagen phase and therefore the hair is shortened. This process may take from only a few years to many decades, but the end result is a hair that has become vellus in character (Fig. 1.2). Eventually even these vellus hairs may be lost, leaving a shiny bald scalp.

## Female Pattern Hair Loss

Accurate identification of the factors that produce FPHL has unfortunately also remained elusive. The failure of finasteride to provide clinical benefit to most women with hair loss reinforces the presumption that a pathway not involving DHT is involved.

Although the subset of women who suffer from hyperandrogenic conditions will experience pattern hair loss, often in a pattern similar to MPHL, and may therefore benefit from antiandrogen therapy, this group does not appear to represent the majority of women suffering from hair loss.

In the absence of a clearly recognized pathway, therapeutic approaches to women have been based less on science and more on experience and tradition (Box 1.1). It is perhaps ironic that minoxidil, which exerts its effects by a mechanism that is poorly understood, does often work reasonably well on FPHL, a disorder with a pathogenesis that is poorly understood. Other therapeutic modalities appear to

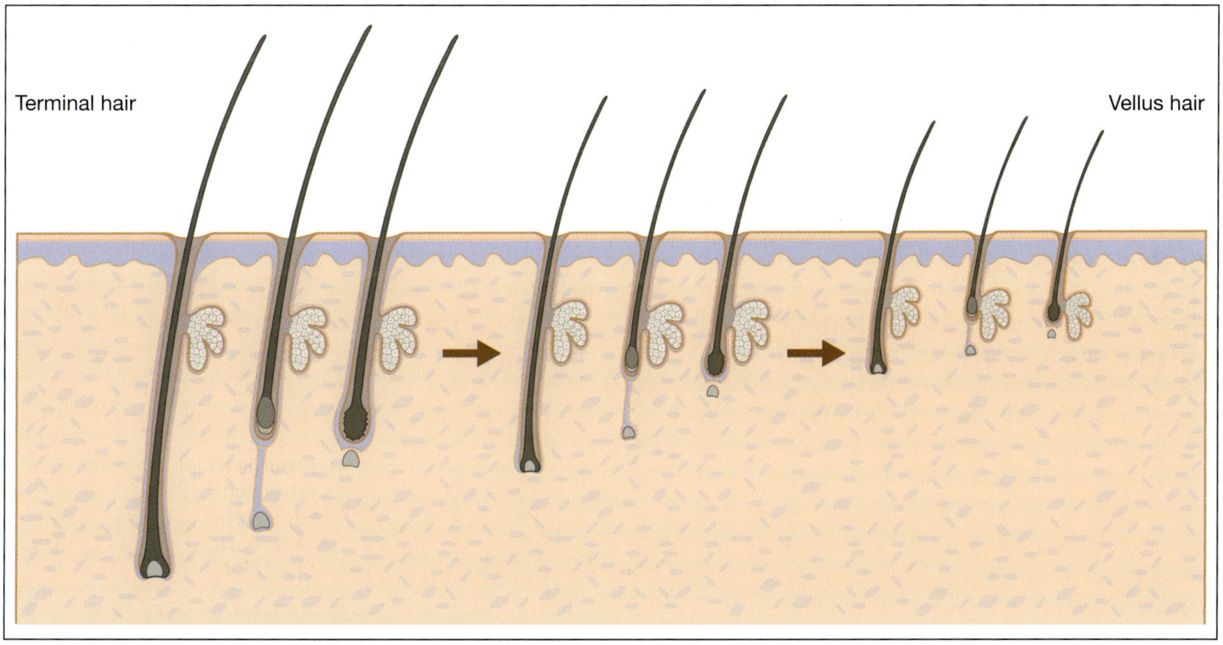


**Fig. 1.2** Miniaturization of the hair follicle in pattern hair loss. Hair grows for shorter periods of time and becomes smaller, finer, and lighter as it approaches the vellus stage (Modified with permission from Stough D, Haber RS 1996 Hair Replacement: Surgical and Medical. Mosby Year Book Publishing Company, St Louis (Modified from Stough D, Haber RS 1996 Hair replacement: Surgical and medical. Mosby Year Book Publishing Company, St Louis, with permission).

**Therapeutic approach to FPHL**

- Careful physical examination, including hair pull and trichogram
- Laboratory evaluation to rule out endocrine disorders, iron deficiency, lupus, other systemic disorders
- Consider scalp biopsy to rule out alopecia areata, telogen effluvium, inflammatory or scarring hair loss processes
- Begin topical minoxidil 2% solution
- Consider vitamin supplementation, including biotin and folic acid
- Consider hair transplantation, if appropriate
- Consider antiandrogen therapy

**Box 1.1** Therapeutic approach to FPHL

Hair growth medications and mechanism of action

| Agent | Mechanism of action |
|---|---|
| Minoxidil | Topical hypertrichotic agent. Calcium channel opener, vasodilator |
| Finasteride | Type II 5AR blockade |
| Fluridil | Topical anti-androgen |
| Dutasteride | Type I and Type II 5AR blockade |
| Flutamide | Systemic nonsteroidal antiandrogen |
| Spironolactone | Systemic weak antiandrogen |
| Cyproterone acetate | Systemic potent antiandrogen |
| Inocoterone acetate | Topical antiandrogen |

**Table 1.1** Hair growth medications and mechanism of action

be based on poorly substantiated beliefs in the prevalence of excess androgen in women, thereby relying on antiandrogens such as spironolactone, flutamide, and others.

## Treatment Overview

Thus far, only two classes of medications have demonstrated efficacy in the treatment of pattern alopecia: direct hypertrichotic agents, and agents that affect the androgen pathway (Table 1.1). In each category, only one medication has demonstrated sufficient efficacy to gain approval from the US Food and Drug Administration (FDA), namely minoxidil and finasteride, respectively.

## Minoxidil

Minoxidil, a potassium channel opener and vasodilator, was initially approved for use as an antihypertensive agent, and a notable side effect was hypertrichosis. The FDA approved a 2% minoxidil solution in 1988 for the treatment of pattern hair loss after studies demonstrated significantly improved hair counts in treated men, with an excellent safety profile. In 1996 2% minoxidil solution was approved as an over-the-counter medication for use in men and women who have pattern hair loss. In 1997, in an action rarely taken, the FDA approved a 5% solution of minoxidil as an over-the-counter preparation without initially approving the formulation as a prescription product.

Early speculation that topical minoxidil produced hair growth by way of vasodilation does not appear to be correct. Minoxidil enhances hair survival in tissue cultures even in the absence of a blood supply. Topical minoxidil is considered to be a nonspecific biologic response modifier with an unknown mechanism of action in hair growth.

A 48-week, double-blind, placebo-controlled, randomized, multicenter trial was undertaken to assess the efficacy and safety of a 5% minoxidil solution compared with 2% minoxidil and placebo in men. Results demonstrated a significant superiority of the 5% topical solution over the 2% topical solution and placebo, with the 5% group enjoying 45% greater hair growth and earlier onset of hair growth than those with the 2% topical solution or placebo. Notably, this study also demonstrated a greater improvement in the psychosocial perceptions of the 5% group compared with the 2% group or placebo. In women, minoxidil 2% solution increased hair counts by 29% and hair weight by 42% compared with –2.6% and 1.9% for controls, respectively, over a 32-week test period. After discontinuation of minoxidil 2% and 5% solutions, hair weight and number counts returned to placebo levels in 24 weeks. Side effects were infrequent, consisting principally of contact or irritant dermatitis in 6% of patients treated with 5% minoxidil topical solution and 2% of patients treated with 2% minoxidil topical solution. Facial hypertrichosis was reported in 3–5% of women treated with 2% minoxidil topical solution and was somewhat more frequent in the 5% minoxidil topical solution group.

Minoxidil can be an important adjunct in the treatment of patients who have MPHL who are undergoing hair transplantation surgery. Use of 2% topical minoxidil solution decreased the usual shedding seen after surgery and shortened the period required for grafted hairs to begin regrowth in a significant percentage of patients. Most, if not all, experienced hair transplant surgeons recommend the use of minoxidil or finasteride to many of their patients.

### *How to use minoxidil*

Men should be instructed to use the 5% topical solution, not the 2% topical solution, unless side effects require a change (Box 1.2). Women should be instructed to use the 2% topical solution, not the 5% topical solution, to minimize side effects, particularly hypertrichosis. The medication should be used twice daily, not once, to maximize efficacy. Patients should be instructed to use the dropper, not the spray attachment, to deliver the medication to the scalp, not the hair. A foam-based delivery vehicle is under development.

**Tips on using minoxidil**

- Men should use 5% solution
- Women should use 2% solution
- Use **twice daily** to maximize efficacy
- Apply to *scalp*, not hair
- Apply to **all thinning areas**, not just the crown
- Use **dropper**, not spray attachment
- If scalp irritation develops, consult dermatologist
- **Transient** hair loss can occur 4–8 weeks after initiation. Reassure patient about this, and **continue** medication

**Box 1.2** Tips on using minoxidil

## Blockage of Androgen Effects

Of the potential sites for androgen blockade, only two have thus far been fruitful, namely inhibition of 5AR (Fig. 1.1, Step 3) and competitive inhibition of the cytosol androgen receptor (Fig. 1.1, Step 10). Thus, medications can be broadly placed into these two categories.

## 5AR Inhibition

There are two isotypes of 5AR: type I, found throughout the body, including the skin, kidney, liver, and brain; and type II, located in scalp hair follicles, prostate, and liver. Both isotypes convert testosterone to dihydrotestosterone, the hormone responsible for MPHL in genetically susceptible men.

## Finasteride

Finasteride is a competitive inhibitor of type II 5AR (Fig. 1.1, Step 3), the isotype most common in hair follicles. Finasteride is administered orally at a dose of 1 mg/day. Several studies have demonstrated clinical efficacy of finasteride in men who have MPHL. Finasteride slowed the progression of hair loss and increased hair growth in 1553 men aged 18–41 years who were treated with finasteride 1 mg/day vs. placebo, and continued improvement was seen in an extension study of 1215 men. These patients were then followed for 5 years to evaluate the long-term safety and efficacy of finasteride. Endpoints evaluated included vertex hair counts, patient self-assessment questionnaires, investigator assessment, and global photographic assessment. Statistically significant improvement over placebo was seen for all endpoints. The long-term safety profile was excellent, with 0.3% of patients reporting loss of libido or erectile dysfunction at 5 years. Mean finasteride semen levels were 0.26 ng/mL, and the maximum level was 1.52 ng/mL – well below levels required to produce any risk to a developing fetus. No other side effects and no drug interactions have been reported. Whiting established the efficacy of finasteride in older men (aged 41–60 years) in a 24-month double-blind, randomized, placebo-controlled study of 424 men. A significant difference was seen between treated men and controls in the measured parameters of global photography, patient self-assessments, and investigator assessments. Sexual side effects were more common in this age group, with an overall incidence of 8.7% vs. 5.1% in controls, and it increased in men from the ages of 41–50 years to ages 51–60 years.

Further evidence of the effectiveness of finasteride came from a unique prospective, double-blinded study in which nine pairs of identical twins received finasteride or placebo for 12 months. Evaluations of global photographic assessments, hair counts, and patient self-assessments revealed statistically significant improvement in the treated group when compared with placebo.

Because finasteride is known to reduce serum prostate-specific antigen (PSA) levels by 30–50%, men over the age of 40 are advised to have their PSA levels doubled for interpretation (drug label data); however, because this correction might not adjust the PSA accurately, an over- or under-correction can occur, potentially resulting in unnecessary or missed diagnostic procedures. More data will be helpful in following PSA in the at-risk population.

## How to use finasteride

Finasteride works best to prevent ongoing hair loss; therefore, patients should be encouraged to begin treatment as soon as hair thinning is noted (Box 1.3). Finasteride is approved for men aged 18–41 who have mild-to-moderate MPHL in the midfrontal area, but it is widely used in men over 41 by prescribing physicians. It is crucial to stress that no change in hair density over time is not a treatment failure but rather a treatment success because ongoing hair loss could be predicted to result in significant thinning over time. Lack of clear communication of this fact to the patient is a significant cause of premature discontinuation of finasteride. It is also important to stress that although women should not take finasteride or handle crushed or broken tablets, there is no risk to a developing fetus exposed to the semen of a man on finasteride. Finasteride is not indicated in women, and it is contraindicated in women who are or might potentially become pregnant because it might cause abnormalities of the external genitalia of a male fetus (drug label data), including hypospadius and undervirilization.

**Tips on using finasteride**

- Begin use at **earliest signs** of hair loss
- Take baseline photos for future comparisons
- No change in hair density over time is **success**, not failure!
- Discuss sexual concerns at **each visit**
- If needed (rarely), prescribe sildenafil, tadalafil, or vardenafil to enhance sexual performance
- Women **should not handle** crushed or broken tablets
- Women **should not use** finasteride
- **No risk** to developing fetus exposed to semen of man on finasteride

**Box 1.3** Tips on using finasteride

## Dutasteride

Dutasteride is a potent inhibitor of type I and type II isoenzymes of 5AR (Fig. 1.1, Step 3). As a dual-blocking agent it is effective at reducing serum levels of DHT. Dutasteride was approved by the FDA in 2002 for use for benign prostatic hypertrophy (BPH), but it does not have an indication for treatment of hair loss. At the recommended dosage of 0.5 mg/day, dutasteride produces a greater than 90% reduction in serum DHT compared with finasteride, which decreases DHT by about 70% at the recommended 1 mg daily dose. Dutasteride appears to be pharmacologically more potent than finasteride, but there is no evidence yet that there is a corresponding long-term clinical benefit from this increased potency for the treatment of BPH or MPHL.

The safety of dutasteride used for MPHL has not been established. No human model exists for the blockage of type I and type II 5AR, and type I 5AR might have unknown functions thus far not identified that could have unintended untoward consequences if blocked. In fact, while type II 5AR is absent in the brain, type I 5AR is found throughout the brain tissue in children and adults of both sexes, possibly indicating an essential role in nonsex-related functions including the synthesis of neuroactive steroids or the catabolism of neurotoxic steroids. Researchers have also discovered that type I 5AR tissue levels are inversely related to tumor size in human breast cancer, suggesting a beneficial effect at least in this common malignancy.

Pharmacologic data demonstrate a half-life for dutasteride of more than 240 hours, compared with finasteride, which has a half-life of 6–8 hours. Any unacceptable adverse event would therefore be expected to persist for a considerably longer time period compared with finasteride. The potential risks of dutasteride when used for men who have MPHL should be considered.

## Systemic Androgen Receptor Blockers

Cyproterone acetate is a potent antiandrogen with a strong affinity for the androgen receptor. It exerts its effect by competing with DHT for androgen receptor binding (Fig. 1.1, Step 10). Cyproterone acetate is approved for use in Europe and has demonstrated some effectiveness for FPHL, particularly for women who have high ferritin levels. When compared with minoxidil, cyproterone acetate was found to be more effective only in women who had clinical evidence of hyperandrogenism, including acne, hirsutism, menstrual irregularities, and a high body mass index. Potential side effects, including menstrual irregularities, weight gain, breast tenderness, and the potential feminization of a male fetus, necessitates the concomitant use of oral contraceptives in women of childbearing potential.

Flutamide 250 mg, a pure nonsteroidal antiandrogen, was compared with cyproterone acetate 50 mg, finasteride 5 mg, and controls in 48 hyperandrogenic women treated daily for 1 year. Flutamide produced a reduction in Ludwig scores of 21%, whereas finasteride and cyproterone acetate did not produce statistically significant changes.

Spironolactone is a potassium-sparing diuretic with antiandrogen properties that has also demonstrated some effectiveness for FPHL (Fig. 1.1, Step 10). Its antiandrogenic properties are weak, and high dosages and long-term therapy are necessary to see any clinical benefit. Recommended doses for FPHL are in the range of 100–200 mg/day, and even at this dose, stabilization of hair loss is more likely than an increase in hair density. Spironolactone can cause menstrual irregularities and feminization of a male fetus, necessitating the concomitant use of oral contraceptives in women of childbearing potential. Hyperkalemia can also complicate treatment, and baseline and monthly monitoring of electrolytes and avoiding potassium supplements are important preventive measures.

## Topical Androgen Receptor Blockers

The development of an effective topical antiandrogen has been elusive, but the promise of a powerful medication that blocks androgen-mediated effects but has no systemic manifestations has been a much sought after 'magic bullet.' A recent report by Sovak described a new compound, fluridil, identified as a de novo synthesized topical androgen blocker with no systemic absorption (Fig. 1.1, Step 10). In a 3-month prospective study, 43 men were given 2% fluridil or placebo. Endpoints evaluated included phototrichogram, hematology, and blood chemistries at 3 months and a phototrichogram at 9 months. In subjects treated with fluridil, the anagen percentage increased from 76% to 85% at 3 months and was 87% at 9 months. No changes were noted in the placebo group and no fluridil was detected in the serum. Although exciting conceptually, additional studies are needed to confirm its efficacy and safety.

## Summary

In spite of many years of research and investigation into the pathogenesis of pattern hair loss, current understanding of this very common and unwanted condition remains incomplete. It is nonetheless crucial for the practitioner to fully understand the identified elements of the process, in order to comprehend the available therapeutic remedies, and to be able to recognize where newly identified pathways and treatments will help in the future.

Pharmacologic management of pattern hair loss is an active area of research. Understanding the proper role of pharmacology as it relates to surgical hair transplantation and nonmedical options is crucial to provide patients with the best clinical, esthetic, and psychological benefits.

## Further Reading

Anderson WR, Harris NM, Holmes SA 2002 Hormonal treatment for male-pattern hair loss: implications for cancer of the prostate? British Journal of Urology International 90:682–685

Avram MR, Cole JP, Gandelman M, et al 2002 The potential role of minoxidil in the hair transplantation setting. Dermatologic Surgery 28:894–900

Carmina E, Lobo RA 2003 Treatment of hyperandrogenic alopecia in women. Fertility and Sterility 79:91–95

Graul A, Silvestre J, Castañer J 1999 Dutasteride. Drugs of the Future 24(3):246–253

Haber RS 2004 Pharmacologic management of pattern hair loss. Facial Plastic Surgery Clinics of North America 12:181–189

Levy-Nissenbaum E, Bar-Natan M, Frydman M, Pras E 2005 Confirmation of the association between male pattern baldness and the androgen receptor gene. European Journal of Dermatology 15:339-340

Olsen EA 2001 Female pattern hair loss. Journal of the American Academy of Dermatology 45(Suppl):S70–S80

Price VH 1999 Treatment of hair loss. New England Journal of Medicine 341:964–973

Price VH, Roberts JL, Hordinsky M 2000 Lack of efficacy of finasteride in postmenopausal women with androgenetic alopecia. Journal of the American Academy of Dermatology 43:768–776

Roehrborn CG, Fuh V, Ruane P, et al 2000 Effect of finasteride 1 mg versus placebo over 48 weeks of serum PSA in men age 40–60 years with androgenic alopecia and no known prostatic disorder. Journal of Urology 163(Suppl 4):220

Sovak M, Seligson AL, Kucerova R, et al 2002 Fluridil, a rationally designed topical agent for androgenetic alopecia: first clinical experience. Dermatologic Surgery 28:678–685

Steckelbroeck S, Watzka M, Reichelt R 2001 Characterization of the 5α-reductase-3α-hydroxysteroid dehydrogenase complex in the human brain. Journal of Clinical Endocrinology and Metabolism 86:1324–1331

Stough DB, Rao NA, Kaufman KD, et al 2002 Finasteride improves male pattern hair loss in a randomized study in identical twins. European Journal of Dermatology 12:32–37

Suzuki T, Darnel AD, Akahira JL 2001 5α-reductase in human breast carcinoma: possible modulator of in situ androgenetic actions. Journal of Clinical Endocrinology and Metabolism 86:2250–2257

Vexiau P, Chaspoux C, Boudou P, et al 2002 Effects of minoxidil 2% vs. cyproterone acetate treatment on female androgenetic alopecia: a controlled, 12-month randomized trial. British Journal of Dermatology 146:992–999

Whiting DA, Olsen EA, Savin R, et al 2003 Efficacy and tolerability of finasteride 1 mg in men aged 41 to 60 years with male pattern hair loss. European Journal of Dermatology 13:150–160

# 2 Classification Systems of Alopecia and Scalp Laxity

*Russell Knudsen, Bernard Cohen*

## Introduction

Standardized descriptions of hair distribution in male pattern hair loss (MPHL) were introduced in 1941 by Hamilton, who classified the more common patterns into eight major types using a formal series of simple drawings. The system was further refined by Norwood in 1975 with four additional variations (Fig. 2.1). The Norwood scale has dominated the literature as the standard system for describing MPHL but it does not address the wide variations in hair distribution and density that actually exist.

The most popular and standard classification of female pattern hair loss (FPHL) was first introduced by Ludwig in 1977 (Fig. 2.2). It is also a series of simple drawings and has been followed by other classifications that are in disagreement. In spite of the differences between these and other classifications, it must be emphasized that MPHL and FPHL are progressive conditions and *any* classification will only, at best, describe a transient anatomic appearance.

## Norwood Classification

The Norwood classification categories are as follows:

1. Type I depicts the normal mature hairline. It pictures minimal temporal recession.
2. Type II depicts mild temporal recession with thinning along the anterior margin of the forelock. The recession is pictured as symmetrical.
3. Type III depicts the minimal amount of hair loss required for the definition of **balding** and demonstrates deep frontal recession with few or no remaining hairs.
4. Type III Vertex depicts hair loss confined to the vertex with deep frontal recession (no greater than the recession in Type III).
5. Type IV depicts significant frontal and temporal recession and frontal thinning together with sparse or absent hair in the vertex. The bridge between the frontal area and the vertex is still retained.
6. Type V depicts larger areas of frontotemporal and vertex alopecia than Type IV and only a narrow and sparse bridge separating both areas.
7. Type VI depicts **loss** of the bridge that separates the frontal and vertex areas with lateral and posterior progression of alopecia.
8. Type VII represents the most severe form of balding. The remaining horseshoe-shaped band of hair in the lower scalp is narrow. It begins anterior to the ear and extends posteriorly and bilaterally to a low point in the occiput. The preauricular hairs have receded both posteriorly and inferiorly. The remaining hair band is frequently of lower density with evidence of some miniaturization. Hair is sparse on the nape of the neck and in some cases the inferior occipital border is significantly raised.

Type A variants (Fig. 2.1) on the Norwood scale present two significant variations to the normal scale. First, recession involves the entire frontal border with no sparing of the mid-frontal zone. Second, there is no simultaneous vertex balding. Vertex balding develops from continuous posterior progression of the anterior recession.

## Less Common Patterns of Alopecia in Men

Transplant surgeons routinely see variations of MPHL that fall outside of the Norwood classification. These are usually of two types: (1) those in which a generalized thinning occurs, or (2) those in which hair persists within a single zone in spite of nearby hair loss.

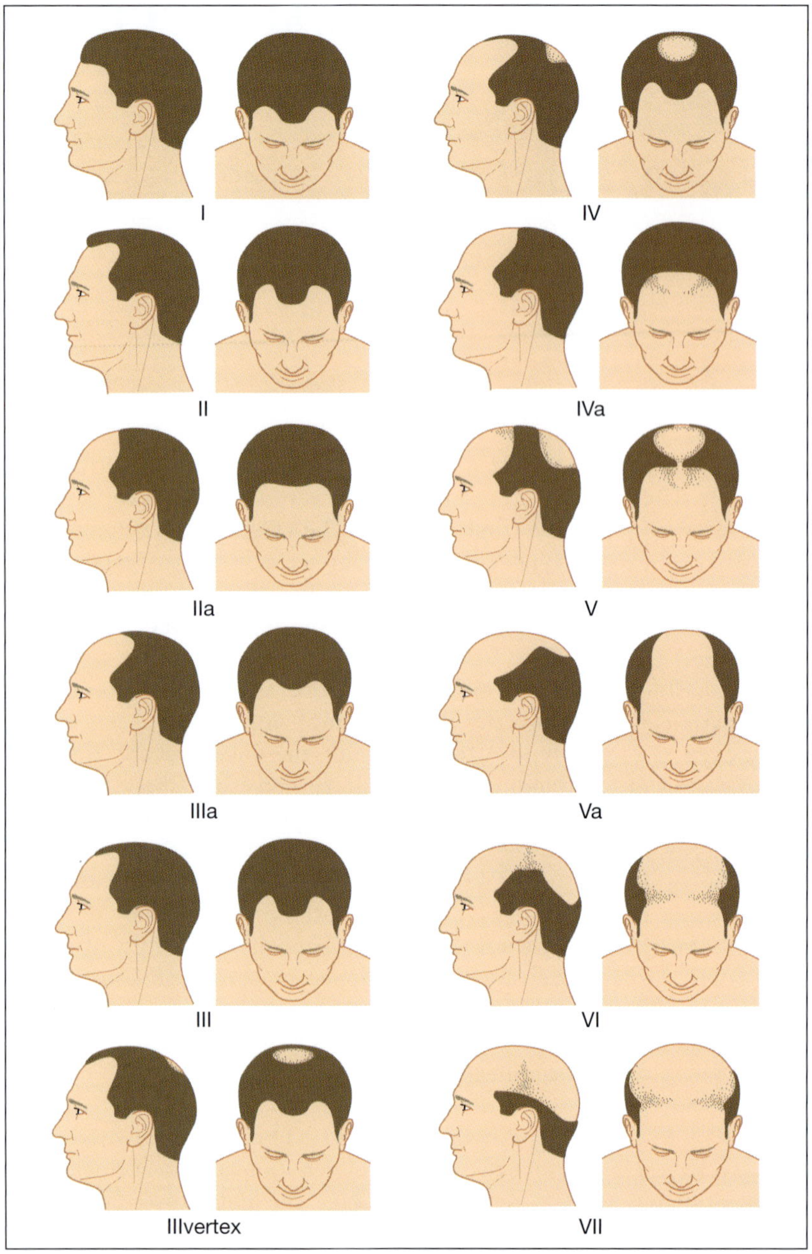


**Fig. 2.1** Male pattern hair loss. The Hamilton–Norwood system, which has been the standard for MPHL classification since first introduced by Hamilton in 1941. From Olsen EA, Weiner MS, DeLong E, Pinnell SR 1985 Topical minoxidil in early male pattern baldness. Journal of the American Academy of Dermatology 13:185–192 with permission

## Diffuse patterned alopecia

The patterns resemble the common Norwood scale but involve thinning without true balding.

## Diffuse unpatterned alopecia (DUPA)

This pattern shows a general thinning, usually of the entire scalp, though frequently more severe in the vertex and frontal regions.

## Persistent frontal forelock

This pattern can occur in combination with any pattern of balding but retains at least medium density in the mid-frontal forelock region (Fig. 2.3).

## Persistent frontal fringe

This pattern presents as total, or near-total, preservation of the frontal fringe with significant thinning

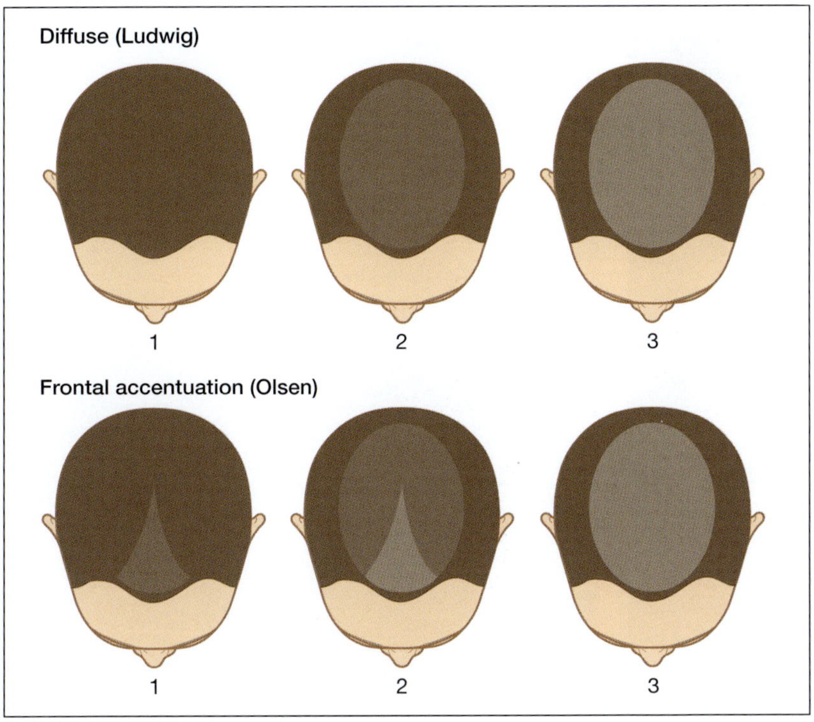


**Fig. 2.2** FPHL. The Ludwig (diffuse) and Olsen (frontal accentuation) patterns both evolve to the same configuration as they progress to stage 3. From Olsen EA 1999 The middle part: an important physical clue to the diagnosis of androgenetic alopecia in women. Journal of the American Academy of Dermatology 40:106–109 with permission

or balding occurring behind. The balding can be quite extensive (Fig. 2.4).

## Classification of FPHL

Four unique patterns of hair loss have been described in women:

1. Hamilton described a pattern that is essentially similar to the male pattern he previously defined. It is seen more commonly in postmenopausal women and does not progress past Type IV, except in conditions of significant androgen excess. Temporal recession is present. This pattern was also later described by several others, namely Venning, Dawber, Maguire, and Kligman (Fig. 2.5).
2. Ludwig described a diffuse pattern of hair loss in the superior scalp with three degrees of severity. Unlike the Hamilton classification, the frontal fringe is retained and there is no temporal recession (Figs 2.2, 2.5).
3. In 1999, Olsen described a frontal accentuation pattern in the shape of a 'Christmas tree.' As the stages advance in severity, the pattern eventuates in an endpoint similar to that of the Ludwig diffuse pattern. Olsen believes this to be the most common pattern of female hair loss (affecting 70% of women with FPHL). It may be seen in its early stages as a widening of the part (Figs 2.2, 2.5).
4. In 2001 Olsen suggested a classification that was not based on anatomic and quantitative elements. She defined FPHL as loss primarily on the superior scalp, with a decrease in anagen hairs and miniaturization of hairs in the involved areas, then expanded the classification to include age of onset and hormonal status (Box 2.1).

## Savin Hair Loss Scale

In the mid 1990s, Savin designed a system of eight computer-generated pictures of hair loss with progressive severity. The pictures were simply the top view of the scalp with hair parted down the midline. By comparing the width of the patient's part to one of the eight examples, the system could be adapted to clinical trials and serve as a method by which practitioners could quantify their patient's hair loss and growth. Unfortunately, the Savin scale does not represent the typical patterns of hair loss

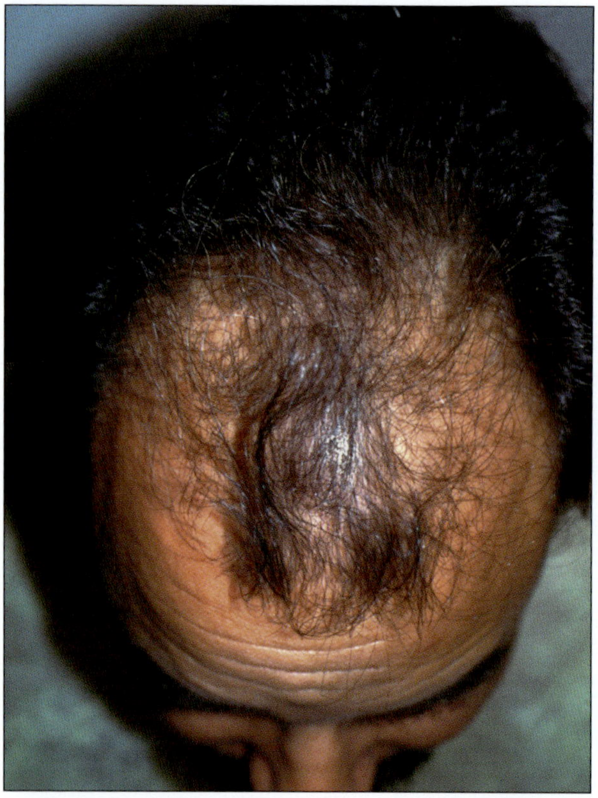

Fig. 2.3 The persistent frontal forelock. The persistent medium density frontal forelock is an uncommon variation of MPHL. Transient frontal forelocks that rapidly disappear are not uncommon in typical MPHL.

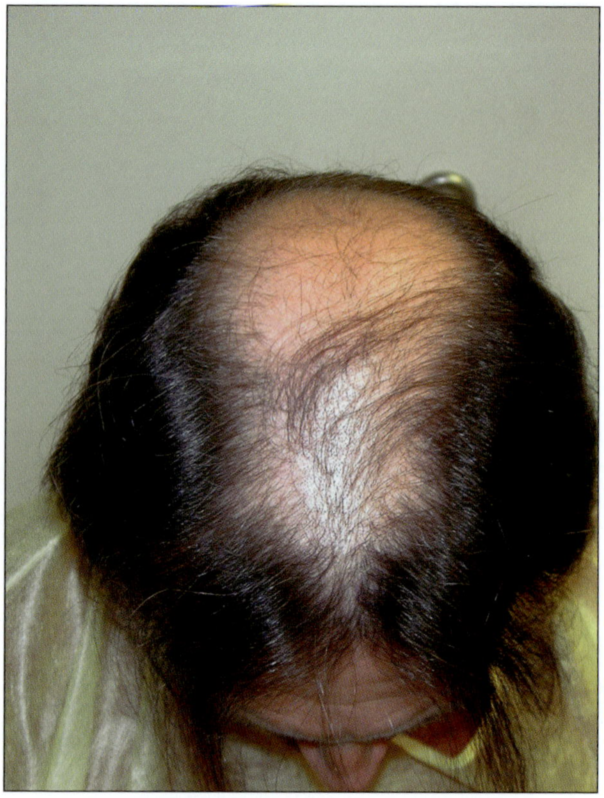

Fig. 2.4 The persistent frontal fringe. One of the least common variations of MPHL.

experienced by most patients, and it has not been widely accepted by hair transplantation surgeons.

## Hair Loss Index, Profile and Severity Scale

In 2002, one of the authors (Cohen) published a comprehensive system as an alternative to the Hamilton–Norwood and Ludwig classifications. It was specifically designed to describe an individual patient's hair distribution and density. Unlike the Olsen's Regional Scalp Hair Density system, it was intended to be a communication tool for those treating patients with pattern loss, and not a method for evaluating therapeutic efficacy. The system has three essential components – a surface map, display chart, and severity scale. Each of the components may be used separately or in conjunction with each other. When all three components are used together, a comprehensive Hair Loss Profile and Index are generated. The **profile** is a graphic display of the loss in each of 10 zones. The **index** is a score for the cumulative loss in all 10 zones.

The surface map is a three-view graphic of the scalp with 10 zones that correspond to the sequence of MPHL (Fig. 2.6A). The zones are weighted according to anatomic size and designed so that mosaic combinations of each closely resemble the Norwood patterns. The display chart (Fig. 2.6B) contains 100 blank cells and corresponds to the 10 zones on the surface map.

Three sets of dots define the position of significant measurable landmarks such as the forehead, bridge and vertex dimensions (if discernible). A simple visual examination is performed at arms length with the hair combed to expose the scalp surface. The hair loss severity is determined by the visual ratio of hair to skin. The Severity Scale has six categories (Fig. 2.7A–D; Table 2.1).

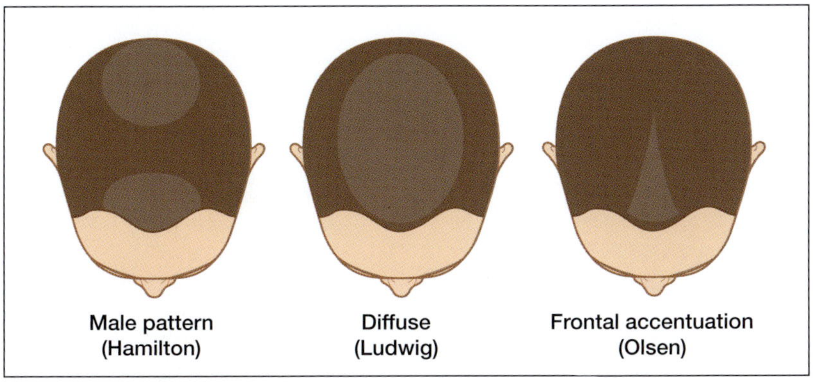


**Fig. 2.5** Variants of FPHL. Of the three variants, the frontal accentuation pattern is the most common, perhaps representing 70%. See Figure 2.2 for the progression of stages in the Ludwig and Olsen patterns. From Olsen EA 1999 The middle part: an important physical clue to the diagnosis of androgenetic alopecia in women. Journal of the American Academy of Dermatology 40:106–109 with permission

**Olsen's description of FPHL**

- Early onset
  - With androgen excess
  - Without androgen excess
- Late onset/postmenopausal
  - With androgen excess
  - Without androgen excess

**Box 2.1** Olsen's description of FPHL

The method for creating the Profile display and calculating the Index is shown (Fig. 2.8A–F). The system communicates clinical data in a concise and comprehensive manner and is valuable for tracking a patient's response, or lack of response, to medical or surgical treatment. The data may be digitized for computer analysis. The Hair Loss Index is a single value that represents the amount of original hair that still remains in spite of the balding process.

## Regional Scalp Hair Density Scale

In 2003, Olsen adapted her 5-zone scalp map (published in 2001) to be used as a method for assessing the efficacy of hair growth promoters in pattern hair loss. Each zone is assigned a terminal hair density value from 0 to 6, where 0 = 100%, 1 = 50%, 2 = 25%, 3 = 12%, 4 = 6%, 5 = 3%, and 6 = 0% (Fig. 2.9).

## Scalp Laxity Classification

The measurement of scalp laxity is useful in two settings: firstly to estimate the amount of tissue that can be safely removed during alopecia reduction procedures, and secondly to estimate the maximal donor strip width that can be safely removed during hair transplantation.

Bosley described a technique for alopecia reduction suitability assessment involving two dots placed 100 mm apart in the balding area that was remeasured after medial compression using the thumbs and index fingers. He classified laxity in five classes sequentially representing up to 5 mm of compression (e.g. Class 3 represents 10–15 mm compression). Class 1 is regarded as unsuitable for alopecia reduction because of insufficient laxity.

Mayer and Paul have presented, but have not published, a similar technique that expresses scalp elasticity as a percentile. This is used primarily to safely estimate donor strip width but is applicable to all areas of the scalp. Two marks are placed 50 mm apart and compressed by thumb pressure. The resulting measurement between the dots is subtracted from the original measurement and expressed as a percentile (Fig. 2.10). For example, the 50 mm marks have moved to 38 mm after compression from the thumbs:

$$\frac{50 \text{ mm} - 38 \text{ mm}}{50 \text{ mm}} \times 100\% = 24\% \text{ scalp elasticity}$$

Mayer and Paul's recommended safe donor width for a **first** surgery varies between the central half and the lateral quarters of the donor strip:

- 10% elasticity = 10 mm central half 8 mm lateral quarters
- 15% elasticity = 15 mm central half 10 mm lateral quarters

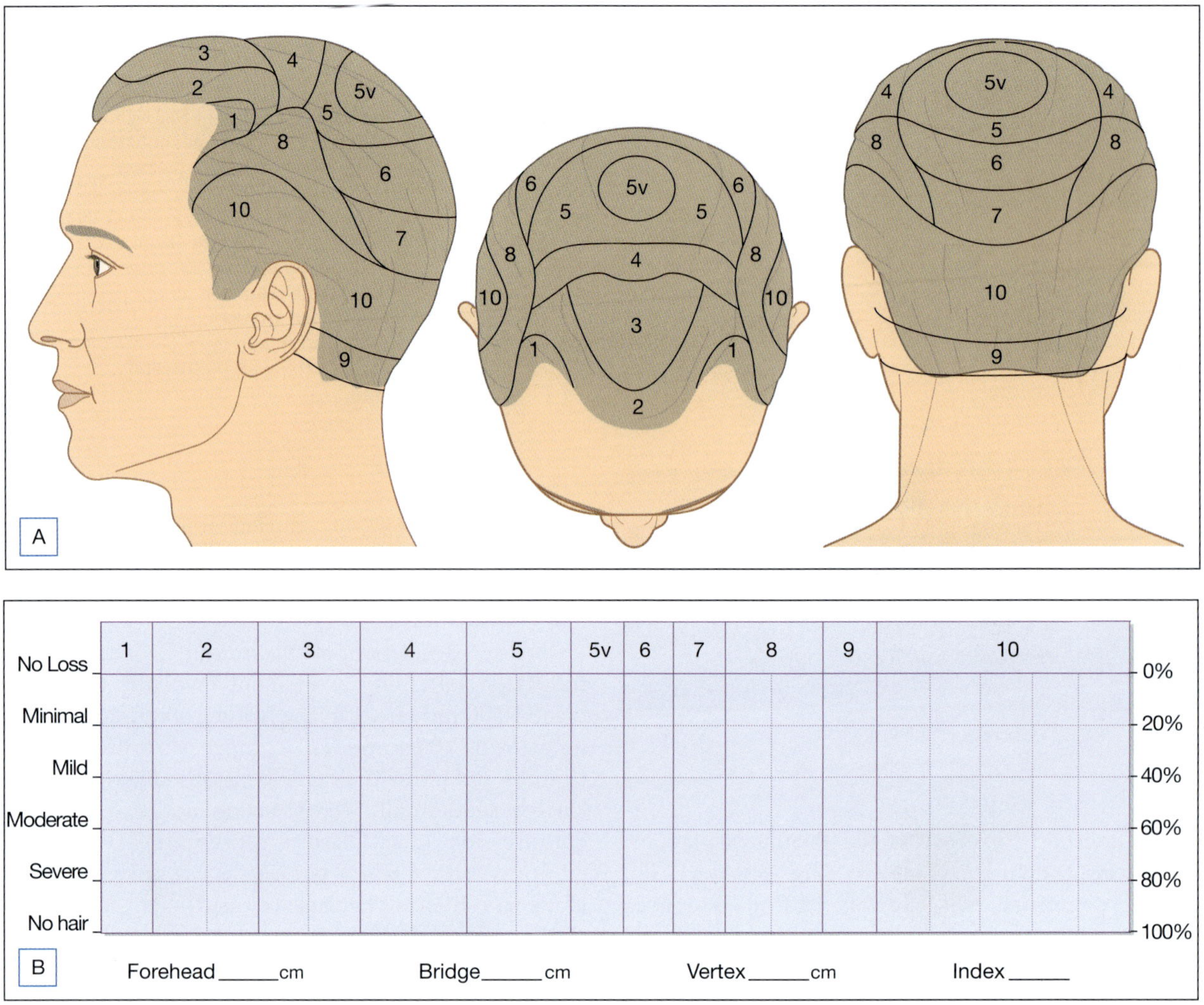


**Fig. 2.6** (**A** and **B**) The hair loss profile and index. The scalp map defines 10 zones numbered to reflect their progressive loss. The blank profile contains 100 cells, each of which is weighted to reflect its relative size.

- 20% elasticity = 20 mm central half 15 mm lateral quarters
- 25% elasticity = 22 mm central half 15 mm lateral quarters
- 30% + elasticity = 22 mm central half 15 mm lateral quarters

Mayer and Paul recommend decreasing these width measurements by 20% for subsequent surgeries to achieve fine donor scars.

## Conclusion

The classification of hair loss has been approached from many perspectives—the graphic, pictorial, and cognitive. Some have approached it from the male pattern point of view, and others from the female pattern. The offerings have ranged from the quantitative complexity of the Hair Loss Profile and Index to the simplicity of Savin's midline part. As the medical science of hair transplantation becomes more sophisticated, so should the manner in which it communicates. The 30-year-old Norwood system remains the most popular classification in use.

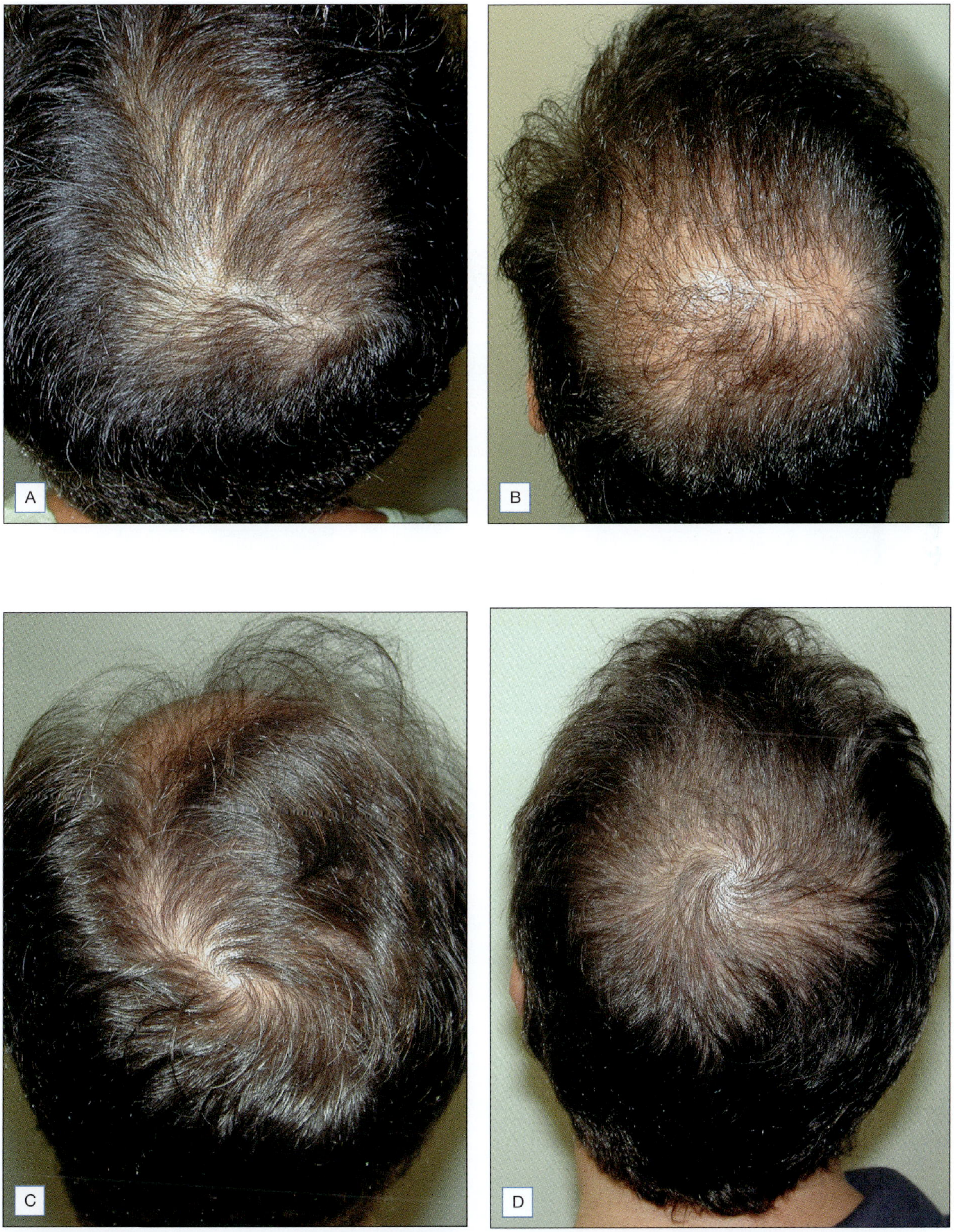


**Fig. 2.7** The Hair Loss Severity Scale. The visual ratio of hair to skin is used to measure the severity of loss in each zone. Photographs show examples of each category.

| Severity scale | |
|---|---|
| **Clinical appearance** | **Hair-to-skin ratio** |
| No loss | All hair |
| Minimal | Much more hair than skin |
| Mild | More hair than skin |
| Moderate | More skin than hair |
| Severe | Much more skin than hair |
| No hair | All skin |

**Table 2.1** Severity scale

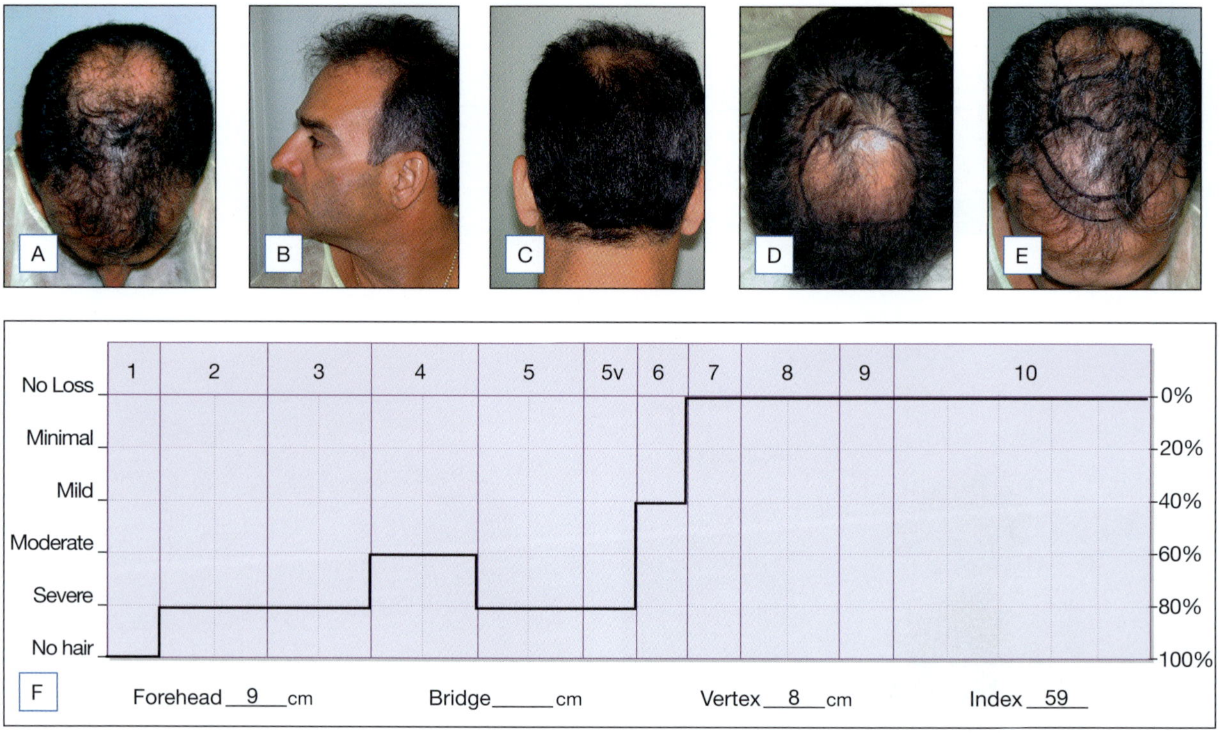


**Fig. 2.8** (**A–F**) The completed Hair Loss Profile and Index. An individualized graphic profile defines the density and distribution of hair loss on the entire scalp. The Index measures the total hair loss on a scale of 1 to 100.

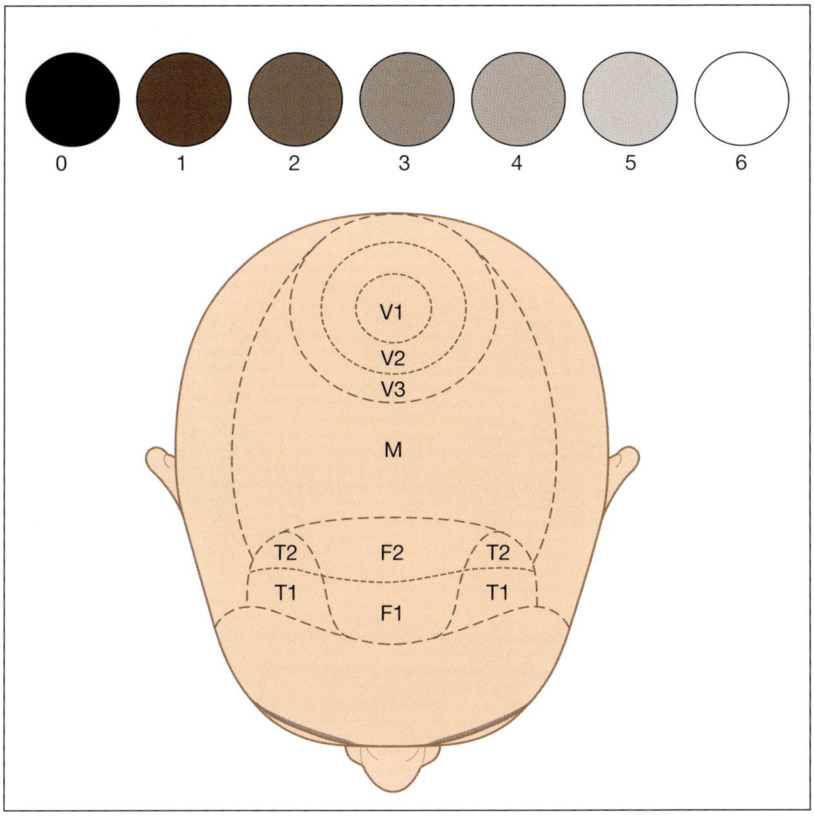


**Fig. 2.9** The Regional Scalp Hair Density Scale. The terminal hair density is determined by direct hair count in each zone. The percentage of original terminal hair still present in each zone is given a corresponding value on a scale of 1 to 6. From Olsen EA 2003 Current and novel methods for assessing efficacy of hair growth promoters in pattern hair loss. Journal of the American Academy of Dermatology 48:253–262 with permission

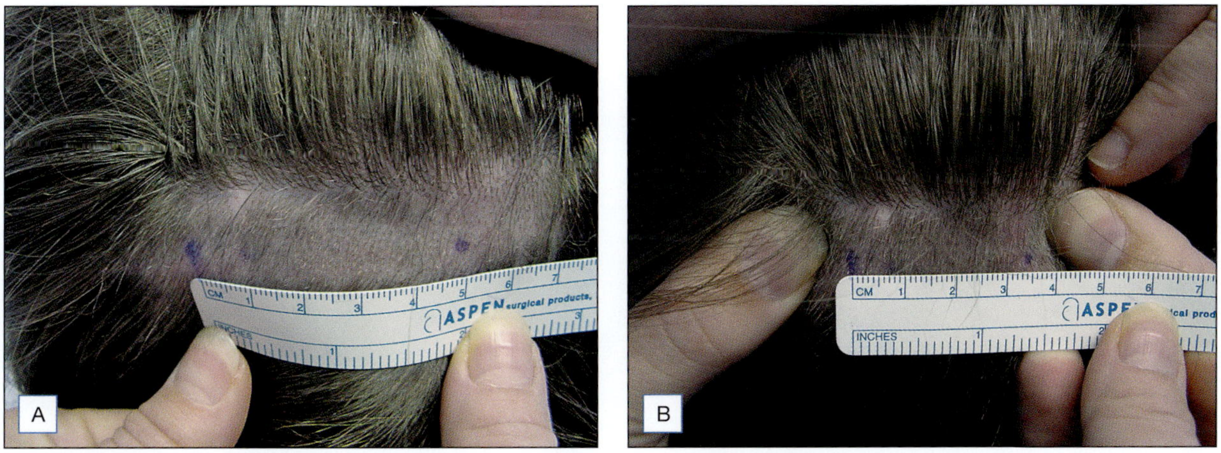


**Fig. 2.10** Scalp Laxity Classification. (**A**) Initial measurement of 50 mm. (**B**) Compressed scalp measurement of 35 mm.

## Further Reading

Bosley LL 1980 Reduction of male pattern baldness in multiple stages: A retrospective study. Journal of Dermatologic Surgery and Oncology 6:498

Cohen BH 2002 The Hair Loss Profile and Index. Journal of Cosmetic Dermatology 15:19–23

Ludwig E 1977 Classification of the types of androgenetic alopecia (common baldness) occurring in the female sex. British Journal of Dermatology 97:247–254

Norwood OT 1975 Male pattern baldness: classification and incidence. Southern Medical Journal 68:1359–1365

Olsen EA 1999 The middle part: an important physical clue to the diagnosis of androgenetic alopecia in women. Journal of the American Academy of Dermatology 40:106–109

Olsen EA 2001 Female pattern hair loss. Journal of the American Academy of Dermatology 45:570–580

Olsen EA 2003 Current and novel methods for assessing efficacy of hair growth promoters in pattern hair loss. Journal of the American Academy of Dermatology 48:253–262

Unger W, Shapiro R 2004 Hair Transplantation. Marcel Dekker, New York, pp 49–56

# 3 Anatomy and Anatomical Landmarks

*Michael Beehner*

## Introduction

The hair transplant surgeon must be familiar with the anatomy of the scalp and its neurovascular supply. Also, for uniformity in communication, a common language in describing the various zones of male pattern baldness and landmarks of the scalp must be used. This nomenclature will be listed and described in this chapter, and will, to the extent possible, be used consistently throughout this text.

## Layers of the Scalp

The scalp consists of five layers: the epidermis, dermis, subcutaneous layer, galea aponeurotica and periosteum (pericranium) (Fig. 3.1). There are also multiple fibrous septa, which traverse the width of the skin, extending from the galea to the dermis, which help hold the skin's layers together as a unit.

The **galea** combines with the frontalis muscle anteriorly and the occipitalis muscle posteriorly to

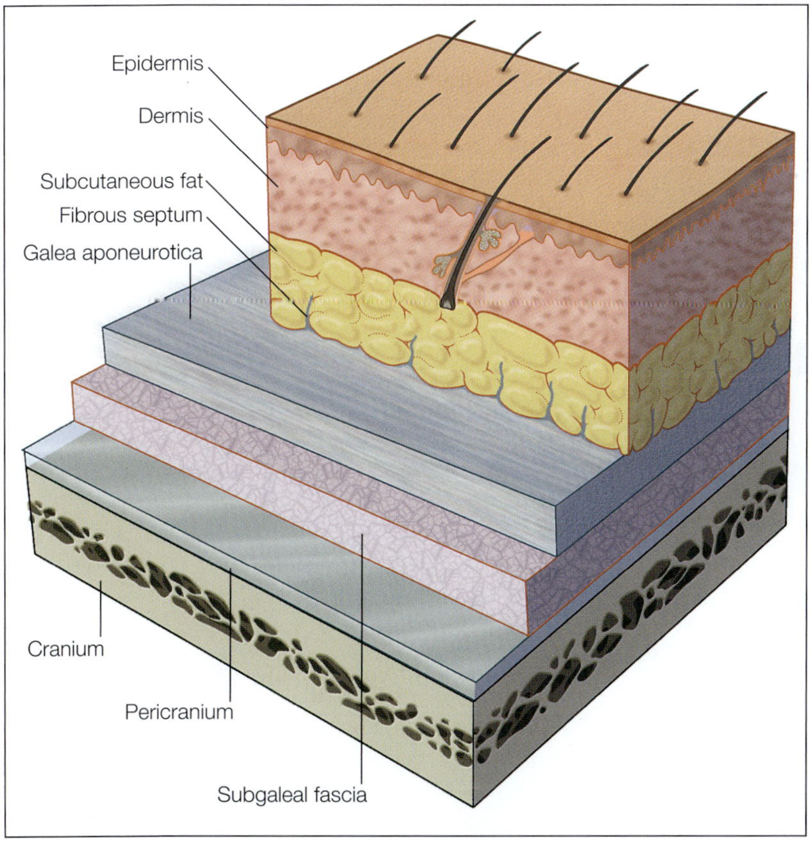


**Fig. 3.1** Layers of the scalp

form the **epicranius muscle**. Laterally, in a nearly circumferential distribution around the ear, are three muscles: the anterior auricular, superior auricular, and posterior auricular.

The **subgaleal plane** (Space of Merkel) is the potential space between the galea and periosteum. Loose areolar tissue in this space allows the upper layers to all flexibly move as a unit. This space also allows fairly bloodless dissection to be carried out when performing alopecia reduction or flap surgery.

A network of small arterial vessels, which richly anastamose and provide the scalp's blood supply, reside in the deep subcutaneous layer, just above the galea.

## Neurovascular Supply of Scalp

### Scalp vasculature

The arterial supply to the scalp is provided by five pairs of arteries: the supraorbital and supratrochlear arteries in front, the superficial temporal and posterior auricular arteries laterally, and the occipital arteries posteriorly (Fig. 3.2). There are no arteries traversing from the cranium into the scalp. All of the scalp's arteries anastamose generously with each other, both ipsilaterally and contralaterally, so much so that it is claimed the scalp tissue will remain viable if only two of the 10 arteries remain intact.

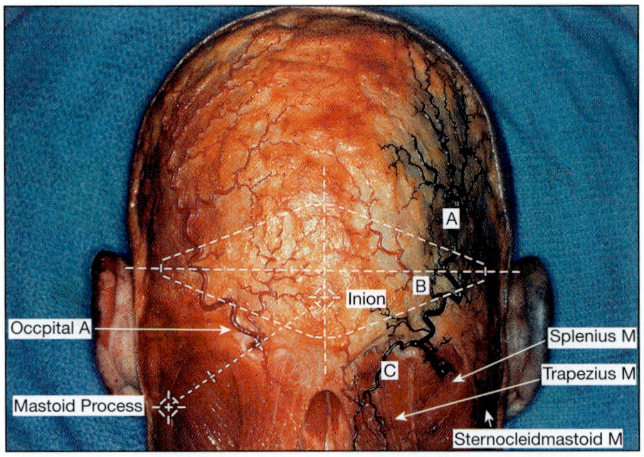


**Fig. 3.2** Occipital artery anatomy. Often ignored in the description of scalp arterial anatomy is the occipital artery. Note the ascending and transverse branches and robust anastomoses across the midline. (Reproduced from Stough D, Haber RS 1996 Hair replacement: Surgical and medical. Mosby Year Book Publishing Company, St Louis. Plate I, p 135, with permission. Courtesy of Dr Hani S. Matlob)

The **veins** of the scalp basically follow the same network as the arteries and drain from the scalp into the jugular veins. There are a few emissary veins, which pass from the scalp through the cranium into the deep intracranial veins.

### Scalp nerve supply

#### *Motor nerve supply*

The scalp is supplied with both a sensory and a motor nerve supply. The motor nerves supply the various muscles adjacent to and contiguous with the galea. The frontalis muscle receives its motor nerve supply from the temporal branch of the facial nerve, the occipitalis muscle from the posterior auricular branch of the facial nerve, and the temporalis muscle from the anterior and posterior deep temporal branches of the mandibular division of the trigeminal nerve. The anterior and superior auricular muscles are supplied by the temporal branch of the facial nerve, and the posterior auricular muscle by the posterior auricular branch of the facial nerve.

#### *Sensory nerve supply*

The anterior regions of the scalp and forehead are supplied by the supraorbital and supratrochlear nerves, which are the terminal sensory branches of the ophthalmic division of the trigeminal nerve (Fig. 3.3). The anterior temporal scalp region is supplied by the zygomaticotemporal nerve, which comes from the maxillary division of the trigeminal nerve. The temporoparietal, and a portion of the temporal, regions are supplied by the auriculotemporal nerve, which is a branch of the mandibular (inferior) division of the trigeminal nerve. The postauricular area receives its sensory innervation from the greater auricular nerve, which is an extension of the cervical plexus. Most of the posterior occipital scalp receives its innervation from the lesser occipital nerve.

## Topographical Zones of the Balding Scalp

The traditional horseshoe-shaped area of hair loss seen in MPHL is divided into three **major zones**: (1) the frontal region; (2) the midscalp; and (3) the vertex (crown) (Figs 3.4 and 3.5).

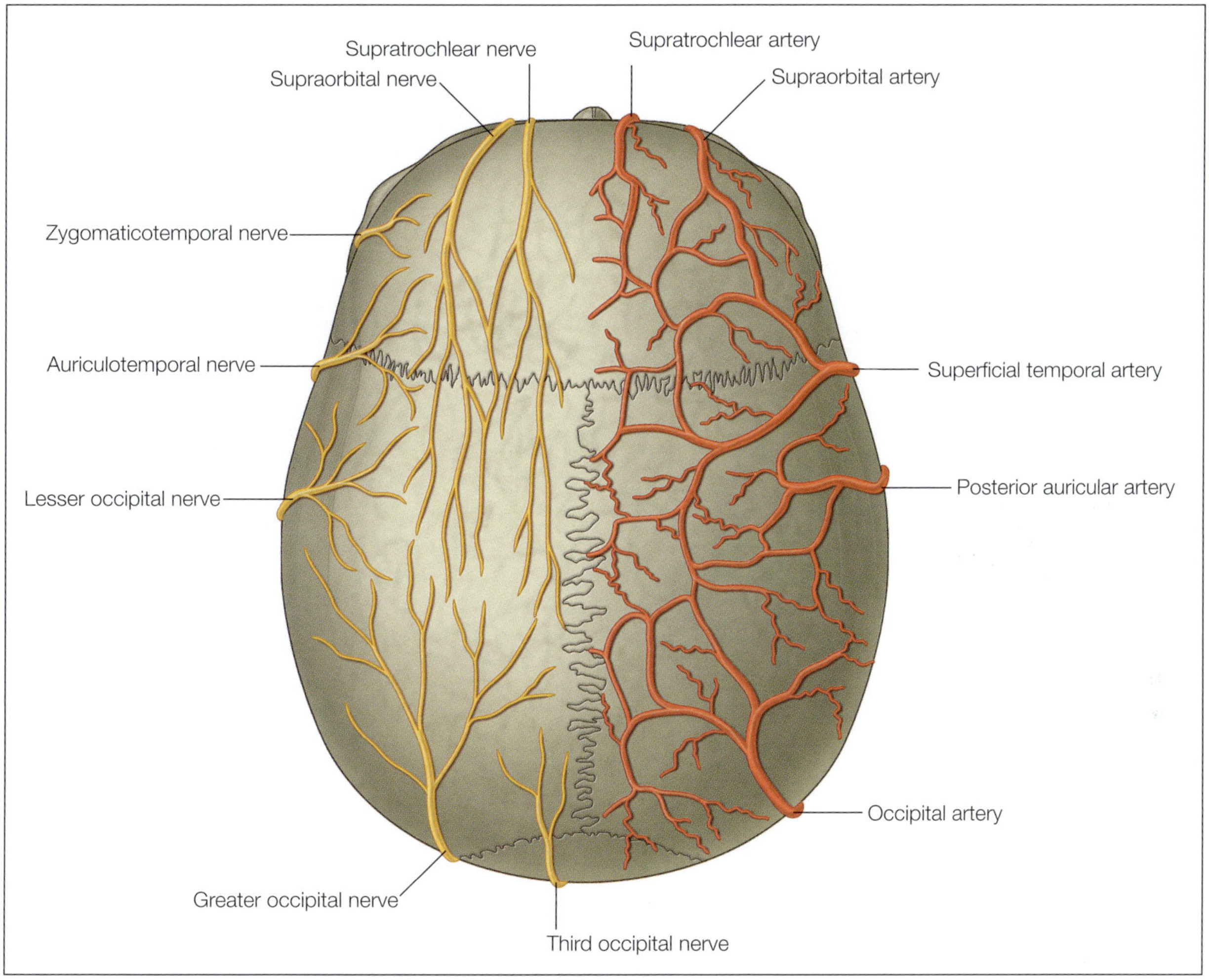


**Fig. 3.3** Neurovascular supply of the scalp

## Frontal region

This zone extends from the front hairline back to a horizontal line drawn between the frontotemporal corners. A modification of this designation, termed the *frontal transplant zone* (Unger) (Fig. 3.6), combines this frontal region with a small portion of the anterior midscalp, such that a naturally curved, esthetic rear border results when transplanting the frontal region only.

## Mid-scalp

This is the relatively horizontal area at the top of the head. It is bordered laterally by the temporal and parietal hair-bearing fringes, anteriorly by the line connecting the two frontotemporal corners, and posteriorly by the anterior border of the vertex.

## Vertex (crown)

This refers to the most posterior area of MPHL. It is generally round or oval in contour and is characterized by a whorl arrangement of the hairs present. Its posterior border is the upper margin of the occipital fringe hair. This curve is then projected anteriorly to form and complete a mirror image. Its size can range from the small early central thinning of MPHL to the large vertical wall of baldness seen in a Norwood Class VII patient.

## Lateral ledge (crease zone)

This refers to the narrow zone along the lateral midscalp, within which both a transition of plane and a transition of hair direction occur (Fig. 3.7). A patient's 'natural part' normally occurs here, and its

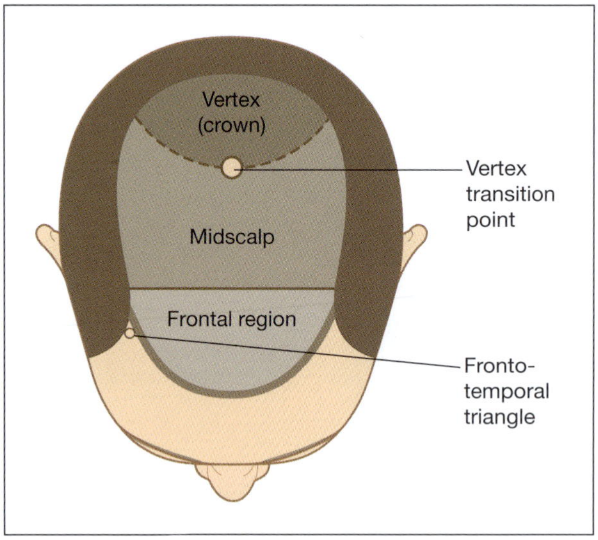


**Fig. 3.4** Three major zones of the alopecic scalp

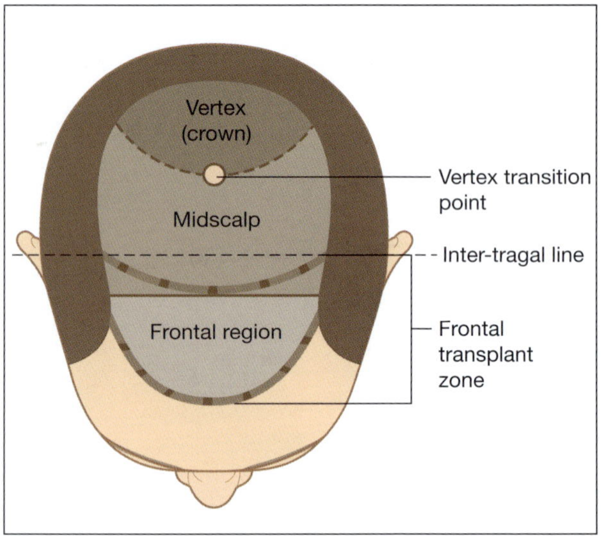


**Fig. 3.6** Frontal transplant zone

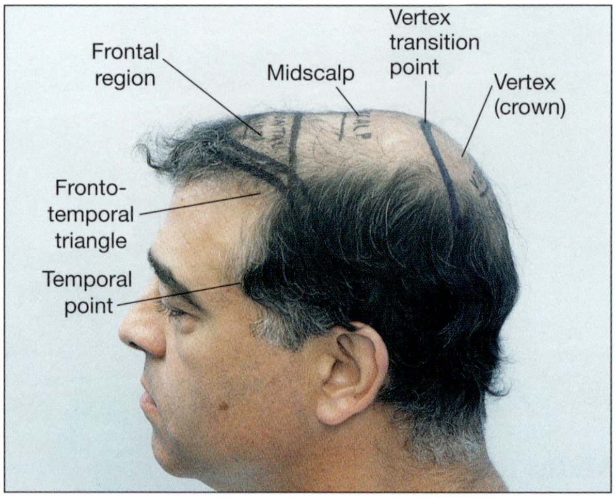


**Fig. 3.5** Major zones and reference points, as seen from the side view of patient

location usually is directly aligned with the lateral canthus of the eye. The lateral ledge straddles the horizontal and vertical planes. Also, residual hairs, if present, are directed antero-inferiorly in its lower aspect, straight anterior in the very center, and anteromedially in the upper portion.

## Frontal hairline zone

This area is self-explanatory. It serves as a transitional zone from the hairless forehead into the relatively denser hair located posterior to it.

## 'Frontal core' zone

The **frontal core** is a relatively small circular zone in the front-central aspect of the frontal region, just behind the front hairline zone. Its importance derives from the fact that the hair in this area is the focal point for 'framing' the face, and thus must receive the highest density in the hair transplant plan for most patients.

## Posterior-parietal triangle zones

These are the two triangular areas in the lateral-posterior mid-scalp region where the relatively level surface of the mid-scalp begins to 'tilt' downward toward a slightly more vertical plane.

## Vertex transition point

This is the mid-line point on the posterior scalp where the horizontal scalp starts to become vertical (Figs 3.5, 3.7). In most patients, it also happens to be the point where the hair's direction starts to become enveloped in a 'whorl' orientation.

## Anterior temporal points

These are the sharply angulated projections of hair at the anterior aspect of each anterior temporal fringe (Fig. 3.5).

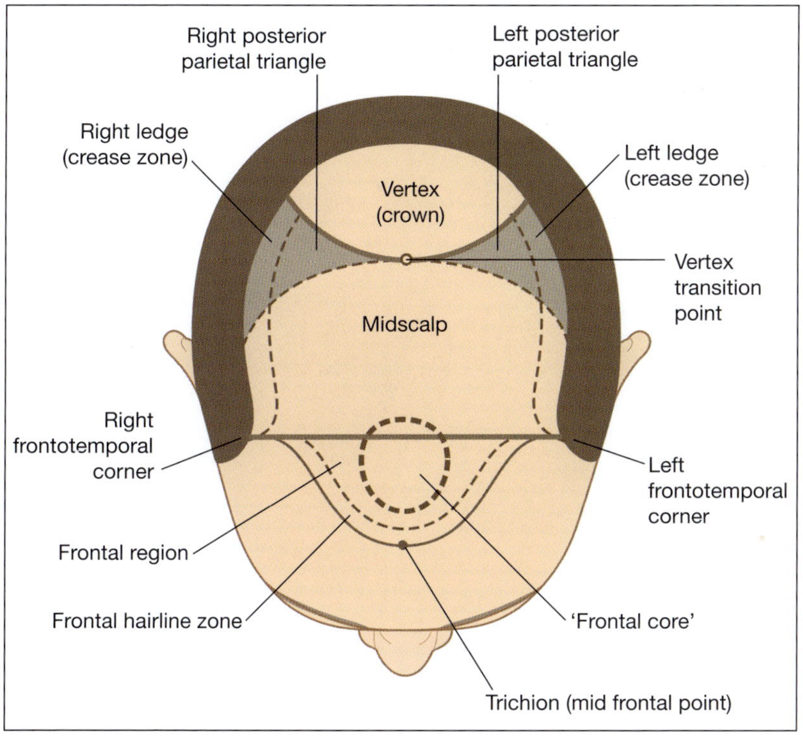


**Fig. 3.7** Various zones and landmarks of the scalp

## Frontotemporal recession (gulf or triangle)

This is the normally alopecic area that lies between the lateral aspect of the frontal hairline and the anterior temporal fringe.

## Anterior temporal fringe

The anterior fringe of temporal hair is situated inferior to the frontotemporal corner and vertically aligned (Fig. 3.8).

## Superior temporal fringe

The superior border of the temporal hair (classically depicted on a Norwood VI Class alopecic male) extends from the frontotemporal corner to a point vertically aligned with the tragus of the ear (Fig. 3.8).

## Parietal fringe

The superior border of fringe hair (again, on a Norwood VI patient) extends from a point aligned vertically with the tragus of the ear and back to the beginning of the occipital fringe (Fig. 3.8).

## Occipital fringe

The occipital fringe is the border of hair that surrounds the alopecic or thinning vertex inferolaterally and posteriorly (Fig. 3.8).

## Trichion (mid-frontal point)

This is a designation for the central-most point of the anterior hairline (Fig. 3.7).

# Measuring Height of Hairline

In designating the height of the frontal hairline, whether natural or transplanted, either the **glabella** or the **supra-eyebrow line** can be used as the lower reference point from which the hairline is measured (Fig. 3.9). Whichever reference point is used should be clearly stated, as the supra-eyebrow line is usually almost a full cm higher than the glabella. This author prefers to use the supra-eyebrow line as the more precise reference point for this measurement.

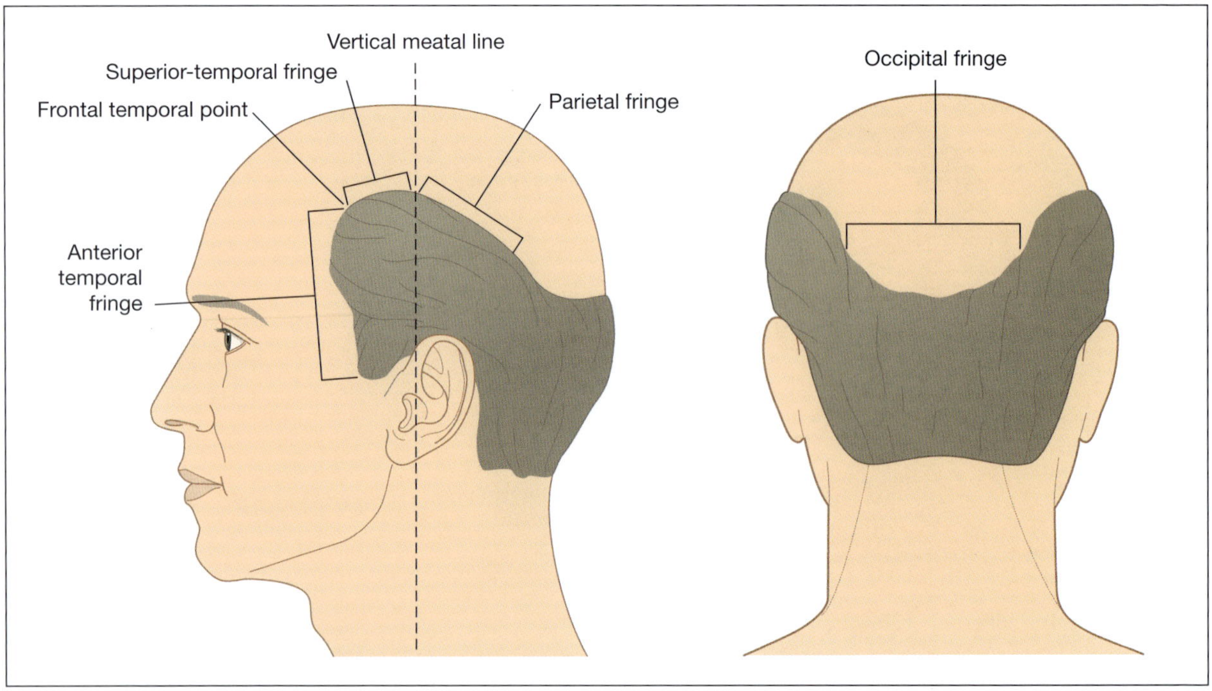


**Fig. 3.8** The various fringe designations of the alopecic scalp

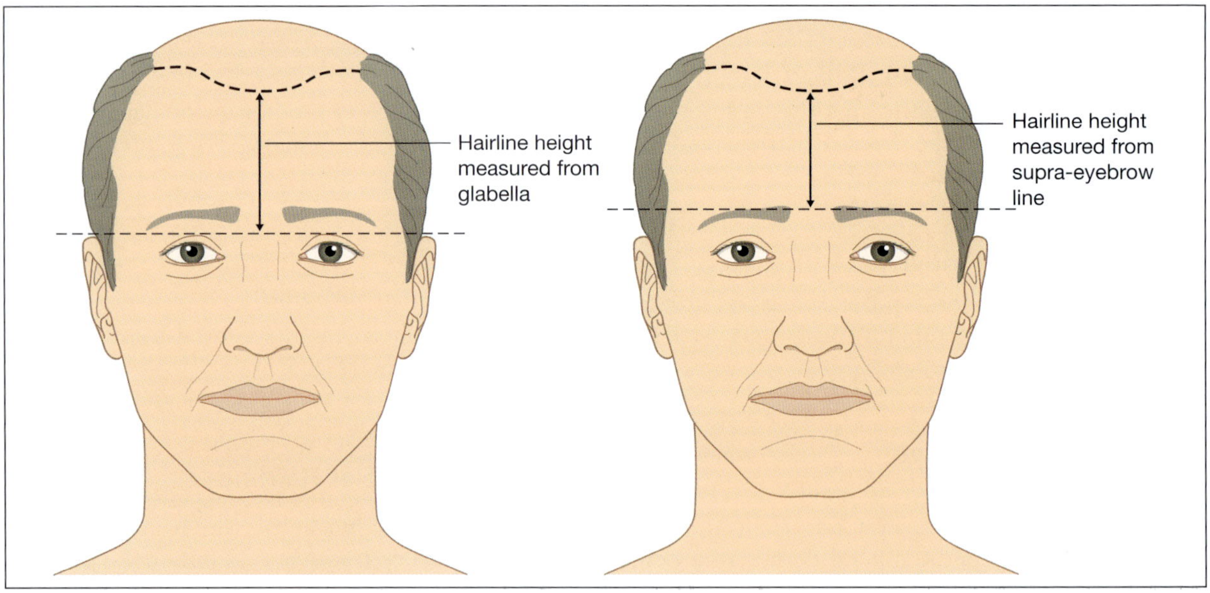


**Fig. 3.9** Measuring height of the hairline

## Summary

Although hair surgeons will often differ in their artistic patterns and areas of emphasis in transplanting any given patient, it is important that they all use a common language when referring to the various landmarks and zones of the scalp in the patient with hair loss. This chapter attempts to provide a nomenclature system to accomplish this task.

## Further Reading

Beehner M, Unger W 2004 Hair transplantation. In: Unger W, Shapiro R (eds) Basic principles and organization. Marcel Dekker, New York, p 85–91

Beehner M 2001 Nomenclature proposal for the zones and landmarks of the balding scalp. Dermatologic Surgery 27:375–380

Bouhanna P, Dardour JC 1996 Hair replacement surgery. Springer Publications, Berlin/New York, pp 10–20

Lewis W 2000 Gray's anatomy of the human body. 20th edn. Bartleby Publications, New York,

Matloub H, Molnar J 1996 Anatomy of the scalp. In: Stough D, Haber RS (eds) Hair replacement: Surgical and medical. Mosby Year Book Publishing Company, St Louis, pp 20–26

# 4 Terminology in Hair Transplant Surgery

*Michael Beehner*

## Introduction

Each subspecialty of medicine possesses its own unique language of commonly used terms with which its practitioners communicate. This section will briefly summarize some of the more important ones in our specialty.

## Designated Terms of Grafts Used in Hair Transplant Surgery

### Follicular unit graft (FU)

The naturally occurring 'bundle' of hair follicles found on the human scalp, each consisting of one to three hairs (uncommonly four to five) (Fig. 4.1).

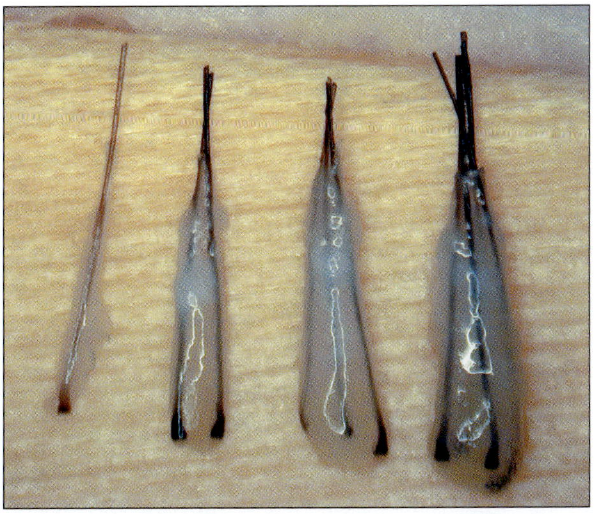

**Fig. 4.1** Examples of follicular units (Photo courtesy of Bill Parsley, MD)

### Multi-FU graft (MFU)

A graft containing either two or three FUs (alternately called either DFUs or TFUs) and which usually consists of three to seven hairs. An MFU can also be described as being a graft that has not been dissected down to a single follicular unit, and has been contoured into a desired shape and size (Fig. 4.2).

### Follicular family graft

A hybrid of the above two grafts designates a three-to-five-hair graft, composed of two adjacent FUs residing closer together than the others (Fig. 4.3).

### Micrografts

In modern transplantation, 'micrograft' primarily refers to a single-hair graft that is dissected out from a two-to-three-hair FU, usually for a purpose such as eyebrow transplantation or for producing the necessary one-hair FUs for the front hairline edge in a patient with too few natural single-hair FUs.

### Minigrafts

The minigraft historically was any graft smaller than the original 4 mm 'standard' large graft and larger than a one-to-two-hair 'micrograft.' At this time, 'minigraft' most commonly refers to four-to-eight-hair grafts that are not cut with microscopes, and that are contoured to fit into slit, slot, or small round recipient sites ('cut to size') (Table 4.1).

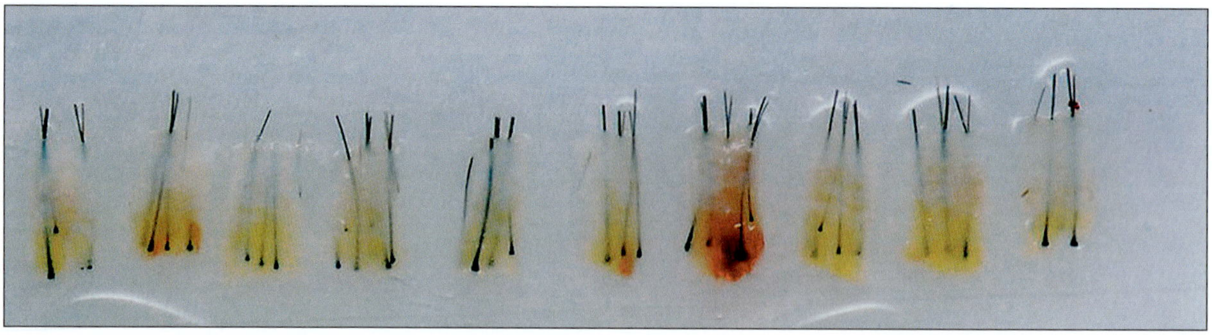

**Fig. 4.2** Multifollicular unit grafts

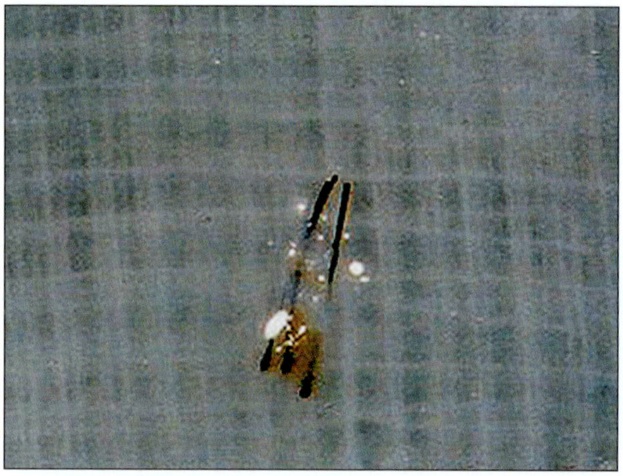

**Fig. 4.3** Follicular family graft

## Hair Transplantation Methods

### Follicular unit transplantation (FUT)

This refers to the exclusive use of follicular unit grafts to accomplish hair transplantation. There is debate as to whether such grafts must be dissected with microscopes, but most would accept FUT as applying to any magnification system that clearly allows the cutter to isolate intact FUs. The 'slivering' step in graft dissection of a thick ellipse must be done with stereoscopic microscopy, if the donor tissue is harvested in this manner.

### Follicular unit extraction

This entails harvesting individual FU's in the donor area one at a time, utilizing a small sharp punch superficially, and then, with gentle traction, pulling the graft free. Occcasionally a freeing up of the deeper fibrous attachments is necessary. An alternate FUE technique utilizes first a sharp superficial cut, followed by a second deeper cut with a dull-edged punch.

### 'Mixed' or 'combination' grafting

This includes the use of **both** FUs and multi-FU grafts (or minigrafts), the latter usually being used centrally for density.

### Laser hair transplantation

This refers to making recipient sites with lasers and is uncommon today. It can be confused with **laser therapy**, which involves administering laser beams to the scalp with either a 'wand' or a hairdryer-like apparatus in an attempt to stimulate hair growth.

### Stick-and-place technique

This technique involves the simultaneous creation of recipient sites with the immediate insertion of the grafts. The recipient site is made, and then as the needle or blade is withdrawn, a graft is immediately placed into the hole.

### Buddy technique

This refers to a team of two people working together to accomplish graft insertion. If the "buddy system" is applied to the 'stick-and-place' technique, then one person makes the site and briefly holds it open, while the other person inserts the graft, with the first person then usually helping to stabilize the graft's position. If all the sites are pre-made, then the person inserting the grafts is assisted

| Graft | Cross-section shape | Usual recipient sites | Hairs per graft |
|---|---|---|---|
| Micrograft | Trimmed and narrow | Tiny needle hole | 1–2 |
| Follicular unit graft (FU)[a] | Usually elongated and narrow | Needle hole, or small slit | 1–4, usually |
| Follicular family graft (FF)[a] | Trimmed to fit arrangement of hairs in FU (varies) | Small slit | 3–6 |
| Multi-follicular unit graft (MFU)[a] | Usually elongated and narrow; varies, but can also be square-like in configuration | (i) Tissue displaced: Slot or round holes | Commonly 3–6 |
| | | (ii) No tissue displaced: slits | Theoretically 2–9 |
| Double FU graft (DFU)[a] | Varies; most commonly narrow and elongated | Same as for MFU | 3–6 |
| Triple FU graft (TFU)[a] | Same as MFU usually | Same as for MFU | 4–9 |
| Minigraft | Varies with relationship of FUs to each other; narrow or roundish | Same as for MFU; sometimes described as 'cut to size' | Varies; usually 3–8 |

[a]*For purposes of definition, it is assumed that all these grafts are dissected microscopically*

**Table 4.1** Terminology of grafts in hair transplantation

by a second person, who either hands the first person each graft or simply holds each site slightly open and then assists in stabilizing the graft during insertion.

## Some Existing Hair Patterns and Variations

A **frontal tuft** is a narrow projection of hair in the front-central scalp. The deep recessions to either side are the **fronto-temporal recessions** (Fig. 4.4).

A **frontal forelock** is an isolated collection of hair, either natural or transplanted, that is usually located in the front-central region of the scalp (Fig. 4.5). An important component of the forelock is the relatively small circular or oval collection of hairs in the front center of the forelock, which is described as the 'frontal core.' Obviously, if the forelock is small, they are one and the same.

In hair transplantation, expanded variants of the 'forelock concept' include various other forelock patterns. Two notable ones are the oval- and the shield-shaped collections of hair, which extend back to the vertex transition point and have the lateral 'alleys' between the forelock and the side fringes blurred with small FU grafts. The large oval forelock was first proposed by Bluford Stough and given the title 'cadre de cheveaux,' (Fig. 4.6). Beehner has designed a 'shield' contoured larger forelock design that has a flared front hairline and a convex posterior border. But, a 'paradox of curves,' which is seen in the natural state, is imitated in the posterior aspect, in which the posterior parietal triangle zones to the rear on each side are filled with sparse FUs, thus giving a concave appearance to the rear hairline when viewed from behind (Fig. 4.7).

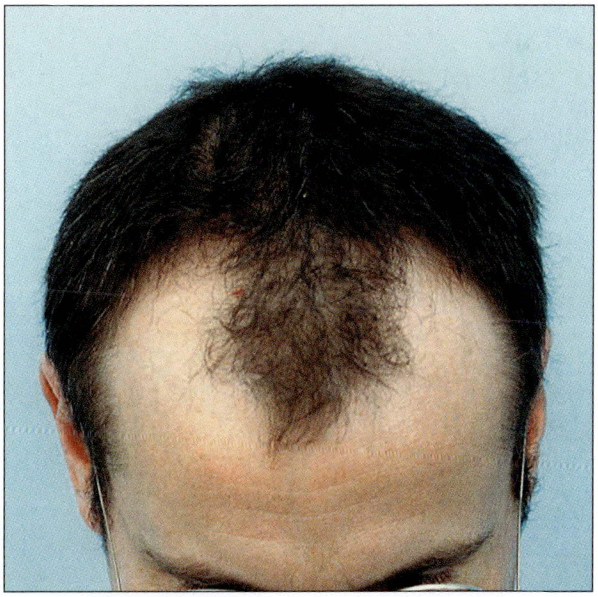

**Fig. 4.4** The frontal tuft

A **scatter zone** is the term given by Beehner to the sparse FU zone to the side of a forelock design that serves to 'blur' the connection between the forelock and fringe hair.

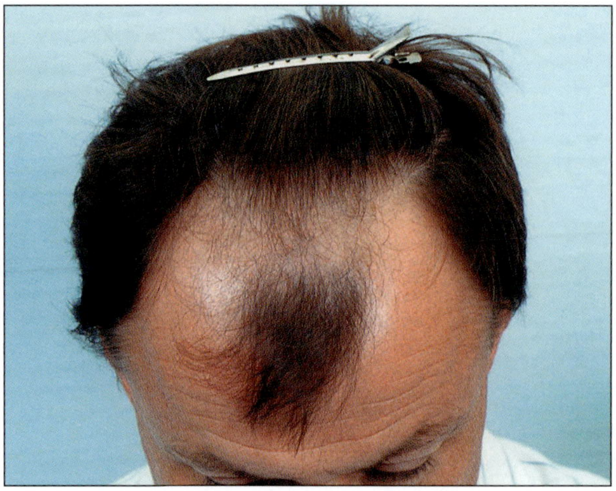

Fig. 4.5 The isolated frontal forelock (natural)

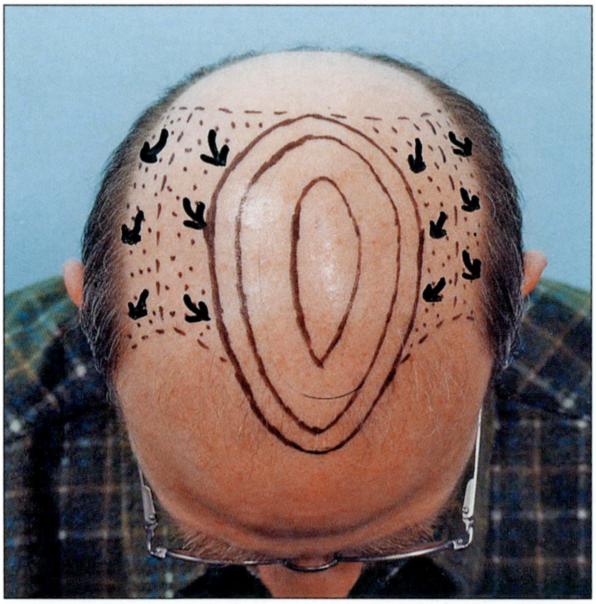

Fig. 4.6 Oval-shaped frontal forelock design

The **mid-parietal bridge** is a band of hair that extends across the mid-scalp.

A **cowlick** refers to an area of the scalp in which the direction of a group of hairs abruptly changes from the direction of those around it.

The **residual anatomic plug** (RAP) is a 3–4 mm area located in the vertex of the scalp that is relatively uncommon and; when present, is consistently depressed and is usually more resistant to the effects of male pattern loss (Fig. 4.8A and and B). The RAP area is generally the last hair in the vertex to be shed due to male pattern baldness. The **vertex dimple** is the depressed remnant of the RAP after all hair has been shed. The **surgical effluvium** – the patient's pre-existing hair in and around the transplanted area – is at risk of being shed as a result of the transplant procedure. The hair that is at greatest risk of being lost is the hair that has already begun the process of miniaturization. The miniaturized hair is termed **vellus** or **indeterminate hairs** (see Chapter 5, p. 35.)

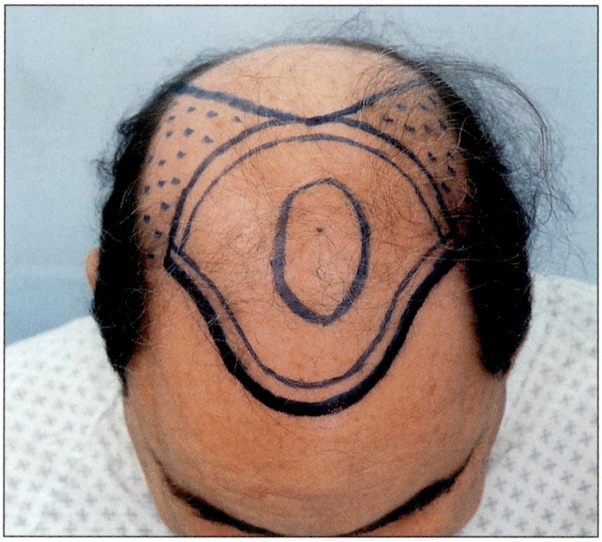

Fig. 4.7 Shield-shaped frontal forelock design

## Instrumentation and Some Specific Surgical Maneuvers

### Strip harvesting

This is a technique for harvesting donor hair which involves excising a horizontal section of 'safe' donor hair from the occipital, parietal, and occasionally, temporal regions. It is the commonest method used in hair transplantation today. The resulting wound is easily sutured or stapled and leaves a relatively undetectable linear scar.

### Multi-blade knife

This is an instrument that holds a number of blades, with various-sized spacers between them, and which cuts one or more horizontal strips of donor hair simultaneously.

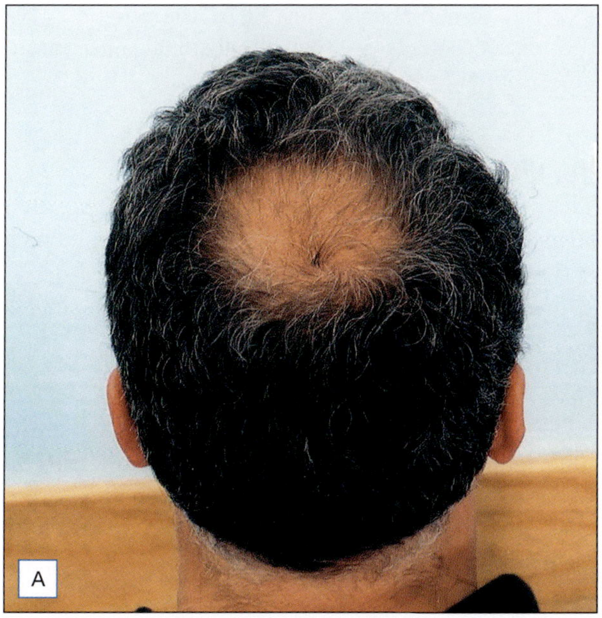


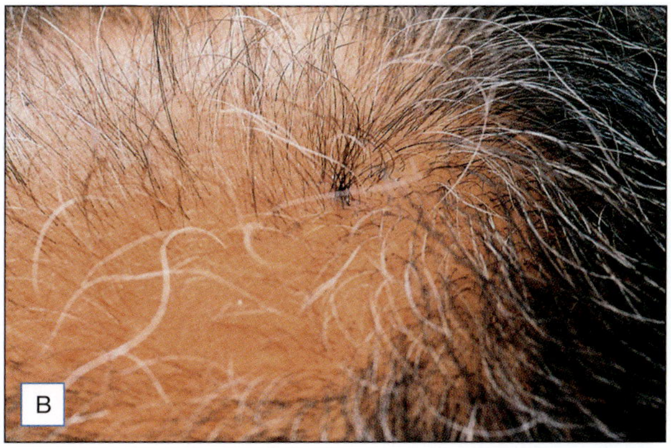


**Fig. 4.8** (**A**) The vertex showing the residual anatomic plug. (**B**) Close up

### Free-hand excision

A single scalpel blade is used to accomplish excision of a single elliptical strip of donor hair. The surgeon first draws out the margins to be excised and then cuts the upper and lower edges separately, varying the angle with that of the hairs present.

### Undermining

In donor harvesting, undermining refers to incising within the subcutaneous layer, between the dermis and galea layers, for the purpose of closing the wound under less tension. In alopecia reductions and flap surgery, however, undermining is carried out in the subgaleal plane between the galea and periosteum.

### FUE instruments

These are being developed presently. Recently, 0.75, 0.9, 1.0, and 1.1 mm diameter sharp hand punches have been used to make the initial shallow cut around the FU. Slightly duller cutting instruments are presently being proposed and developed for the deeper dissection, some with a slight conical shape. Small hypodermic needles have also been used to free up the deep attachments during the 'gentle traction' step of graft removal.

## Instruments For Making Graft Sites

### Hand punch

Made of stainless steel or titanium, the hand punch is used for cutting circular **round graft** holes of various sizes (the ones used most commonly today are 1, 1.25, 1.3, and 1.5 mm in diameter). Larger ones are available, up to 4 mm in diameter, and are primarily used for 'corrective' work removing old, large grafts. When used for this purpose, they accomplish their task more precisely in the chuck of an electric rotary hand engine.

### Scalpel blades (in donor area)

In strip harvesting, No. 10 blades, and occasionally No. 15 blades, are used to excise the donor strip. The blade can be used singly in free-hand excision or inserted into a multi-blade holder.

### Blades for making slit grafts

These come in a range of sizes and shapes. Those with flat bottoms feature either a very thin, sharp blade (MinDe Blade) or have a slightly thicker blade with a sharper 'chisel' or 'pointed chisel' bottom (SP90 Blade). Most of the thin, sharp ones are slightly angled at the bottom to allow for a level floor to the site when the instrument is inserted at an angle.

Some blades are thin and narrow at the bottom, such as the No. 11 blade and the SpearPoint Blade, which comes in various angles (one edge of the 'spear' is straight and the other is angled from it, with the greater angle creating a longer slit site).

Examples of blades used to make recipient sites, which have a slightly rounded bottom, are the Beaver Blade and the No. 15 blade.

### Needles

These may be standard cored hypodermic needles, NoKor needles, or 'solid core' needles, and are used for making FU graft recipient sites.

### Custom blades

Very small, custom-cut, squared-off or tapered blades (Hasson and Wong) are also used for FU graft recipient sites. Generally a precise cutting apparatus, which is commercially available, is necessary to produce these blades.

## Graft Dissection Terminology

### Loupe magnification

This refers to using a magnifying lens, either attached to the head, the practitioner's glasses, or as a fixed large lens over the field.

### Back-lighting

Back-lighting is a further modification that provides an illuminated translucent background during graft cutting.

### Stereoscopic microscopes

Usually 10× magnification is commonly used for dissecting FUs and MFUs. The more ergonomic, upright **Mantis Scope** is 6× magnification.

### LCD monitor with video magnification

This is a setup that features a camera that looks down on the dissection field and transmits the image to a flat screen that is viewed by the person doing the dissecting. It is two-dimensional not three-dimensional.

### Impulsive-force graft preparation

This refers to using sudden impact on a long, thin strip of donor hair by a fixed multi-blade cutting surface.

## Recipient Site Orientation

### Coronal slits

Slits made with the thin blade surface oriented in the coronal plane from side-to-side (parallel to the inter-tragal line) and usually leaning anteriorly.

### Sagittal slits

Slits made with the thin blade surface oriented in the sagittal plane (from the anterior–posterior axis).

### Perpendicular (lateral) slits

Refers to recipient sites in which the incised slit is perpendicular to the direction of the hair. In the central scalp, many of these happen to be 'coronal' (Fig. 4.9).

### Parallel slits

Refers to recipient sites in which the incised slit is parallel with the direction of the hair. In the central scalp, many of these are 'sagittal' in orientation (Fig. 4.10).

## Conclusion

The equipment and techniques of hair transplantation have been improving and changing at a dizzying pace since 1990. More refinements and changes are inevitable. The earlier-mentioned terminology represents the current understanding of what is available and creates a common language for all to use in discussing the particulars of this specialty.

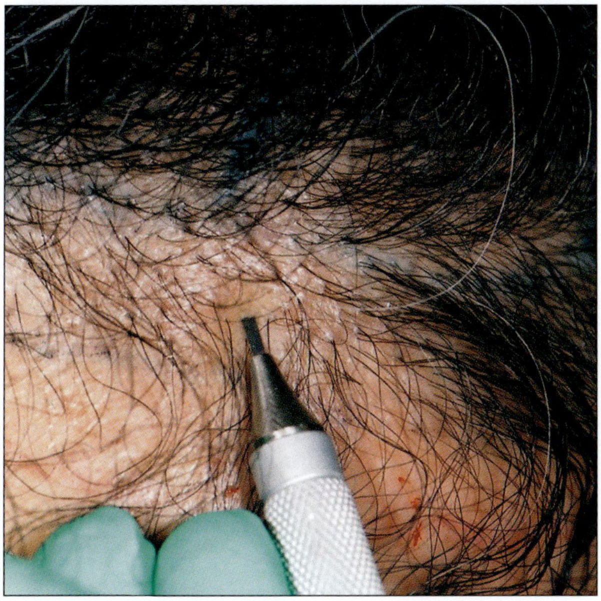

**Fig. 4.9** Front hairline recipient microslits, being made with a **perpendicular** orientation in relation to the direction of the patient's pre-existing hair in the area

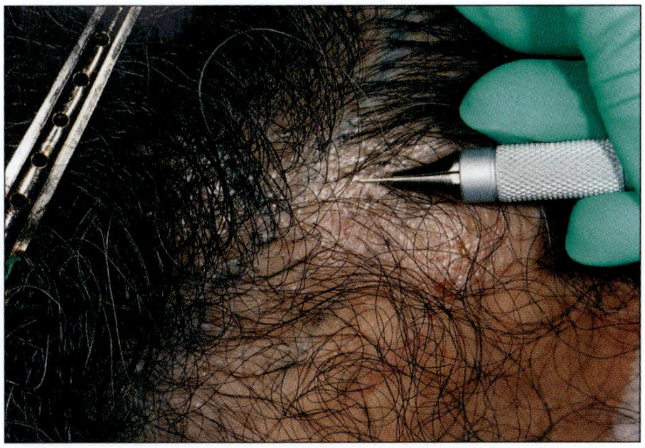

**Fig. 4.10** Front hairline recipient microslits, being made with a **parallel** orientation in relation to the direction of the patient's pre-existing hair in the area

## Further Reading


Bernstein R, Rassman WR, Seager D, et al 1998 Standardizing the classification and description of follicular unit transplantation and mini-micrografting techniques. Dermatologic Surgery 24:957–963

Bouhanna P, Dardour JC 1996 Hair Replacement Surgery, Textbook and Atlas. Springer, Berlin

Epstein ES 2004 Hair restoration and removal. Facial Plastic Surgery Clinics 12:

Seager D 1998 Dense hair transplantation from sparse donor area-introducing the "follicular unit family". HT Int 8:21–22

Stough D, Haber RS 1996 Hair replacement: Surgical and medical. Mosby Year Book, St Louis (Especially chapters 1–6)

Unger W, Shapiro R 2004 Hair Transplantation. Marcel Dekker, New York, (Especially chapters 2, 3, 5, 8, 10, 11, 12, 13)

# 5 Gross and Microscopic Anatomy of the Follicular Unit

*Francisco Jiménez, Enrique Poblet*

## Introduction

### Hair follicle development

Hair follicles develop from ectodermal and mesenchymal cells. The first morphological sign of hair follicle development is the appearance in the fetal epidermis of regularly spaced thickenings of epithelial cells known as 'placodes.' The formation and regular spacing of the placodes result from a competition between promoting and inhibitory dermal signals. The placodes then signal back to the underlying mesenchyma to form a cluster of dermal cells known as 'dermal condensate,' which will develop into the dermal papilla. The proliferation and growth of placode cells into the dermis will form the 'hair germ.' Along the length of the primitive hair follicle, two bulbous formations will be formed: the uppermost, which will give rise to the sebaceous gland and the lowermost, which will be the insertion site of the arrector pili (AP) muscle as well as the presumptive site of the hair follicle stem cells (Fig. 5.1).

## Macroscopic Anatomy of the Scalp Human Hair

### Types of hair

According to the diameter and length of the hair shafts, two types of hairs can be recognized: vellus and terminal. Vellus hair replaces lanugo hair in postnatal life. They are spread over the body surface and are difficult to visualize unless appropriate magnification is used. Vellus shafts are soft, hypopigmented, unmedullated, less than 0.03 mm in diameter and less than 1cm in length. Terminal hair shafts are longer, coarser, often medullated and pigmented. They exceed 0.06 mm in diameter and 1 cm in length. Indeterminate hairs are intermediate in size between terminal and vellus hairs. The bulb of the terminal follicle is located in the subcutaneous tissue or deep dermis. The bulb of the vellus follicle is located in the upper dermis.

Roughly 5 million hair follicles cover the human body at birth. After birth, no additional follicles are formed, although the size of the follicles can change with time, primarily under the influence of androgens. The scalp contains approximately 100,000–125,000 terminal hairs.

## Hair Distribution in Follicular Units

Under appropriate magnification, it can be seen that hair shafts exit the scalp as groupings (Fig. 5.2). Each of these hair groupings represents the visible, superficial portion of a more complex, but well-defined, histologic structure known as the follicular unit (FU). Each FU may contain one to five terminal hairs, but the majority of them (approximately 80%) are composed of two or three terminal hairs.

It is important to differentiate between FU density (number of FU per $cm^2$) and hair density (number of hairs per $cm^2$). It is the distribution of natural hair groupings in each FU that determines the patient's hair density. For example, individuals with low hair density may have a FU density within the normal range, the difference being that their one-hair FUs are more abundant than their three-hair FUs.

There are significant racial differences in FU and hair density. Asians and Blacks have a lower density than Caucasians. The FU density in the donor occipital scalp of Caucasians ranges from 60–100 FU/$cm^2$, and the average hair density around 260 ± 30 hairs/$cm^2$. As a rule of thumb the hair density is about 2.5–3.0 times the FU density. Due to the

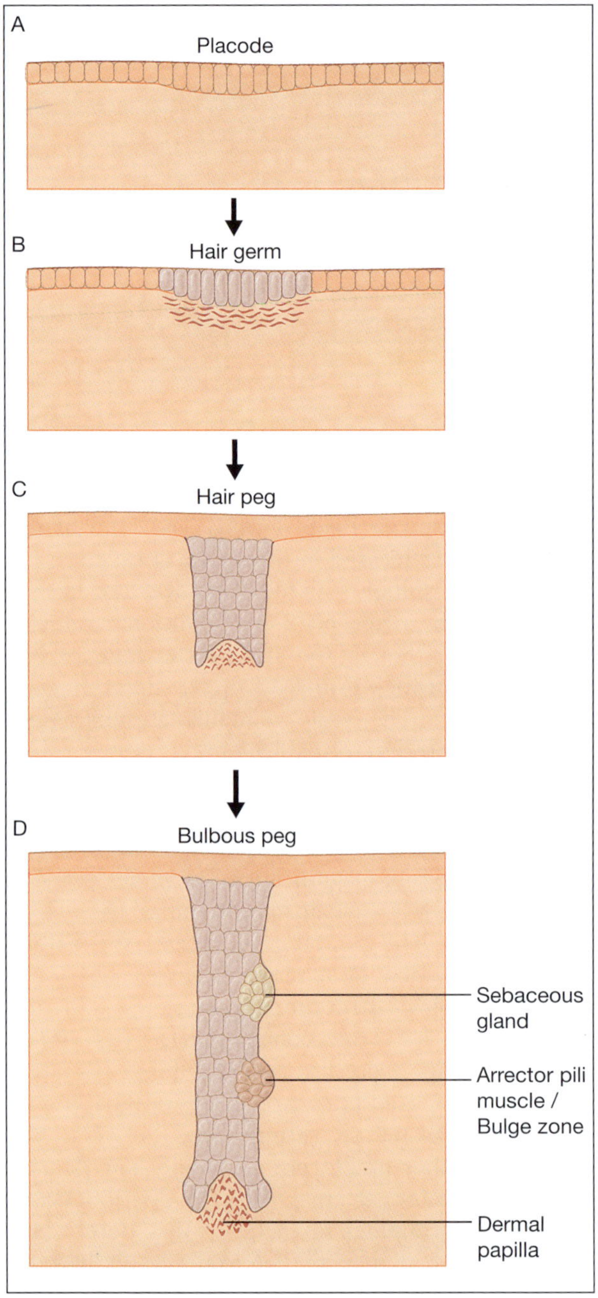


**Fig. 5.1** Schematic drawing of hair follicle embryogenesis

patient-to-patient variability in densities, the current authors encourage making measurements in each patient, so that the hair transplant surgeon can predict the total number of FUs to be obtained from the donor area (Fig. 5.3).

The FUs tend to maintain a certain distance between each other. This distance correlates with

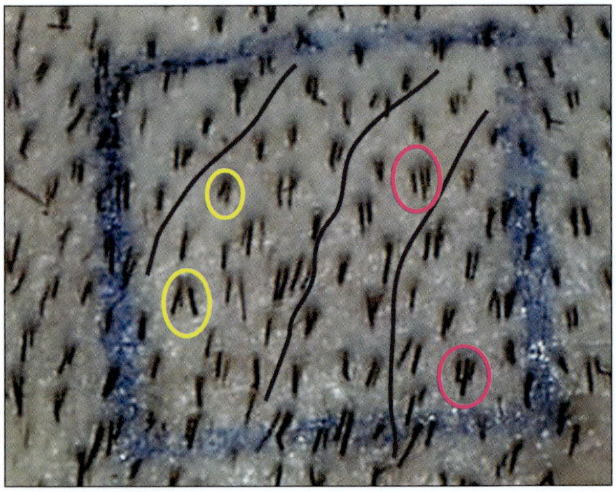

**Fig. 5.2** Photograph of occipital scalp, showing hair exiting the skin in groupings (follicular units). The blue ink outlines a 1 cm by 1 cm square. Note that follicular units are aligned in rows according to the pattern of spirals (black lines). The orientation of the hair shafts at the skin surface tend to be perpendicular to the direction of the hair flow (pink circles). Some hair shafts splay out above the level of the epidermis (yellow circles).

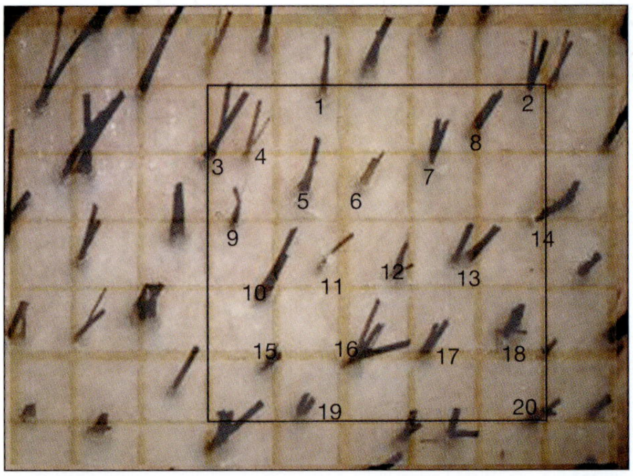


**Fig. 5.3** Close-up photograph (original magnification × 9) of donor occipital scalp showing hair exiting the skin in groupings (FUs). A total of 20 FUs are counted in a 5 × 5 mm square. The FU density will be around 80 FUs/cm$^2$. Most FUs in this area are composed of 2-terminal hairs. FUs 1 and 11 are one-hair FUs. FUs 16 and 18 are three-hair FUs. It is not possible to discern whether 3 and 4 are single four-hair FUs or two different two-hair FUs close together (serial histological sections down to the isthmus level need to be done to answer this question). This figure also demonstrates how hair shafts are bunched at their point of epidermal origin, but splay out above the level of epidermis (see 16, 3, 4 and others)

the FU density according to the formula described by Jiménez and Ruifernandez $L = 10/\sqrt{n}$, where L represents the average distance between FU expressed in millimeters, and n the number of FUs per square centimeter.

## Microscopic Anatomy of Follicular Unit

### Histology of follicular units

The FU as an independent histologic structure was first described by the pathologist John T. Headington in 1984 by analyzing transverse (horizontal) histologic sections of punch biopsies from the scalp. The reason why the FU has taken so long to be characterized is because pathologists use vertical skin sections in which the whole structure of the FU cannot be properly visualized.

Follicular units are composed of terminal hairs, vellus hairs, their associated sebaceous glands and the insertions of the AP muscles, surrounded by a circumferential band of collagen known as perifolliculum (Fig. 5.4).

The grouping of hair follicles in FUs is more pronounced above the insertion of the AP muscles (in the 'permanent portion' of the hair follicle). Below that level, the hair follicles tend to be dispersed in the subcutaneous fat, losing their grouping distribution. Serial horizontal sections show that the AP muscles originating from their respective hair follicles join together, forming a single muscular structure per FU. This evidence supports the notion that the AP muscles contribute to the anatomical integrity of the FU by holding together each of the hair follicles contained in the FU at the isthmus level 'like a ribbon on a bunch of flowers' (Fig. 5.5).

### Histology of hair follicles

The histology of a hair follicle changes according to the stage of growth cycle it is going through. A typical terminal hair follicle in anagen stage can be divided in three vertical segments (Fig. 5.6):

1. The upper portion or **infundibulum**, extending from the follicular orifice to the entrance of the sebaceous duct.
2. The middle portion or **isthmus**, extending from the entrance of the sebaceous duct to the insertion of the arrector pili muscle (bulge region).
3. The lower or **inferior** portion, extending from the insertion of the arrector pili muscle to the base of the follicle. The bulbous portion at the base of the follicle is known as the hair bulb, and is composed of the hair matrix and the dermal papilla (Fig. 5.7).

The infundibulum and the isthmus constitute the **permanent portion of the hair follicle** because they remain intact throughout the entire hair cycle. In contrast, the lower portion of the hair follicle suffers periods of regression and regeneration during the hair cycle.

The hair follicle is composed of epithelial and dermal components (dermal papilla and dermal sheath). The dermal sheath, which surrounds the follicle, is made of connective tissue. The dermal papilla is an oval mass of extracellular matrix harboring spindle-shaped fibroblasts. Its size apparently controls the size of the follicle. The dermal papilla is connected to the surrounding dermal sheath at its lower pole, and surrounded on its top and sides by the hair matrix.

The epithelial components of the hair follicle are the hair matrix and a number of different concentric layers (from inside to outside): hair shaft, inner root sheath (IRS), companion layer, and outer root sheath (ORS) (Fig. 5.7). The hair matrix is the actively growing portion of the hair. It consists of rapidly proliferating epithelial cells that differentiate and move upward, producing the hair shaft. The hair shaft consists of a narrow central medulla (only present in terminal hairs), a thick cortex, and a cuticle made of a single layer of overlapping cells. The hair shaft is composed of specific 'hard' $\alpha$-keratins.

The IRS is composed of three cylindrical cell layers: the cuticle of the internal sheath, Huxley's layer, and Henle's layer (Fig. 5.8). A multistep differentiation program characterizes the IRS, resulting in a rigid structure that may serve as a guide and mold to the growing shaft. The ORS lies in continuity with the epidermis and is composed of multiple layers of epithelial cubical cells, containing large quantities of glycogen. In between the ORS and the IRS, there is a single layer of flattened cells, known as the companion layer. The slippage plane at which the IRS-packaged hair shaft moves distally up to the skin surface is at the level of the companion layer, which moves in conjunction with the Henle's layer while adjacent ORS cells remain stationary.

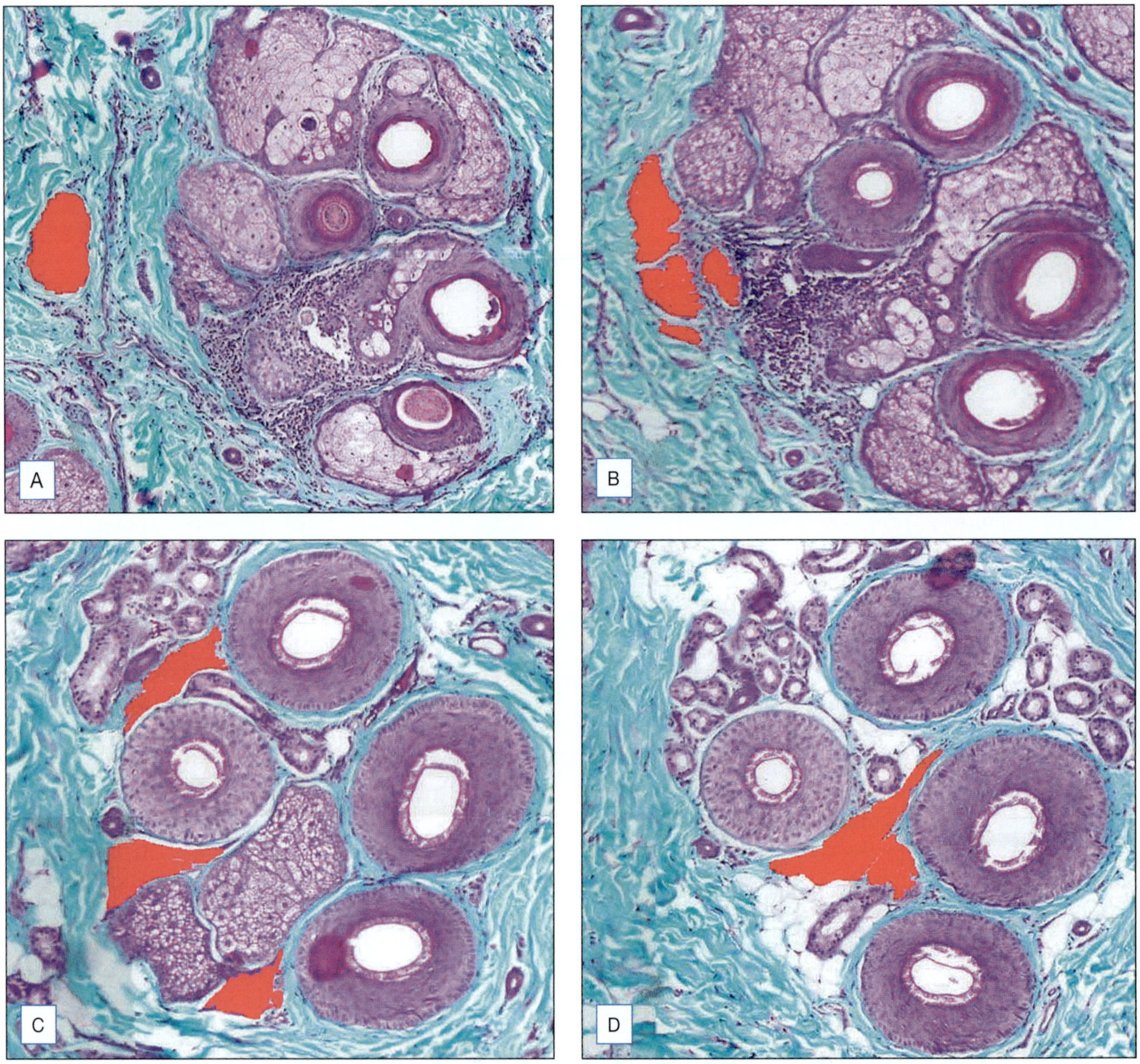


**Fig. 5.4** Horizontal serial sections through a FU showing four terminal hairs, sebaceous glands, and arrector pili muscles (in red). Sections are ordered sequentially from the upper isthmus (section A) down to the lower isthmus (section D). Sebaceous glands are seen mainly at the upper and mid-isthmus level (sections A and B). The attachment of the arrector pili muscles to the hair follicles indicate that sections C and D are made at the lower isthmus level. This photograph shows the concept of 'one arrector pili muscle serving one follicular unit.' In photomicrograph A, a thick, single, arrector pili muscle bundle appears at the left margin of the follicular unit. Deeper sections show how this muscle bundle divides into fascicles, which are going to attach to each one of the four hair follicles that constitute the FU.

Pigment in the hair shaft is produced by numerous dendritic melanocytes interspersed among the matrix cells. They extend their dendrites into the matrix cells to which they transfer melanosomes.

In the ORS, at the level of the isthmus, Langerhans cells and Merkel cells are also present. Their roles in hair physiology are still unclear.

## Follicular stem cells

A hair follicle is a regenerating system, and as with any cellular structure that periodically renews itself, it depends on stem cells that retain the ability to divide over the lifetime of the individual and regenerate that structure.

The presumptive location of the hair follicle stem cells is in the so-called 'bulge region' of the ORS, at

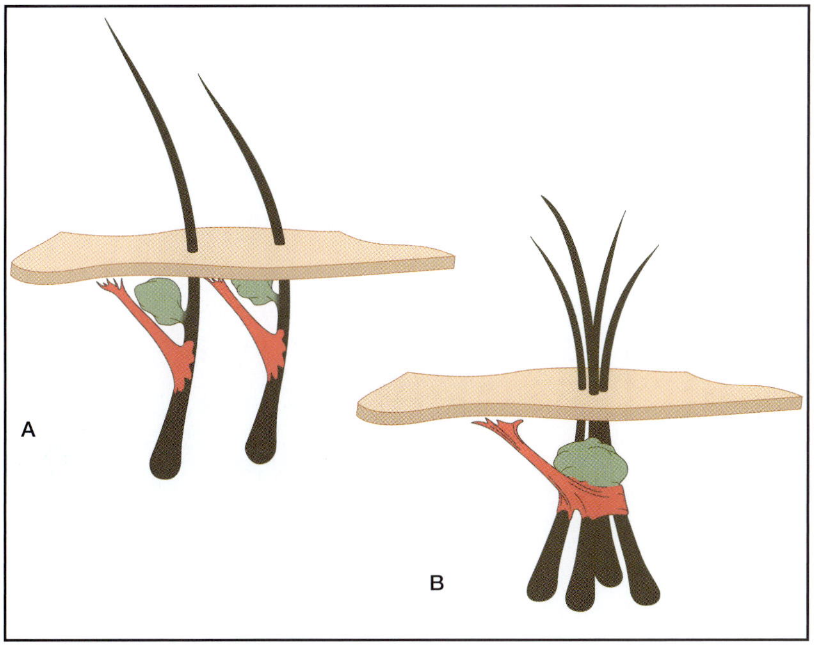


**Fig. 5.5** Drawing **A** shows the traditional anatomy of human scalp hair. Drawing **B** shows a more accurate representation of the FU. The epidermis is drawn in yellow, the arrector pili muscle in red, and the sebaceous glands in green. (Reprinted from Poblet E, Jimenez F, Ortega F 2004 The contribution of the arrector pili muscle and sebaceous glands to the follicular unit structure. Journal of the American Academy of Dermatology 51:217–222, with permission)

the level of the arrector pili muscle insertion. In the adult human hair follicle the bulge is not visible. Immunohistochemical studies using presumptive stem cell markers (keratin 15, keratin 19, or CD34) suggest that epithelial stem cells in human hair follicles may be more widely spread along the ORS.

Recent evidence supports the multipotentiality of the hair follicle stem cells, which can give rise not only to the different hair follicle layers but also, in certain conditions, to epidermal cells and the sebaceous glands. Grafting experiments performed in a mouse model have shown that bulge stem cells isolated by cell sorting analysis and expanded in vitro are able to induce new hair growth when reinjected into the animal's skin. By improving methods to isolate and culture follicular stem cells, a number of research teams are trying to reproduce these striking results in humans, which may open new treatment strategies in hair transplantation.

Although most investigators have focused on 'epithelial' stem cells, recent evidence also indicates the existence of 'mesenchymal' stem cells in the dermal sheath. These stem cells could play a significant role in the dermal wound healing process.

## Hair Growth: The Hair Cycle

The hair cycle can be divided into three phases: anagen, in which a fully formed hair follicle is producing a mature hair fiber at a continuous rate of 0.35 mm/day; catagen (involution stage); and telogen (resting stage) (Fig. 5.9). The hair cycle duration differs in different regions of the body. In the adult human scalp the anagen stage lasts on average around 3 years, catagen 3 weeks, and telogen 3 months.

During catagen, the inferior portion of the hair follicles goes through a process of involution driven by programmed cell death (apoptosis). At the end of catagen, the dermal papilla condenses and moves upward, coming to rest underneath the base of the telogen follicle. During telogen the hair follicle matures into a 'club hair', which is eventually shed (exogen). Sometimes, a recently described 'lag phase' can occur. The follicle is empty and no hair shaft is growing. Its duration varies from 2–5 months but not all follicles are affected.

What initiates a new anagen stage from telogen and from where that stimulus comes from is currently unknown. The induction of anagen is associated with the enlargement of the dermal papilla and a burst of proliferation in the lower portion of the telogen hair follicle ('secondary hair germ'), which grows down into the deep dermis and subcutaneous fat.

It is important to note that in humans the follicular activity is asynchronous and neighboring follicles are normally at different stages of the cycle,

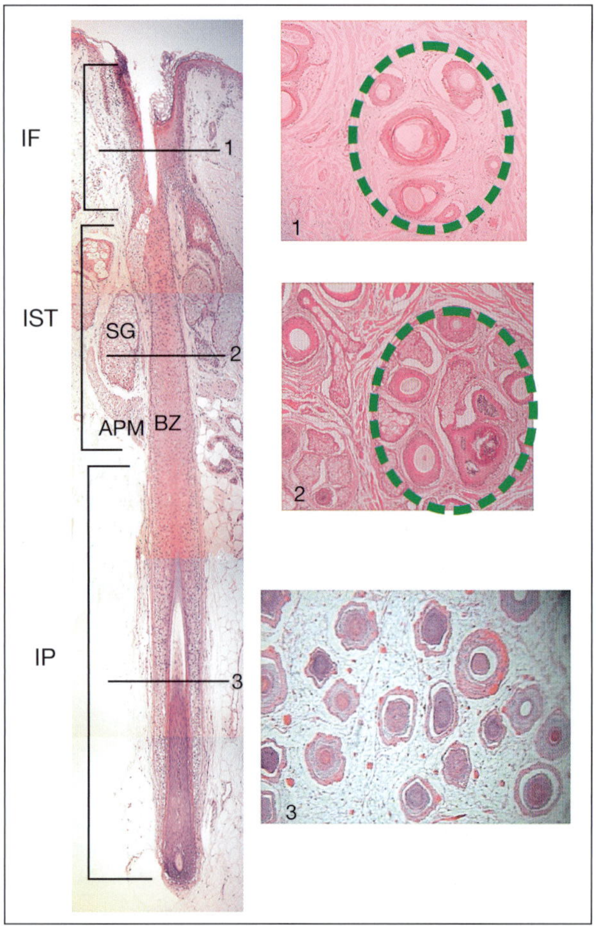


**Fig. 5.6** Vertical histologic section of a terminal anagen hair showing the three segments in which a hair follicle can be divided: the infundibulum (IF), the isthmus (IST), and the inferior portion (IP). The bulge zone (BZ) corresponds to the region of the arrector pili muscle (APM) insertion. The upper and middle figures on the right show horizontal sections made through the infundibulum (1) and isthmus (2) levels, respectively. At these levels of depth the hair follicles are distributed in follicular units (green circles). Figure 3 shows a horizontal section made at the level of the inferior portion (3), in which the hair follicles are disposed in an irregular arrangement surrounded by subcutaneous tissue. The follicular units cannot be identified at this level. SG: sebaceous gland.

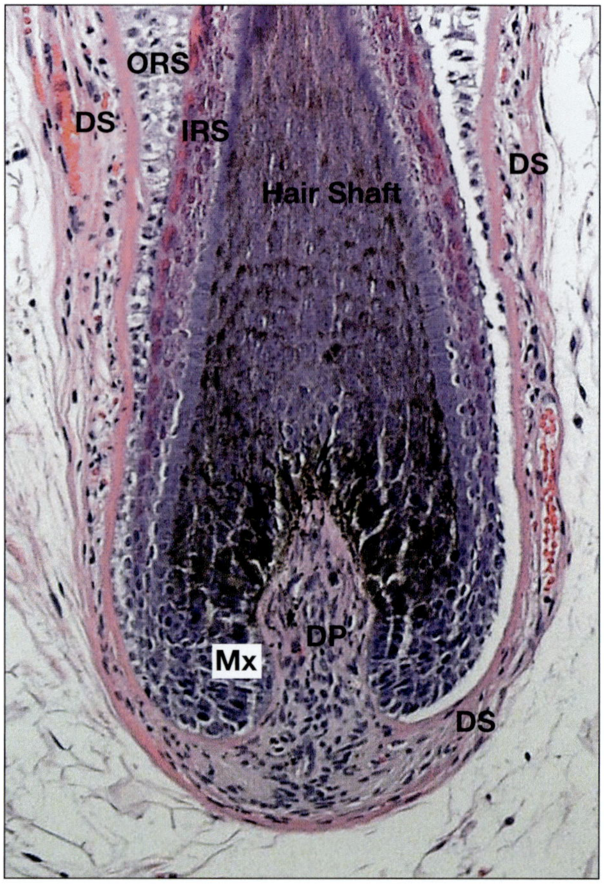


**Fig. 5.7** The hair bulb of a terminal anagen hair follicle. DS = dermal sheath, DP = dermal papilla, Mx = matrix, IRS = internal root sheath, ORS = outer root sheath. Note the continuity between the dermal papilla and the dermal sheath. Dendritic melanocytes can be seen within the hair matrix

the so-called mosaic cycle. At any given time, approximately 84–90% of scalp hairs are in anagen, 2% in catagen, and 10–16% in telogen (Fig. 5.10). Thus, assuming 100,000 scalp hairs with 10% in telogen, the average hair loss equals 100 hairs per day.

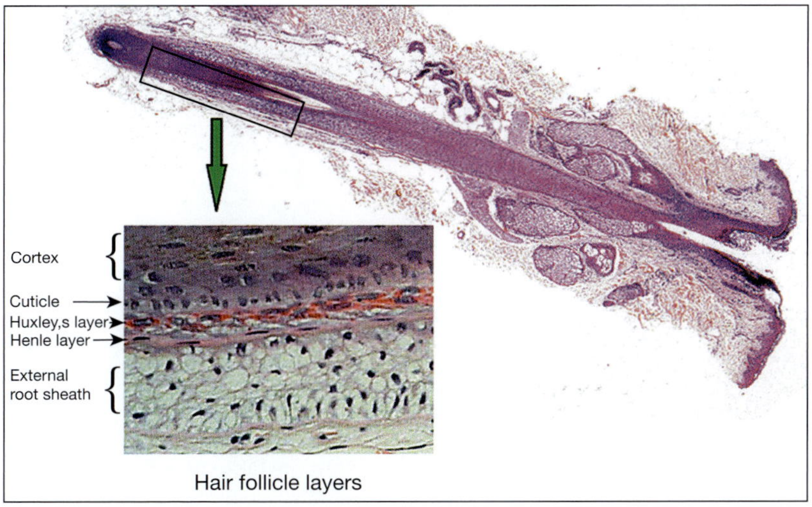


**Fig. 5.8** Vertical section of the suprabulbar region of a terminal anagen hair showing the different hair follicle layers

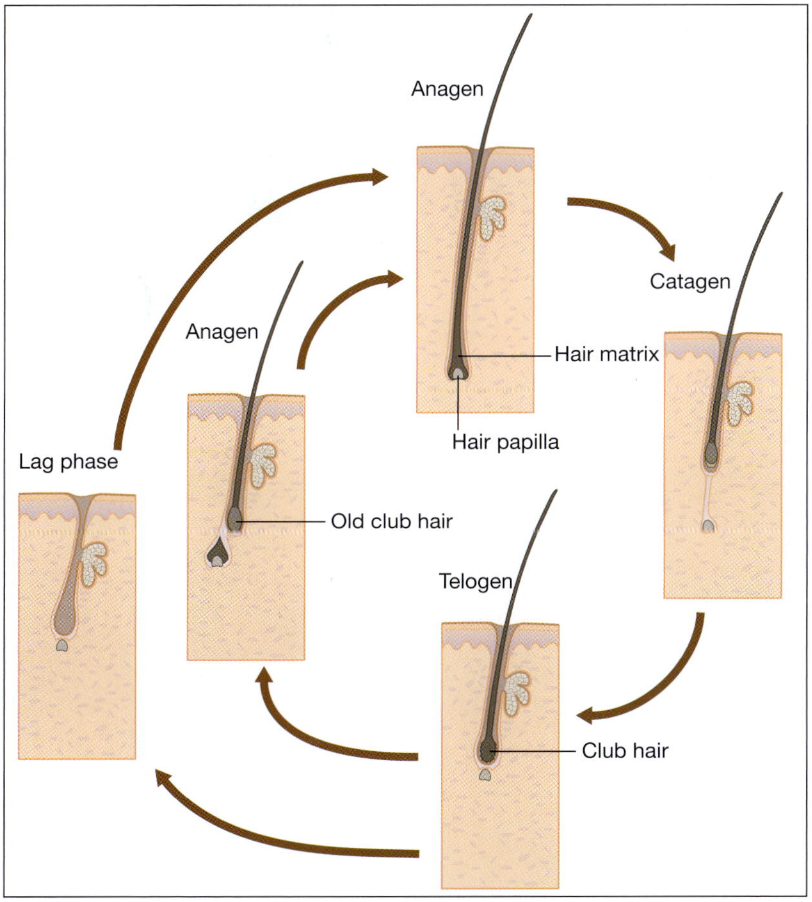


**Fig. 5.9** A schematic drawing of the hair cycle representing the different stages: anagen, catagen, telogen, and lag phase

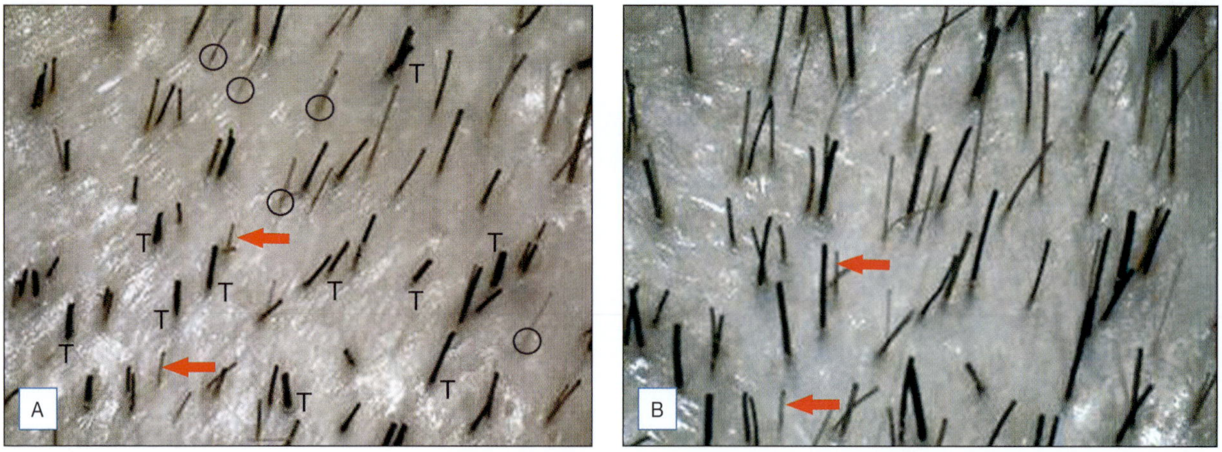


**Fig. 5.10** Phototrichogram, a noninvasive method to evaluate the hair cycle. Two photographs are taken from the same donor scalp site immediately after clipping (**A**) and 48 hours later (**B**). Hairs that have grown (the great majority in this picture) are in the anagen phase; those that have not grown are in telogen (red arrows). In this patient with androgenetic alopecia, numerous thin, hypopigmented, miniaturized hairs can be seen along with thick terminal hairs (T)

## Summary

This chapter gives an introductory review of the anatomy and physiology of the human hair follicle, emphasizing different aspects particularly useful for the hair transplant surgeon. This organelle of mammals has unique characteristics that allow it to serve as a model for unveiling some of the most challenging topics in modern biology, including organogenesis, stem cell biology, epithelial–mesenchymal interactions, and cell differentiation.

## Further Reading

Balplain C, Lowry WE, Geoghegan A, Polar L, Fuchs E 2004 Self-renewal, multipotency, and the existence of two cell populations within an epithelial stem cell niche. Cell 118:635–648

Dámico D, Vaccaro M, Guarneri F, et al 2001 Phototrichogram using videomicroscopy: a useful technique in the evaluation of scalp hair. European Journal of Dermatology 11:17–20

Headington JT 1984 Transverse microscopic anatomy of the human scalp. Archives of Dermatology 120:449–456

Jahoda CAB, Reynolds AJ 2001 Hair follicle dermal sheath cells: unsung participants in wound healing. Lancet 358:1445–1448

Jimenez F, Ruifernández JM 1999 Distribution of human hair in follicular units. Dermatologic Surgery 25:294–298

Lavker RM, Sun TT, Oshima H, et al 2003 Hair follicle stem cells. Journal of Investigative Dermatology Symposia Proceedings 8:28–38

Millar SA 2002 Molecular mechanisms regulating hair follicle development. Journal of Investigative Dermatology 118:216–225

Morris RJ, Liu Y, Marles L, et al 2004 Capturing and profiling adult hair follicle stem cells. Nature and Biotechnology 22:411–417

Paus R, Foitzik K 2004 In search of the hair cycle clock: a guided tour. Differentiation 72:489–511

Poblet E, Jimenez F, Ortega F 2004 The contribution of the arrector pili muscle and sebaceous glands to the follicular unit structure. Journal of the American Academy of Dermatology 51:217–222

Sperling LC 2003 An Atlas of Hair Pathology with Clinical Correlations. Parthenon Publishing Group, New York

Stenn KS, Paus R 2001 Controls of hair follicle cycling. Physiol Review 81:449–494

# 6 The Consultation

*Dowling B. Stough*

"First the patient, second the patient, third the patient, fourth the patient, fifth the patient, and then maybe comes science. We first do everything for the patient ..."

**Béla Schick** (1877–1967) renowned Hungarian pediatrician and bacteriologist

## Introduction

The consultation process involves the patient communicating his or her goals, as well as a discussion of what may be reasonably expected in achieving these goals. The surgeon must refuse a certain percentage of individuals seeking hair transplantation surgery. These individuals either do not meet the necessary criteria, have unrealistic goals of the procedure outcome or cannot be satisfied with current techniques. The experienced surgeon understands this and recognizes the patient who will ultimately not be satisfied with a hair transplant procedure. Decisions made during the consultation have a far greater impact on long-term results and satisfaction of said results than technical nuances employed by various surgeons.

It is difficult for the layperson to comprehend the complexity of choosing the right candidate for the transplantation, how to proceed with surgery based upon the individual's goals and how to produce an excellent long-term result. Patients seek out surgeons based on their technical ability to produce an outstanding result. Their decision is supported by before and after photographs found in brochures, videos, and the Internet, meeting with and examining former patients, and/or referrals from trusted physicians or other resources. The surgeon must place the short-term and long-term goals of the patient first. All decisions regarding whether or not to proceed with surgery, placement of the hairline, and density of grafts must be made in the patient's best interest. The surgeon should disregard any personal and financial goals, or else the very core of doctoring – humanism – is sacrificed and the bond between patient and physician becomes weakened or is never formed. It is only through this approach that the field of hair transplantation will earn its rightfully deserved respect in the field of medicine.

## Key Points of the Consultation (Box 6.1)

It is incumbent upon the physician to identify the patient's spoken and unspoken needs and to make it very clear to the patient the expected and attainable results. The process of consultation is an effort by the physician to communicate his or her knowledge and apply it to the unique needs of each patient. All patients should discuss and comprehend the following points:

| Key points of the consultation | |
|---|---|
| **Patient goals** | The patient must communicate his or her goals to the surgeon |
| **Progressive nature of hair loss** | The patient must understand hair loss is an unrelenting and ongoing process. More than one session will eventually be needed |
| **Facial framing** | The patient should understand the positive aspects of facial framing and that framing restores the central facial features |
| **Natural appearance** | The transplanted pattern must mimic a natural appearance in the short and long term. Long-term vertex transplantation may be discouraged |
| **Permanence** | The patient must understand that transplanted hairlines are permanent |

**Box 6.1** Key points of the consultation

1. **Ascertaining goals**. A consultation flow sheet specifically for hair transplantation should be composed (Fig. 6.1). The simple question: 'What is your goal?' is the single most important question to ask during the consultation. The question should be thoroughly discussed between the surgeon and the patient seeking hair transplantation. The physician should specifically ask what area of loss is the most disconcerting to the patient to determine and understand the motivating factor for seeking hair transplantation. This consideration is of critical significance in the preoperative evaluation since it is the basis from which patient expectations are synchronized with surgical and medical capabilities.

   A history of previous hair transplants or scalp surgeries, both of which factor into preoperative planning from the standpoint of scalp elasticity, recipient site creation, and donor strip harvesting, is imperative. Many patients presenting with a history of round, standard 4 mm punch autografts display an unnatural appearance. Removal of the large, cosmetically unacceptable grafts is often necessary, especially when located in the frontal most hairline. Most patients with standard punch autografts have no comprehension of the degree of refinement and advancements in modern hair transplantation. This should be communicated and explained to all of those with unnatural-standard punch autografts.
2. **The progressive nature of hair loss**. Hair loss is not static. It is an ongoing process that proceeds (albeit slowly in some cases) throughout a person's lifetime. There is a limited ability to predict the extent of a person's baldness.
3. **The importance of framing the face**. Unique facial features are more distinguished by facial framing. A natural facial framing returns the patient's familiar appearance and restores the central face as the focus of attention. This is mostly applicable to bald patients, but anyone undergoing transplantation should understand the concept of facial framing. Patients should understand that the positive aspects of facial framing far exceed the importance of density.
4. **The goal of a natural appearance**. Baldness is a very natural condition. The treatment for hair loss should therefore produce a natural appearance. Utilizing current techniques, hair replacement should never look odd or apparent. Hair transplantation cannot produce an exact duplicate of nature, but it can provide a natural-looking alternative to hair loss. Modern hair transplantation surgery is natural and undetectable. The exception may be transplantation into the vertex. When transplantation is performed in the vertex followed by extensive hair loss, an unnatural result will ensue.
5. **The permanence of the transplanted hairline**. While hair loss is relentlessly progressive, transplanted hairlines are permanent. The creation of a hairline utilizing hair transplantation surgery visually arrests the change in appearance. Hairlines must be acceptable at their initial placement as well as throughout the patient's lifetime. An examination of patients who received wide, rounded, youthful hairlines reveals an odd appearance after the fifth decade of life. A compromise between a low hairline and a natural mature hairline must be communicated during the consultation process. In Chapter 3, p. 23 reference is made to the frontal corners; this area represents the apex of the frontal-temporal triangle. Young men desire a complete fill of this corner area. Older men who are completely bald focus on facial framing and have no desire to recreate troughs, which may look unnatural in the advanced balding state. Thus, a paradox exists. Pleasing the young patient at an early age may ultimately create problems at a later age. There is no textbook solution to solve this problem. It can only be hoped that good judgment by all parties will prevail.

## History

A medical history should include questions regarding previous bleeding problems, prescription medications, current hair loss medications, drug allergies as well as vitamin and herbal supplement intake. Aspirin, Clopidogrel (Plavix), heparin, and Warfarin sodium (Coumadin) are all potentially problematic for the transplant surgeon. Sessions on patients using these medications can become quite vascular, severely limiting the size of the session. If medically acceptable, cease all of these medicines prior to transplantation. Aspirin should be stopped for a minimum of 2 weeks prior to transplantation, Clopidogrel for at least 5 days, and Warfarin sodium and heparin for 24 hours. Vitamin E, garlic, ginseng, and ginkgo have been reported anecdotally to increase bleeding during surgery. Evaluation may

## MEDICAL CONSULTATION FOR HAIR TRANSPLANT

Date ____________________ Time in/out ____________________

Name ______________________________________

Age _____

### MEDICAL HISTORY:

General health ____________________
Drug allergies ____________________
Bleeding tendencies ____________________
Smoking history ____________________
Age hair loss began ____________________
History of diabetes, artificial joints, heart valves, pacemaker ____________________
History of abnormal scarring or keloid ____________________

Current meds ____________________
Family history of hair loss ____________________
Hair loss treatments used ____________________
Vitamin/supplements ____________________

### PATIENT'S STATED GOALS:

______________________________________

______________________________________

### TREATMENT PLAN:

Past scalp reductions ____________________
Previous transplants ____________________
Estimated graft sessions ____________________

______________________________________

Propecia rx ____________________

______________________________________

HIV and Hep B & C blood work explained ____________________

______________________________________

Procedure explained ____________________
Web site reviewed ____________________
Literature reviewed ____________________
Areas of most concern to patient ____________________
Areas to be transplanted ____________________

### HAIR & SCALP EVALUATION:

*Grade ____________________
Current pattern ____________________
Anticipated pattern ____________________
Density ____________________
Scalp thickness ____________________
Hair color ____________________
Skin color ____________________
Curl ____________________
Texture ____________________
Vellous hair ____________________
Terminal hair ____________________
Hair caliber ____________________
Problems ____________________

### COMMENTS / SPECIAL INSTRUCTIONS:

______________________________________

______________________________________

* Hair is graded on a scale of (ABCD) with 'A' having all of the favorable qualities for transplantation, i.e., color, caliber, and curl. 'D' would represent an individual with fine, silky hair devoid of curl and body. See discussion under caliber on page 47.

**Fig. 6.1** Form for hair transplant consultation

also include assessing the need for preoperative antibiotics in select cases, i.e. prosthetic joints, valvular heart disease, diabetes and immunosuppressed patients. Preoperative antibiotics are not recommended on a routine basis.

## Counselor

The role of the hair counselor is indispensable in composing and distributing information concerning the physician and the clinic. The counselor acts as a mediator between the patient and physician. This person is readily available to the patient to answer questions regarding preoperative instructions, tests, and postoperative care. Patients often feel more comfortable speaking with someone other than the doctor about their fears leading up to the procedure as well as during the recovery phase. The proper use of counselors can result in improved communication between the patient and staff. Only the physician should dictate the actual treatment plan, but the counselor may relate the surgeon's common recommendations and document all questions, concerns and discussions between the patient and counselor.

The hair counselor must understand the delicate balance between enthusiastically explaining a procedure to a good candidate and selling a 'medical procedure.' The influence of the hair counselor should be focused on factual information and not on persuasion. It is considered unethical for counselors to act on behalf of the surgeon and present an individualized specific treatment plan without the surgeon's involvement. It is imperative that the counselor not act as 'the physician' in dictating treatment plans. A controversial issue within the world transplant community has been the topic of counselors receiving financial reimbursements for 'signing patients up.'

A patient visiting for consultation should receive frank, open, and honest communication regarding his or her hair loss. The patient should gain a clear understanding of the progressive nature of pattern hair loss with potential complications. It is the counselor's job to reiterate the treatment plan proposed by the surgeon and ascertain any concerns that may be unresolved. The counselor can supply information on websites, review before-and-after photographs, provide brochures, videos, and printed material. Most importantly, the counselor can review the patients' and physicians' stated goals. Appropriate consent and all pre and postoperative instructions can be communicated by this individual.

## Conveying limitations

The rate of hair loss in any given individual is unpredictable, but the success of a hair transplant depends in part on the amount of subsequent hair loss experienced by the patient. Hair loss never becomes static and further transplantation is always a possibility. It is best to avoid quoting the exact number of grafts or procedures required to satisfy an individual. Instead, provide ranges and emphasize that these are estimates only, for example, a 40-year-old man with isolated bi-temporal recession may require only one session of follicular unit (FU) grafts. He may require further grafting 5 years later to prevent the unnatural appearance of a separation between his transplanted frontal hairs and receding parietal hair. If it is not understood at the outset that this progression of loss is likely to occur, the patient may present for further work with the misconception that a 'repair' is being performed due to inadequate surgery during his first transplant session. If however he understands the progressive nature of hair loss, he will rightly view subsequent transplant sessions as maintenance. Medical therapy is helpful in preventing ongoing hair loss, but cannot be relied upon as fail-safe. When predicting how much hair loss an individual will incur, it is safest to assume that all will progress to an advanced stage of alopecia; therefore, surgeons should plan any transplant accordingly. Since the extent of future hair loss cannot be predicted, it is unfair and unreasonable to place the entire burden upon the surgeon. Despite careful planning by the surgeon, some degree of risk must be assumed by the patient.

## Postoperative effluvium

The observation of hair loss in the immediate postoperative period can occasionally be expected and should be communicated to the patient. This post-transplant effluvium is thought to occur as a result of local tissue trauma. This involves loss of nontransplanted hairs. Terminal hairs can be affected, but vellus hair is the most susceptible to this process. Medical therapy, such as finasteride, may help to modify this loss, but there are only anecdotal reports without studies to prove its effectiveness in this situation. Owing to the delay of

6 months between the transplant session and the observed result, patients will frequently be forgetful of their initial counseling and their initial appearance. It is the authors' current practice to take photographs and to incorporate the above-mentioned discussions into the consultation and the informed consent.

## Candidate Selection

Useful criteria for assessing an individual's quality as a candidate for hair transplantation include, but are not limited to, the age, caliber of the hair shaft, donor hair quality, degree of baldness, and patient expectations (Box 6.2).

### Age considerations

Men in good health can be transplanted throughout their lifetime. Men in their late teens and early 20s with the beginnings of frontotemporal recessions often desire transplantation of their hairline to its original location. Such cases are problematic. The fear of future baldness is usually the stimulus in seeking consultation. Surgery can provide a quick fix but may result in an unnatural hairline placement 10–20 years later. Young men in the early stages of hair loss (Norwood stages I and II) who presently maintain facial framing will receive limited esthetic benefit from surgery. This is also true of patients only seeking transplantation in areas of early thinning.

### Caliber

The caliber of hair will directly influence the outcome of transplantation. The caliber should be gauged in each patient at the time of consultation and recorded. The author currently assigns a value rating of A through D at this stage. (A represents hair with the largest caliber diameter, i.e. 100 μ or more; B represents large caliber; C average caliber; and D represents fine, corn silk hair of 60 μ.) Hair transplant surgeons generally speak of hair caliber when discussing the size of the hair shaft. Larger width (> 80 μ) hair is of higher cosmetic value than fine hair. A successful one-session result generally requires individuals with a larger hair caliber. It is difficult to achieve a one-session result in a patient with fine hair despite adequate dense packing. Patients possessing fine

| Five basic criteria for hair transplantation | |
|---|---|
| **Age** | Patients over the age of 30 years are preferable. While patients under 30 often consult, there is a reluctance to operate. The predictive value of future hair loss is much lower for individuals between the ages of 15 and 25 years of age. Even with the theoretical safety net of finasteride, physicians should hesitate and carefully choose candidates under 25 years of age. This subgroup also tends to desire a return to a full head of hair as opposed to a mature pattern of transplantation that is routinely performed in older age groups |
| **Hair shaft caliber** | The caliber of the hair shaft is crucial. Those with large-caliber hair shafts (greater than 80 μ) obtain much denser coverage than individuals with corn silk quality hair. This can be demonstrated mathematically in that very small volume increases in hair shaft diameter result in exponential increases in surface area coverage |
| **Donor hair** | The donor density can be measured using an instrument designed specifically to evaluate hair count. Patients seeking hair transplantation who have greater than 80 FUs per $cm^2$ are excellent candidates. Those with a donor hair density of less than 40 FUs per $cm^2$ are considered poor candidates. A variety of instruments are available to measure donor hair density |
| **Degree of baldness** | The degree of baldness is perhaps the most important criteria in candidate selection. Those with complete baldness in the frontal scalp as opposed to baldness limited to the vertex are excellent candidates. Individuals are rarely transplanted in the vertex, therefore it is preferred that patients possess complete frontal baldness. This area can be corrected and creates the most dramatic positive change in appearance |
| **Patient expectations** | The consultation is important to convey realistic expectations. Most unrealistic expectations occur in the realm of density. Those with fine hair should not expect significant density. Patients should be advised that future grafting may become necessary due to the progressive nature of hair loss |

**Box 6.2** Five basic criteria for hair transplantation

hair (< 60 μ) are certain to have a sparse quality to their transplant. These patients can have 'see through' hair, even with dense packing of more than 25 follicular units per $cm^2$ in the recipient area. Fine hair will always cover less surface area than hair of a large caliber. Sometimes, the results of transplanting these patients can be marginal. Some surgeons will refuse to transplant these individuals since they feel they are poor candidates.

## Donor hair quality

Patients with larger numbers of FUs per $cm^2$ in the occipital scalp yield a greater number of FUs per donor strip. Men require a density count of at least 40 FUs per $cm^2$ in their donor area to be considered for transplants. Fortunately, most men presenting for hair transplantation have greater than 55 FUs/$cm^2$ in the occipital region. FU counts vary among different ethnic groups. Caucasians have higher FU counts than Asians, but Asians have larger caliber hair shafts and often receive excellent coverage. The number of hairs per FU grouping also varies among ethnic groups (Table 6.1). The density of harvestable terminal hair in the occipital region, especially in the central anatomical point of the inion, should be evaluated in every potential candidate. Most transplant surgeons utilize magnification devices to aid with this measurement.

## Patient expectations

The patient's expectations are often the most important consideration when assessing a candidate for hair transplantation. If a patient presents with unrealistic expectations or desires that cannot be modified through careful consultation and explanations, this person is a poor candidate for hair transplantation. Most unrealistic expectations occur in the realm of density and hairline placement. Individuals with fine hair (<60 μ) cannot expect significant density. Patients who wear hair systems may never be pleased with the comparative density achieved with FU grafting. This subset has proved difficult to satisfy. Discussions regarding hair loss, placement of grafts and areas of transplantation may be difficult and time consuming, but are essential to a mutually acceptable outcome.

Follicular differences among people of different ethnic groups

| Factor | Caucasians | Asians | Africans |
|---|---|---|---|
| FU/$mm^2$ | 1 | 1 | 0.6 |
| Average density (hairs/$mm^2$) | 2 | 1.7 | 1.6 |
| Predominant hair grouping | Two | Two | Three |

*(From Tsai R-U, et al 2002 The distribution of follicular units in the Chinese scalp: Implications for reconstruction of natural-appearing hairlines in Orientals. Dermatologic Surgery 28(6):500–503, with permission.)*

**Table 6.1** Follicular differences among people of different ethnic groups

## The Vertex

While some individuals desire full coverage from the vertex to the frontal scalp, this should be discouraged. The vertex is problematic due to the potential consumption of a limited supply of donor tissue. There are two primary reasons for dissatisfaction with vertex transplantation. The first is the inevitable 360-degree progression of baldness, and the second is the central gravity pull that always leaves an area of scalp visible. Therefore adequate density is difficult to achieve in this area; even if high density is achieved in the short term, the patient will risk a poor outcome later in life due to peripheral loss of nontransplanted hair. The vertex area does not become stable with time, and therefore the vertex should be approached with extreme caution. Statistical probability dictates that most individuals will experience significant future vertex hair loss that may result in a deformity and/or an unnatural cosmetic outcome.

## Further Reading


Barrera A 2002 Hair transplantation: The art of micrografting and minigrafting. Quality Medical Publishing Inc. St Louis, USA

Bryan CS, Brett AS, Saunders DE Jr, Khushf G, Fulton GB 2004 Professionalism. In: Medical ethics and professionalism: A synopsis for students and residents. Center for Bioethics and Medical Humanities, University of South Carolina, 13

Leavitt M 1999 Patient Services Survey (post consultation, conducted nationally.) Maitland. Florida Medical Hair Restoration Data on file

Nouri K, Leal-Khouri S 2003 Techniques in dermatologic surgery. Elsevier, p.217–232

Swinehart JM 1996 Color Atlas of Hair Restoration Surgery. Appleton & Lange, Simon and Schuster, Stanford, CT, USA

# 7 International Standards for the Consent Process

*Paul T. Rose*

## Introduction

Inherent to the care provided by a physician is the communication between physician and patient. The physician must relate to the patient various aspects of the patient's medical condition, modalities for treatment and probabilities of a successful outcome. Lapses in such communication can lead to disappointment on the part of the patient and possibly even litigation based on lack of informed consent. For an example of a consent form, see Fig. 7.1.

## Concept of Informed Consent

The concept of informed consent has evolved over time in American jurisprudence and today the need to provide informed consent to patients is shared throughout many parts of the world. Fundamentally, informed consent is based on the belief that every person has a right to autonomy over his or her body and therefore the right to refuse treatment or even information.

Early cases concerning informed consent were often based on a claim of assault and battery. While some jurisdictions still accept such a theory for action, most jurisdictions consider the matter under tort law. Specifically, claims are generally made under a theory of negligence. Under a claim of negligence the defendant may be entitled to substantially more damages as compared to an action based on assault and battery.

In the context of a claim of negligence based on lack of informed consent, the plaintiff would have to show that the physician had a duty to provide information: (1) that a reasonable physician performing the same or similar procedure would provide regarding the procedure or treatment; (2) that the physician failed to do so; (3) that by not having received adequate informed consent the patient suffered an injury (damage); and (4) that had the patient known about the risk of the adverse reaction or complication he or she would not have undertaken the procedure.

It is generally accepted that to provide adequate informed consent the physician is obligated to discuss:

1. The nature of the patient's condition and the advised treatment plan
2. The prognosis or expected outcome
3. The risks, adverse reactions and complications that might occur with the procedure
4. Reasonable alternative therapies and the associated benefits and risks
5. The right to refuse any treatment and the possible consequences of doing so.

Some courts refer to the idea of material risks. Material risks are usually those risks that are important to a patient. Usually these are risks that could cause serious temporary or permanent injury. There are attorneys who would argue that even if a risk is nominal but occurs with some frequency it should probably be disclosed and the physician would be best protected by full disclosure. Furthermore it is felt that the more elective the treatment, the higher the obligation to discuss even the less likely risks. For example, it might be contended that in discussing a blepharoplasty the potential patient should be advised about the possibility of blindness.

While it might seem obvious that there is always a risk of death in any procedure, some attorneys suggest that it is prudent to disclose such a risk. It should be pointed out that what is an irrelevant risk to a physician could actually be a major risk in the patient's mind.

CONSENT FOR HAIR TRANSPLANTATION PROCEDURE'
(Please underline any portion of this consent you want explained)

1. I, ____________, hereby give consent to Dr. ______________ and his/her hair transplantation team to have hair replacement surgery performed upon me. I also consent to any other medical services during the procedure that may become medically reasonable and necessary. This includes, but is not limited to, the administration of anesthetics and/or sedatives necessary to perform a hair transplant procedure.

2. I am aware that good results will depend in part upon my completing the necessary number of operations recommended by the doctor. However, because many variables exist, I have not been promised or guaranteed good results. I also understand that the quality and amount of preexisting hair are major factors in the ultimate result. I understand I will not have hair of the same thickness/density as I had prior to the onset of my hair loss.

3. Prior to my consenting to cosmetic surgery, I state I have read or have been given the opportunity to review literature available to me that may include:

Brochure
Review of websites
List of Complications
Preoperative and post operative instructions
A fee schedule of current charges per session

4. I fully understand the results that I may reasonably expect. I understand hair transplants are not perfect. An explanation of this procedure has been given to me. I have had the opportunity to ask any questions regarding this procedure. I do understand that I will not obtain a full head of hair from the procedure. I understand that visibility of the sites following a transplant surgery can last for a number of days.

5. The pros, cons, and alternatives to hair transplantation have been explained. I have the option of doing nothing, wearing a hairpiece/wig, using prescription medication or having a transplant surgery or other type of scalp surgery procedure. A combination of the above is also possible. I have been informed of all options.

6. It is suggested I receive _________ session(s) of grafts as a minimum. I understand that more operations may be recommended later due to ongoing loss of my non-transplanted hair. I understand that all recommendations made during my consultation and treatment are estimates and may change later. ______. (Initial) If the doctors or I feel an additional procedure is necessary, I understand there will be additional surgical fees.

7. I understand every time an incision is made in the human body, a scar will occur, although every effort will be made to make the scar inconspicuous. Superficial crusting, pinkness, or redness of the incision area may occur, but these will likely be temporary. A thickened or raised scar (a hypertrophic scar/keloid) is possible. This is more likely to occur in patients with a history of this type of scarring. Wide scarring is also possible in the donor area.

8. I have been informed that hair transplantation is generally a safe procedure, however I am aware that complications may occur. The more common complications and a partial list of rare complications of this surgery have been explained to me and/or I have reviewed a list of them provided which I signed and dated. A copy of that list is attached. Unforeseen, rare complications, such as unanticipated reaction to medications and anesthetics, uncommon infections, and unusual healing responses, are possible. Every unforeseen complication may not have been discussed with me in detail, but I do understand that such risks do exist.

9. I consent to and authorize the performance of hair transplant surgery by ____________, associate doctors, and hair transplant technicians.

10. I believe I have been well informed. I understand that good results are expected, but the practices of medicine and surgery are not exact sciences. I understand knowledgeable practitioners sometimes disagree as to the best methods of treatment to achieve desired results.

11. It has been explained to me that the amount and location of future hair loss on the scalp, including the sides and back area cannot be predicted. I do understand it is possible to lose my existing hair at any point in the future. I do understand this may affect the appearance of the grafted area. Hair transplants may not be permanent. They are usually very long lasting, but rarely have fallen out in one to ten years.

12. There is a possibility of some temporary hair loss in the back of the scalp surrounding the area where the donor strip was removed. In rare cases, there may be permanent loss of hair adjacent to the surgical incision. In the transplanted area shedding of existing hair, called surgical effluvium, may occur after the surgery. If this hair is at the end of its normal life span, it may not return.

13. I understand the success of the hair transplant procedure is dependent upon my closely following all instructions. This includes, but is not limited to, pre-operative and post-operative activities and precautions, which have been explained to me. I have also received a written copy of these instructions.

14. This consent was read and signed while I was not under the influence of medications that might alter my mental capacity to understand its contents.

15. I certify this form has been read or it has been read to me, the blank spaces have been filled in, and I understand its contents.

16. I have disclosed all information regarding past and present medical conditions, current medications, and known drug allergies. This information is necessary so that the proper medical treatment is given at all times during the transplant procedure.

Some postoperative discomfort may be experienced. __________ (Initial)

This procedure is offered to obtain the best results for the patient, separate of any profit motive.

I acknowledge I am responsible for payment of these services with no fee reimbursement regardless of procedure results. I understand the fee paid is for the procedure and not for an expected result.

Date: ____________________ Time ________________ AM/PM

______________________________________________

Patient or Other Legally Responsible Person

______________________________________________

Witness

______________________________________________

Patient Name – Printed

______________________________________________

Address

______________________________________________

City State Zip

______________________________________________

Home Telephone Number

POSSIBLE COMPLICATIONS

- Nausea and vomiting from pain medication
- Bleeding (less than 5%)
- Infection (less than 1%)
- Excessive swelling
- A temporary headache
- Temporary numbness of the scalp
- Scarring around the grafts
- Poor growth of grafts
- Reaction to medications (less than 1%)
- Fainting (less than 1%) or syncope episodes
- Occasional small-ingrown hairs – causing a cyst (less than 10%)
- Scarring of the donor area – wide scars are possible (less than 5%)
- Bruising
  Patients who smoke have a higher rate of delayed wound healing and lower graft yield. Smoking not recommended for 2–3 weeks prior to and following the procedure.

RARE COMPLICATIONS (Partial list only)

- Keloid formation
- Complete failure of growth of transplanted hairs
- Persistent scalp pain
- Total loss of donor hair
- Permanent numbness of the scalp
- Noticeable scarring of donor area
- Loss of transplanted hair
- An allergic reaction or medication-related problem

I have read and understand all of the possible complications listed above. I accept the risks of these possible complications and consequences associated with this surgery.

______________________________________

Patient Signature Date

______________________________________

Witness Date

**FOR PATIENTS WHO HAVE HAD PRIOR TRANSPLANTS WITH ANOTHER PHYSICIAN:**

I acknowledge that prior to contacting ____________________, I received transplants or scalp reductions from another physician. I further acknowledge ____________________, its physicians and employees bear no responsibility for my present condition. I have been informed that my condition cannot be completely restored to its original state prior to any transplant surgery. ____________. Initial

**CONSENT FOR ANESTHESIA SERVICES**

1. All forms of anesthesia involve some risk and no guarantees or promises can be made concerning the results of my procedure or treatment. Although rare and unexpected severe complications with anesthesia can occur and include the remote possibility of infection, bleeding, drug reaction, blood clots, loss of sensation, loss of limb function, paralysis, stroke, brain damage, heart attack, or death.
2. I understand the type of anesthesia service (listed below) will be used for my procedure and that the anesthetic technique to be used will be determined by many factors including my physical condition, the physicians' preference, as well as my own desire.
3. Nerve block anesthesia is highly effective and generally safe. In rare cases though, there have been reports of nerve damage. The instances are approximately 1:30,000. Most cases resolve on their own and do not require treatment.

Anesthesia to be used: **Major/Minor Nerve block without sedation**

Expected results: Temporary loss of feeling and/or movement of a specific area.

Technique: Drug injected near nerves providing loss of sensation to the area of the operation.

Risks: Include but are not limited to, infection, convulsions, weakness, persistent numbness, residual pain, injury to blood vessels, or nerve injury.

I hereby consent to the anesthesia service described above and authorize its administration by ______________ ____________ and/or his associates. I also consent to an alternative type of anesthesia if necessary and deemed appropriate.

I certify and acknowledge that I have read this form or had it read to me, that I understand the risks, alternatives and expected results of the anesthesia service and that I had ample time to ask questions and consider my decision.

______________________________________

Patients' signature date/time

______________________________________

Responsible party (if other than patient) date/time

______________________________________

Witness

**Fig. 7.1** Example of consent form for hair transplantation procedure

This argument should be tempered with the view that if most surgeons do not provide such information the 'standard of care' does not require that such a complication or reaction be discussed. In some jurisdictions the degree of disclosure is measured by the local community standards of practice, while in some parts of the United States there are specific statutes that govern the informed consent standard. As mentioned earlier, the level of informed consent is generally that which a 'reasonably prudent physician' would consider in similar circumstances.

## Who Can Provide Informed Consent?

In obtaining informed consent the physician should realize that this duty cannot simply be delegated to another health care provider or lay person without recognizing that the physician still bears responsibility for the consent process. In some jurisdictions the informed consent must be obtained by a face-to-face meeting between the physician and patient. Although health care professionals or ancillary people may provide relevant information such as brochures, videos, etc. or even review the actual consent form, in some jurisdictions the consent can be viewed as invalid if the patient did not have an opportunity to discuss the consent with the physician and have an opportunity to ask questions of the physician. In the case of non-emancipated minors or patients who have been deemed incompetent, consent must be obtained from a parent or legal guardian. It should be noted that a patient who gives consent while on medication that could alter their mental ability may be considered incompetent and therefore the consent would be invalid.

It also follows that the physician should make an effort to thoroughly document the consent process. Even if the patient refuses the treatment the physician should document the consent process to be able to show that the patient's refusal was based on an informed decision.

Some physicians utilize a consent form that can be signed repeatedly as additional procedures are performed. It is probably wiser to utilize a new consent form for each subsequent procedure. The rationale for such an approach is that techniques and risks may change and the patient's medical condition and understanding of the procedure may change.

In an effort to demonstrate that a patient was aware of all of the clauses in a consent form, a physician may require a patient to initial each paragraph of the form. On the other hand if the patient neglects to initial a particular paragraph and the omission is not caught, the patient could allege that the particular clause was not reviewed when in fact it may have been.

## Informed Consent and Hair Replacement

Fortunately hair replacement surgery carries minimal risks. There are few reports of significant bodily injury that could impair a person's life. Rather the cases related to informed consent relate more to expectations not met and promises not kept.

The consent process often begins with the initial meeting with the patient. During this encounter the physician reviews the patient's history, medications and condition. The physician should discuss the process of hair transplantation, available techniques, and advise the patient as to whether he or she is a candidate. Furthermore the surgeon should discuss the results that can be realized. It is crucial to understand the patient's expectations and ensure that such expectations are in line with reality. The surgeon is also obligated to discuss other alternatives such as the medical treatments available to restore or control hair loss.

In the consultation the physician can discuss how the procedure is done and who performs various aspects of the procedure. It is important to recognize that the patient has a right to know who will be working on him or her and what portions of the surgery the assistants perform.

Prior to surgery the physician is expected to discuss the relevant risks of the procedure. It is important to try to discuss the risks in plain language whenever possible. Commonly discussed risks include: poor donor scar formation, infection, pain, altered nerve sensation, infection, shock loss, lack of growth, hematoma and bleeding. If relevant, the physician should review the possible effects of previous surgery on the outcome of the current procedure. The effects of medication and habits such as smoking may also be discussed.

Adequate informed consent calls for discussion of alternative treatments. This may include medications such as finasteride and minoxidil as well as other types of surgical procedures such as scalp reduction. Again it is important to emphasize the need to cover that which would be within the standard of care for a physician performing the procedure.

The physician should obtain an adequate history and should be aware of the patients' existing conditions that may affect the results of their procedure. Recognition of these potential problems demands that the physician discuss risks associated with the problem or problems. These risks may be outside of the risks normally reviewed in hair transplantation procedures. For instance, if a patient has recently had a pin placed in a bone it would be reasonable for the physician to advise the patient about the risk of osteomyelitis.

## Conclusion

In spite of providing informed consent such action does not prevent a person from filing a lawsuit. Rendering adequate informed consent can diminish the chance of a suit being filed. The communication process and relationship between the patient and physician can be enhanced as well as the perception of the outcome of the procedure.

## Further Reading

American Medical Association, Website, Informed Consent, www.ama-assn.org

Berg JW, Appelbaum PS, Parker LS, Lidz CW 2001 Informed consent: Legal theory and clinical practice, Oxford University Press, New York, New York

Bussey GD 1995 Informed consent: Its legal history and impact of medicine. Hawaii Medical Journal 54:472–475

Stough D 1993 Legal obligations of hair transplant surgery: covering the basics. Cosmetic Dermatology 6:10

# 8 Science of Hairline Design

*Paul T. Rose, William M. Parsley*

## Introduction

Hair transplantation has made giant strides since the early 1990's. Large round grafts have given way to smaller and smaller grafts, and finally to follicular unit (FU) grafts. A properly trimmed and placed FU graft is extremely difficult and sometimes impossible to distinguish from the patient's natural nontransplanted hair. These grafts allow the creation of a greater variety of natural patterns, restricted mainly by the patient's donor supply. In creating these patterns, it is imperative that the hair transplantation surgeon understands the predominant pleasing natural patterns and how they relate to facial and scalp landmarks. In this chapter, the most common patterns are discussed along with how they are designed and in what circumstances they should be used.

## Design Zones

### Scalp zones

General scalp zones are well known to all hair transplantation surgeons. The exact borders of these zones, however, are very subjective. In the diagram (Fig. 8.1) a rough consensus of the landmarks is presented on a nonbalding scalp. These zones can become obscured with advancing baldness, so it is important to know their general borders during hair transplantation. The mid-frontal point (MFP) is the most anterior point on the frontal hairline in the sagittal plane. In hair transplantation, it is assumed to be the designed point, even though it is frequently the same as the patient's existing MFP. The term 'apex' will be used in reference to the frontotemporal junction and refers to the designed apex unless otherwise stated. The term 'existing apex' will be used to distinguish the current apex from the 'designed apex' if confusion is possible. These are both distinguished from the 'original apex' before the patient started balding. The vertex transition point (VTP) is the anteriormost point of the vertex and is the point where the sagittal plane of the skull transitions from being mostly horizontal to vertical. As discussed later, the VTP is considered by many to be the most posterior point that can be transplanted without committing to transplantation of the vertex. The 'temporal triangle' is the triangular protrusion of the temple beyond the line

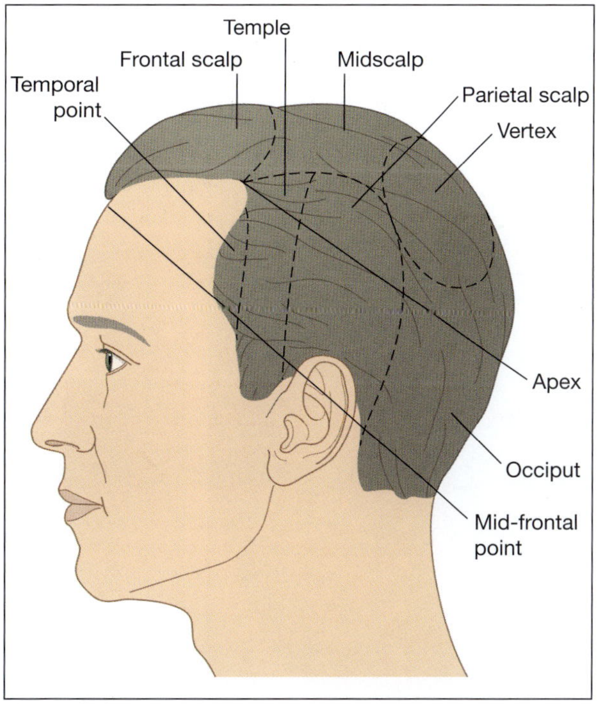


**Fig. 8.1** Scalp zones. Shown are the generally accepted scalp zones of concern in hair transplantation. The mid-frontal point (MFP) can be the original, the current, or the designed (created) MFP

extending from the anterior sideburn border. The 'temporal point' is the anterior point of this triangle, demarcating the border between the upper and lower temporal hairline (Fig. 8.1).

### Frontal zone

The frontal zone is the most commonly designed and is often the only designed zone. It frames the face and certainly has the most impact on a patient's appearance. It ends on each side at the junction with the temporoparietal fringe (the apex). Along the periphery of the frontal hairline is a 'transition zone' of lesser hair density and less hair caliber that creates a narrow irregular border between the hairless forehead and the full density of the frontal scalp.

### Temple

Transplanting the temples requires an ample donor supply and a thorough knowledge of the nuances of reconstructing this area to provide naturalness. Nevertheless reconstruction of this area is gaining popularity. Results can be very rewarding in the properly selected patient, as sparse temples can limit the advancement of the frontal hairline.

### Parietal zone

The parietal zone is the zone between the temple and occipital scalp; it blends superiorly into the mid-scalp. Its superior border is important in hair transplantation in that a high border will not require parietal transplantation, conserving valuable donor hair.

### Vertex

This zone is usually transplanted in more mature patients in order to give the surgeon confidence that there will be an adequate donor supply to support the grafts it will demand. If the vertex is not transplanted, a design is still often necessary to demarcate its anterior border. This design could be considered as a second hairline (the first being the frontotemporal hairline), but on the posterior superior scalp.

## Basic Considerations When Creating Designs

### Age of the patient

The age of the patient is of primary importance. In spite of wishful thinking, the patient's hairline is not static and will generally continue to thin and recede throughout his or her lifetime (Fig. 8.2). Any design

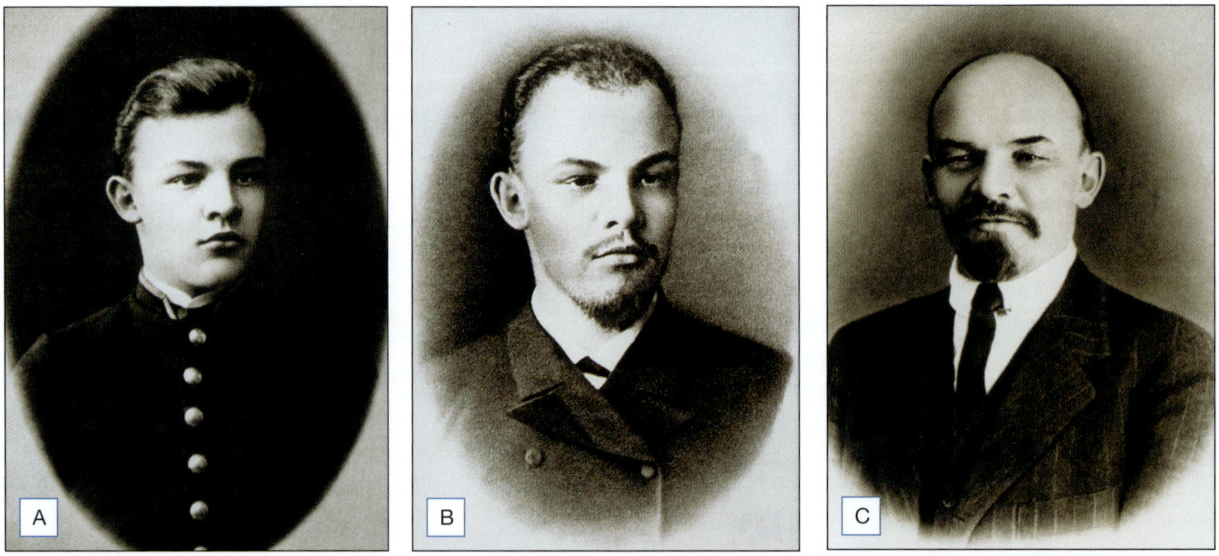


**Fig. 8.2** The hairline of Lenin as an 18 year old (**A**) in comparison with his hairline at 38 years (**B**) and at 58 years (**C**). The physician/artist should consider which hairline will best suit the patient's purposes throughout his lifetime, not just during youth. (Reproduced from Stough D, Haber RS 1996 Hair replacement: Surgical and medical. Mosby Year Book Publishing Company, St Louis. Fig 6.12, p 165 with permission. From Interphoto, Munich)

must take into consideration the forthcoming changes and continue to make a positive contribution as the patient ages (Fig. 8.3). The older the patient, the more predictable the ultimate hair loss (Fig. 8.4). In a young patient, it is advisable to postpone hair transplantation until a clearer picture of the ultimate hair loss emerges. If done, the transplanted hairline should be relatively high (8 cm or more), and the temples and vertex should generally be avoided, or approached with great caution.

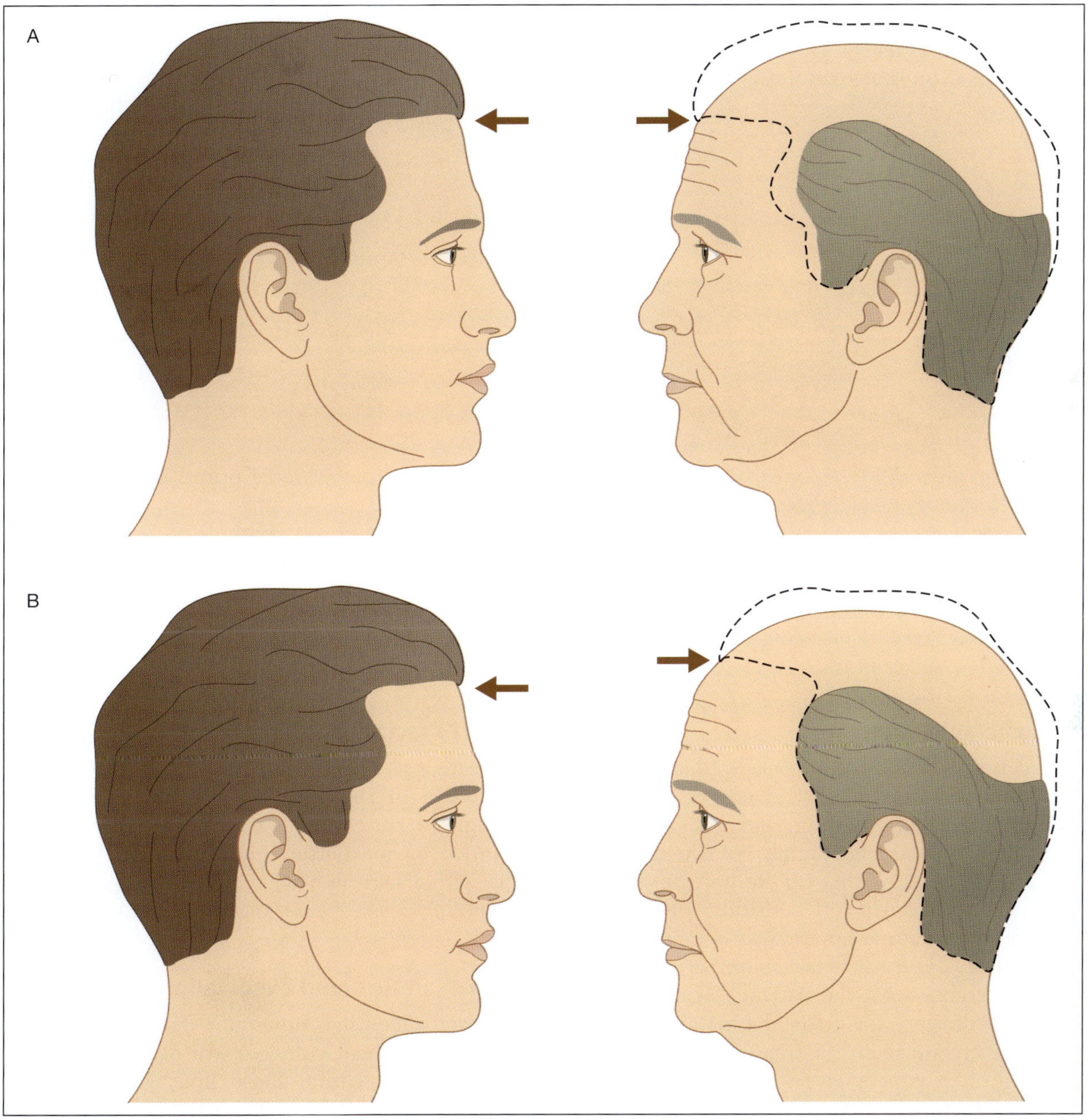


**Fig. 8.3** (**A**) If available hair is transplanted in a limited amount only to the outer margin of the original hairline, an unesthetic relation between the forehead and the remaining bald area will develop with time. (**B**) If, on the other hand, the transplanted hair is placed where the hairline of a middle-aged man would be, an esthetic result that will last for the remainder of the patient's life can be expected. (Modified from Stough D, Haber RS 1996 Hair replacement: Surgical and medical. Mosby Year Book Publishing Company, St Louis. Fig 6.13, p 166, with permission)

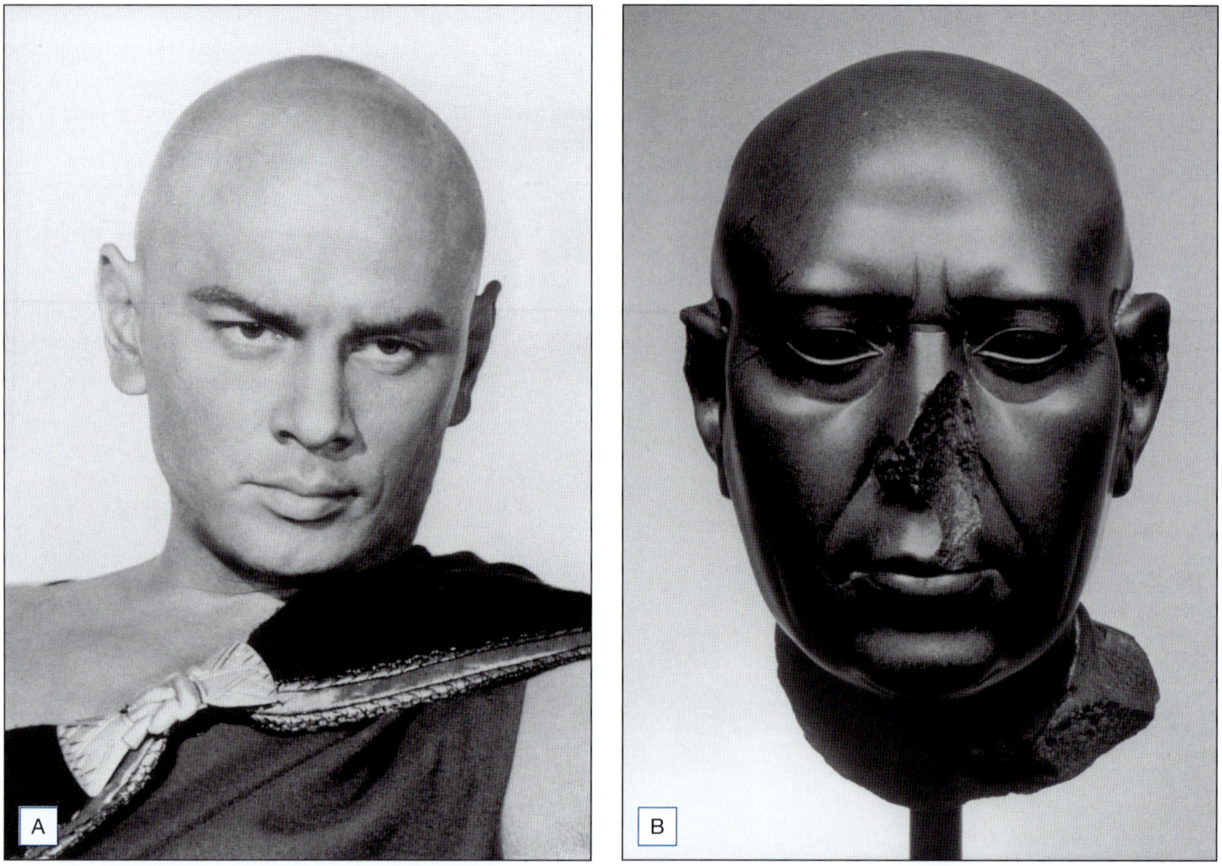


**Fig. 8.4** (**A**) Rather than fighting impending baldness, actor Yul Brenner shaved off all of his hair for the role of the King of Siam in *The King and I*. He continued this practice until his death. (**B**) The pure form of the bald scalp can take on the appearance of a finely crafted sculpture. (Reproduced from Stough D, Haber RS 1996 Hair replacement: Surgical and medical. Mosby Year Book Publishing Company, St Louis. Fig 6.7, p 163, with permission. From Interphoto, Munich)

## Hair characteristics

Hair density (FUs/cm$^2$), coarseness (determined by the combination of hair shaft diameter and average number of hairs/FU), color, and curl all have an effect on hairline design. Simply put, the denser the hair, the more grafts that can be harvested from a given area. Creating a soft transition zone (defined earlier) and a natural appearance is more difficult when using coarse hair. Hair color, particularly the way it matches with the patient's skin color, can affect the design – the closer the match, the fewer worries there are about the transition zones. Darker hair will often visually give a fuller appearance. If, however, there is a great disparity in skin and hair color, such as black hair and very white skin, the hair can appear less dense. Hair curl allows better coverage per graft and therefore allows the illusion of more density with a given number of grafts.

## Patient's facial contours

To create a pleasing result, it is important to match the design to the patient's natural contours. For example, a patient with a wide, round face may require a higher, flatter (more horizontal) hairline. One with a narrow head may require a less flared hairline.

## Patient's desires and expectations

The doctor identifies minimum and maximum safe limits. The patient's desires will determine which hairline design within those limits will be used. There needs to be communication between the doctor and patient so that the patient's expectations and the doctor's plans are similar. Unrealistic expectations are a major reason for patient dissatisfaction.

## Sex

A receded male hairline usually has an enlarging triangular recession at the frontotemporal junction. To diagonally cut across this triangle in restoring a male's hairline is nearly always a mistake. These triangular recessions are not to be confused with the frontal troughs, which are commonly transplanted (Fig. 8.5A and B). On the other hand, in females without hair loss the hairline frequently curves into the temples with no triangular recession.

## Ethnicity

Racial background often influences the hairline. Blacks, Asians and Hispanics, for example, often have broad, flat hairlines. To create a hairline that is inconsistent with their natural ethnic characteristics can draw attention to the transplant.

# Integration of All Areas of Design

All areas of the patient's hair loss must be considered when creating a design so that they coordinate to give the desired result; for example, when a patient has receded temples with loss of temporal points, the frontal hairline design must be conservatively high unless the temples are to be transplanted.

## Frontal hairline

The frontal hairline design is used by most hair transplantation specialists as their framework, with the other patterns being used to fit into its design like hanging ornaments on a tree. Because it frames the face, it generally has the most impact on cosmetic improvement. The design should be considered permanent; therefore, great care should be taken in its creation so that it will be cosmetically acceptable over the life of the patient. As the patient ages, the hairline can easily be lowered, but raising an overly low hairline is difficult. The different frontal hairline designs are considered below.

# Patterns

## Overview of patterns

The designed frontal hairline can connect to the temporal/parietal fringe or to the mid-scalp (natural or transplanted) (Box 8.1).

### *Frontotemporal design patterns (Fig 8.6)*

Frontotemporal design without flare.

A frontotemporal design without a flare allows the frontotemporal junction (apex) to slide posteriorly with the future recession of the temporal border.

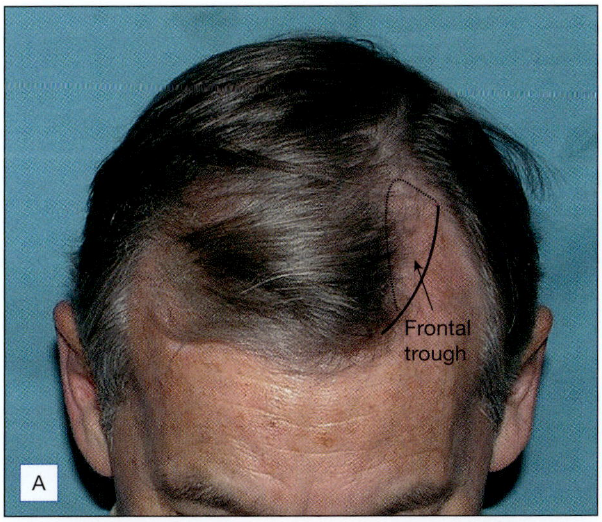


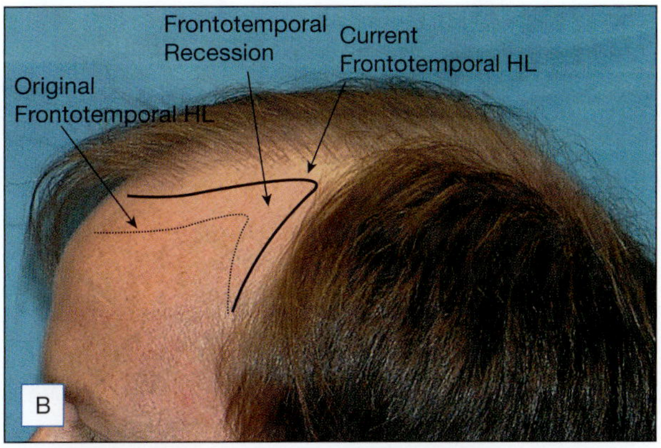


**Fig. 8.5** Natural recessions of the frontal hairline and frontotemporal junction. (**A**) Nearly all men and many women have natural triangular frontotemporal junctions. The angle gets deeper with recession. Troughs are not present at birth but develop in many men with recession. Troughs are concave areas that develop medial to the lateral frontal hairline and medial to a nonflared frontal hairline design. They often are the precursors of an isolated frontal forelock. (**B**) This figure illustrates the deepening frontotemporal triangle with recession

Because it doesn't leave lateral troughs, it gives a somewhat fuller appearance to the hairline when viewed from the side. This design tends to blend better with a straight or convex upper temporal margin. The author finds this nonflared design the most advantageous pattern for a young to middle-aged male, in whom moderate further hair loss is anticipated.

### Frontotemporal design with flare.

Flaring the lateral posterior margin of the hairline makes future posterior sliding of the frontotemporal junction difficult; however, it tends to create a pleasing blend into the temple, particularly if the patient's upper temple margin is concave. A flare should be created by forming a concave trough medial to the nonflared design. A flare should not be created without this medial concavity, or else the created frontotemporal triangle would be violated. Creating a trough is a good technique for patients planning to brush their hair posteriorly toward the vertex. Most naturally balding men brush their hair posteriorly to cover a balding vertex and/or to hide balding troughs. Because the troughs are not transplanted, this technique is also useful in conserving limited donor supplies for use elsewhere on the scalp. When creating this pattern, it is best to start by drawing the frontal hairline to the desired apex without a flare, and then design the flare by creating a trough medial to this line – this will ensure the apex is in its proper position. If the patient is young, it is best to place the apex a centimeter or more posterior to his existing apex to allow for future recession, making sure not to go posterior to a vertical line from the tragus.

The flared and nonflared designs are the predominant designs used in hair transplantation.

**Frontal hairline designs**

1. Frontotemporal design
    a. Frontal hairline design without flare
    b. Frontal hairline design with flare
    c. Frontal hairline design with full sweep into temples
    d. Isolated frontal forelock – unconnected or loose connection
2. Fronto-midscalp design
    a. frontal hairline design without flare
    b. frontal hairline design with flare

**Box 8.1** Frontal hairline designs

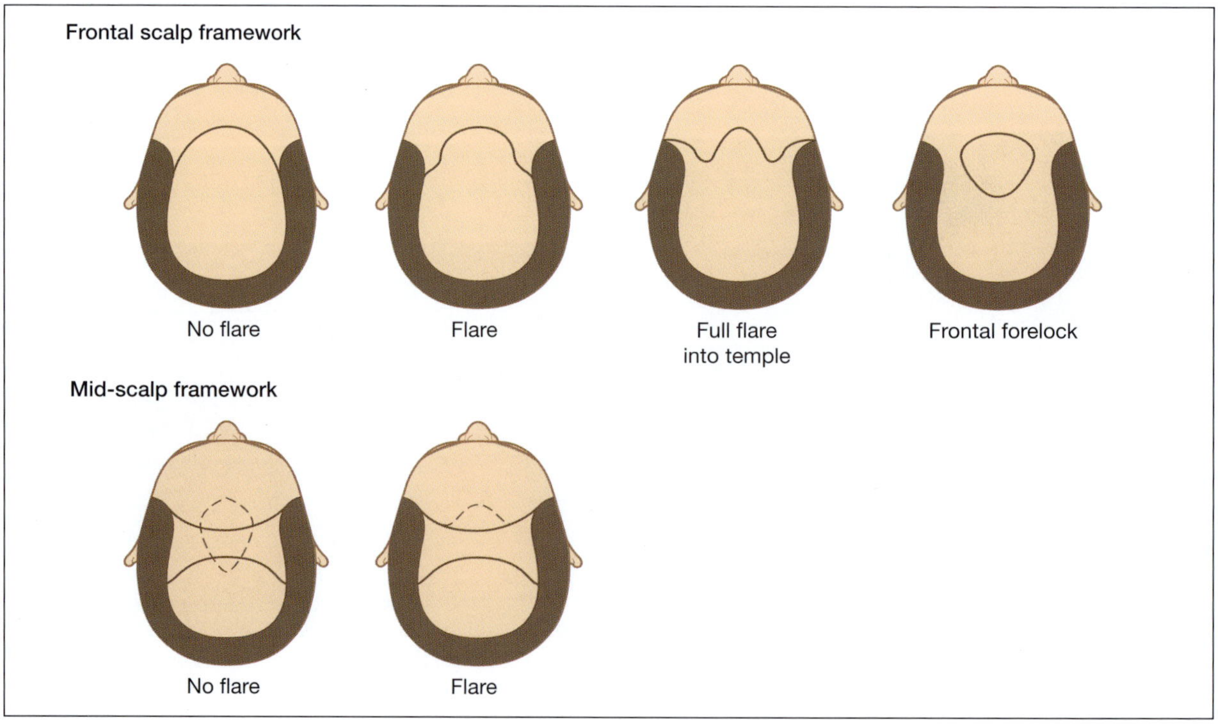


**Fig. 8.6** Frontal hairline design patterns. Listed are the major frontal hairline design patterns. These designs can either be connected to the temporoparietal fringe or a mid-scalp bridge, or be unconnected (frontal forelock)

The other frontal designs will be mentioned only briefly for completeness (Fig. 8.7).

### Frontotemporal design with full sweep into temples.

Sweeping the frontal hairline into the temples is one of the most aggressive designs used by transplant surgeons. This design both fixes the frontotemporal junction (apex) and commits the doctor to transplanting the current recession of the temples and its future recession. This design can create impressive results, but should only be used in patients considered to have a lifelong surplus of donor hair (Fig. 8.8A–C).

### Isolated frontal forelock.

The isolated frontal forelock, popularized by Beehner, is one of the most conservative hairline designs presently used. This pattern, like the other designs, can occur naturally in balding men and can occur in a variety of patterns. As its name suggests, a frontal pattern is designed without connection to the surrounding border of recession, creating a 'moat' of baldness. This moat may be left untransplanted, but is usually filled in with a light 'blur' zone of sparse single-hair grafts in order to create the hint of a connection to temporoparietal fringe (Fig. 8.9).

### *Frontomid-scalp design patterns*

This connection can be made either to a naturally retained or to a created mid-scalp.

### Frontomid-scalp design without flare.

This is essentially an isolated frontal forelock design that blends into a created or natural mid-scalp bridge. It is very useful when there is a limitation of donor hair, and is particularly good for patients planning to brush their hair posteriorly.

### *Frontomid-scalp design with flare.*

This allows a much higher than normal mid-frontal point, thus conserving hair in patients with limited donor supplies, yet mimics a pattern commonly seen in balding men. Cosmetically, it looks better on a patient with a broad scalp.

## Placement of Hairline

Once the desired pattern has been selected, the placement and dimensions of the pattern need to be made – the mid-frontal point, mid-frontal hairline, lateral frontal hairline and connection to the temporoparietal zone. Great care must be taken to keep the hairline symmetrical on the head. The below measurements help but should not be totally trusted. After a preliminary hairline is drawn, a

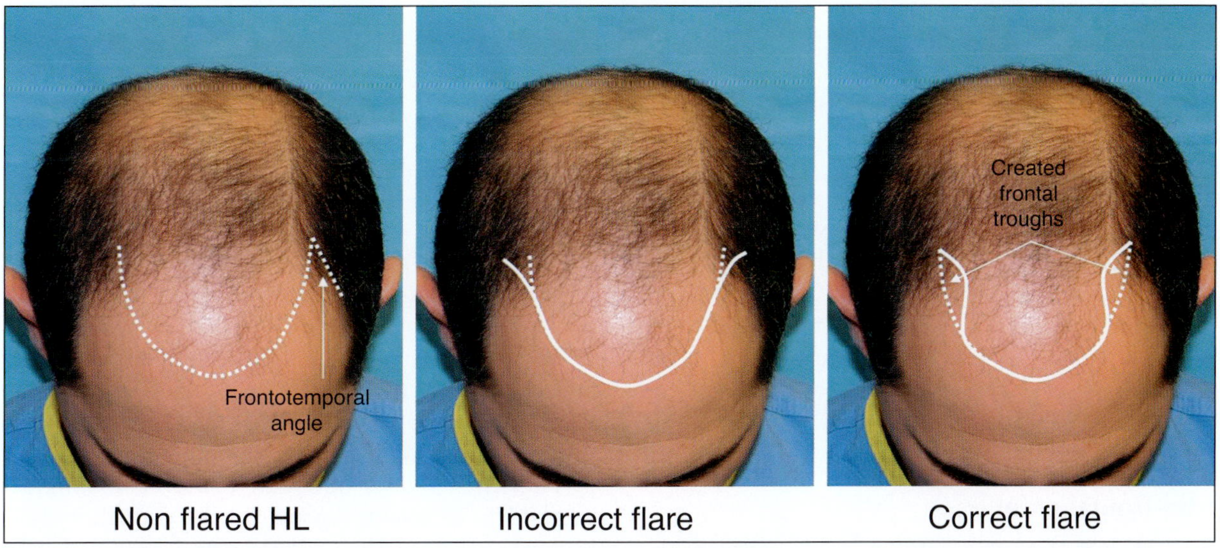


**Fig. 8.7** Creating a flare. Creating a flare should begin by drawing a nonflared hairline, which also creates a frontotemporal angle. A correct flare is designed by creating a concave area medial to this line, talking care not to cross the natural nonflared hairline

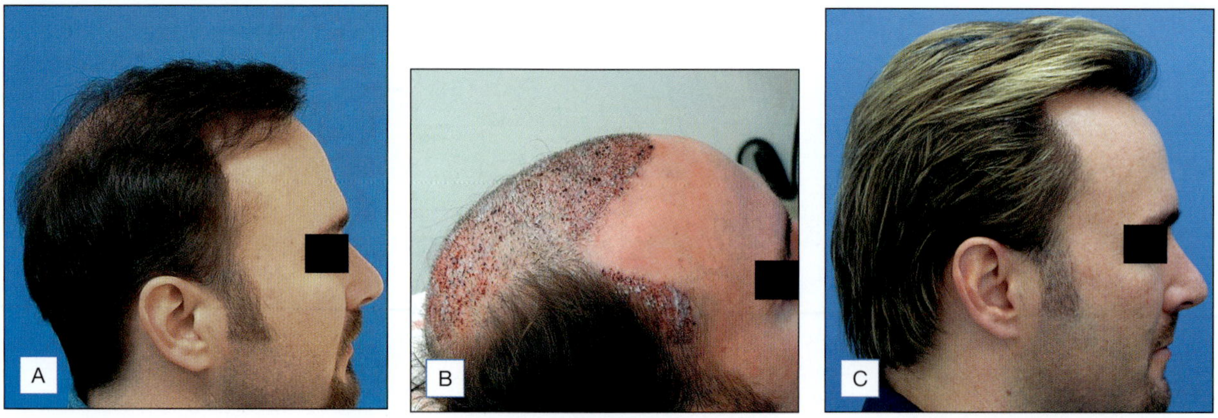


**Fig. 8.8** Fontotemporal design with full sweep into temples. This is an aggressive design that fixes the apex and obligates one to transplant any further temporal recessions. Generous donor supplies are required but results can be very satisfying. (**A**) Before. (**B**) Immediately postoperatively. (**C**) With one session's growing. (Photos courtesy of Dr Jerry Wong)

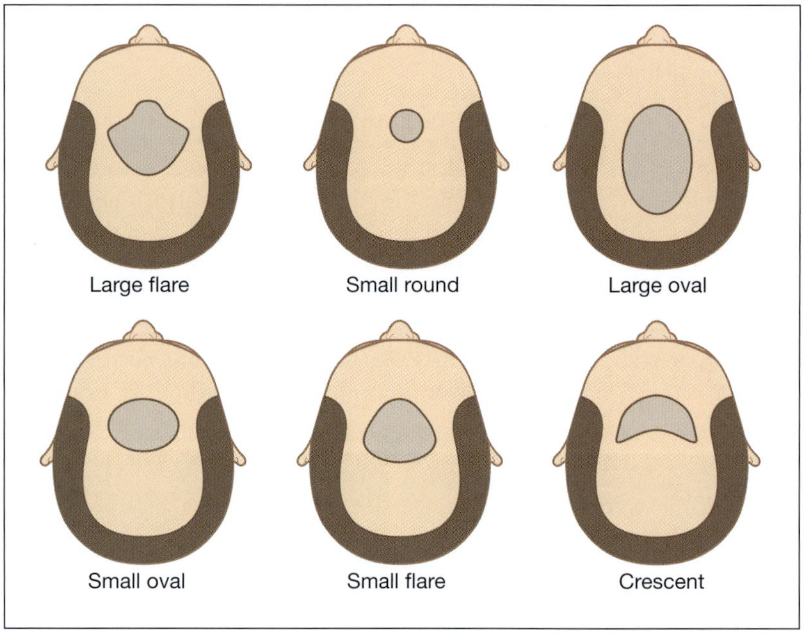


**Fig. 8.9** Frontal forelock designs. Popularized by Beehner, a variety of natural designs can be created for use as a frontal forelock. Expertise of the doctor is required to create a design that will work well for a given patient. A lightly planted 'blur' zone of single haired grafts can give it a hint of attachment to the temporoparietal fringe

helpful technique is to stand behind the patient with a mirror placed in front of the patient, and angled to provide a good view of the hairline. It is also helpful to assess the hairline from several vantage points and request input from any assistants.

## Mid-frontal point

The MFP is the most anterior point of the frontal hairline. If one follows the artists' 'Rule of Thirds' – an ideal face should have equal distance from: (1) the MFP to the glabella; (2) the glabella to the base of the nose; and (3) the base of the nose to the tip of the chin (mentum) (Fig. 8.10). While this may be ideal, most patients do not have enough hair to allow this pattern or have an oval or round face, which would not fit these dimensions; therefore, a more posterior MFP must be created.

The MFP should be created first. The simplest method is to select a point on the glabella that is midway between the eyebrows and centered over the nose. The created MFP is usually 7–11 cm above this point (Fig. 8.11). At a later date, this point can

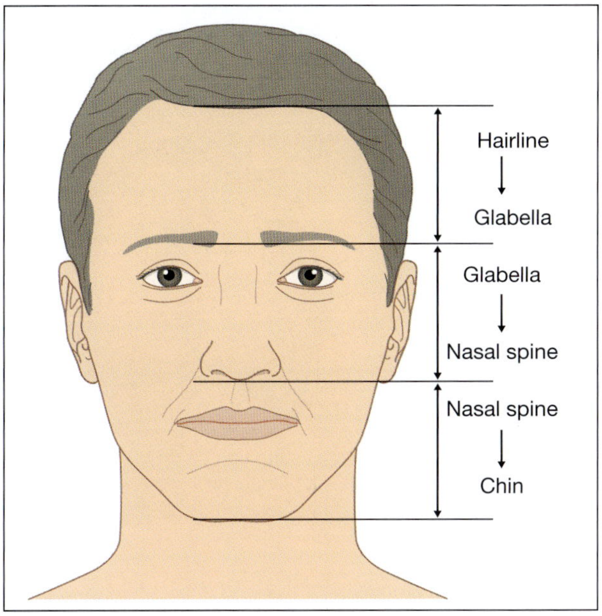


**Fig. 8.10** Rule of thirds. This old artistic principle relates to ideal facial proportions and should only be used as a general guideline. Few people naturally have these exact proportions

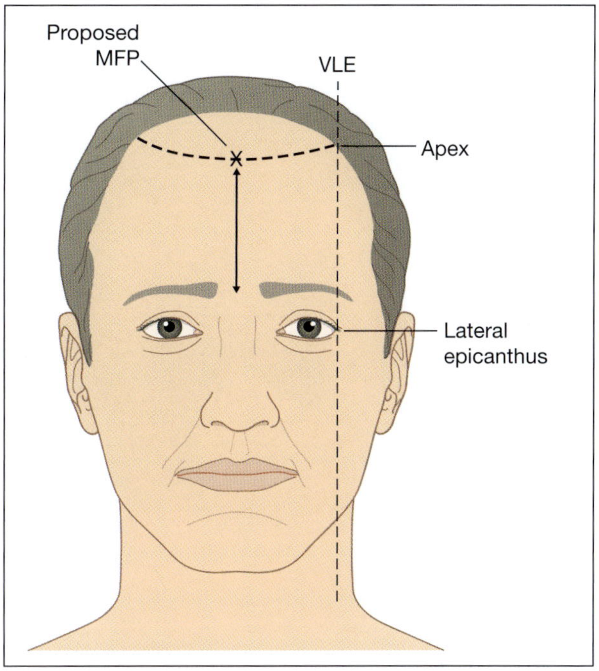


**Fig. 8.11** Locating the MFP and the apex from frontal view. The mid-frontal point is normally located 7–11 cm vertically from the mid-glabella. The apex is usually placed at or medial to a point projected posteriorly from a line drawn vertically from the lateral epicanthus (VLE). At the point this line meets the temporoparietal fringe is roughly where the apex is placed

easily be lowered (but never below the Rule of Thirds line); however, it is difficult to raise, making it necessary to be conservative, particularly on a young patient. At least three situations call for a higher MFP: (1) recessed temples; (2) limited donor hair; and (3) present or anticipated advanced baldness in the future.

## Frontotemporal junction: the apex

Placement of the frontotemporal junction (FTP – apex) is subjective, and a common mistake is to make the apex too low (lateral). This creates a problem that often later needs repair, while using up valuable donor hair. A commonly used guideline is to draw a line vertically from the lateral canthus (visually extending it posteriorly toward the upper temporal hairline), and placing the permanent apex along this line. If the temples are not to be transplanted, it is often best to place the permanent apex at least 1 cm posterior to the present border of hair to allow for future recession.

A useful technique for creating the lateral portion of the frontal hairline is to find a point 1 cm lateral to the mid-point of the outer orbital rim (horizontal with the lateral canthus); the lateral hairline should be roughly 9–11 cm vertical to this point. Measure the distance of this point from the MFP, then repeat the process on the other side, thus creating a mirror image. Once the MFP and these lateral markings have been made, draw a curved line on each side, connecting the MFP to the lateral marks; then simply continue this line without allowing it to drop inferiorly until it reaches the temporal fringe. This junction will be the **apex**. Most experts recommend that the apex not be placed posterior to a line drawn vertically from the pretragal border. Stough feels the apex should generally be placed 4–7 cm posterior to the MFP (Fig. 8.12A and B).

These are just guidelines and the final pattern must be customized so that it is pleasing in appearance.

## Transition zone

When designing the hairline, a 6–10 mm transition zone of gradually increasing density should be created to match natural hairlines. This should be done with random hairs, gaps and clusters (see

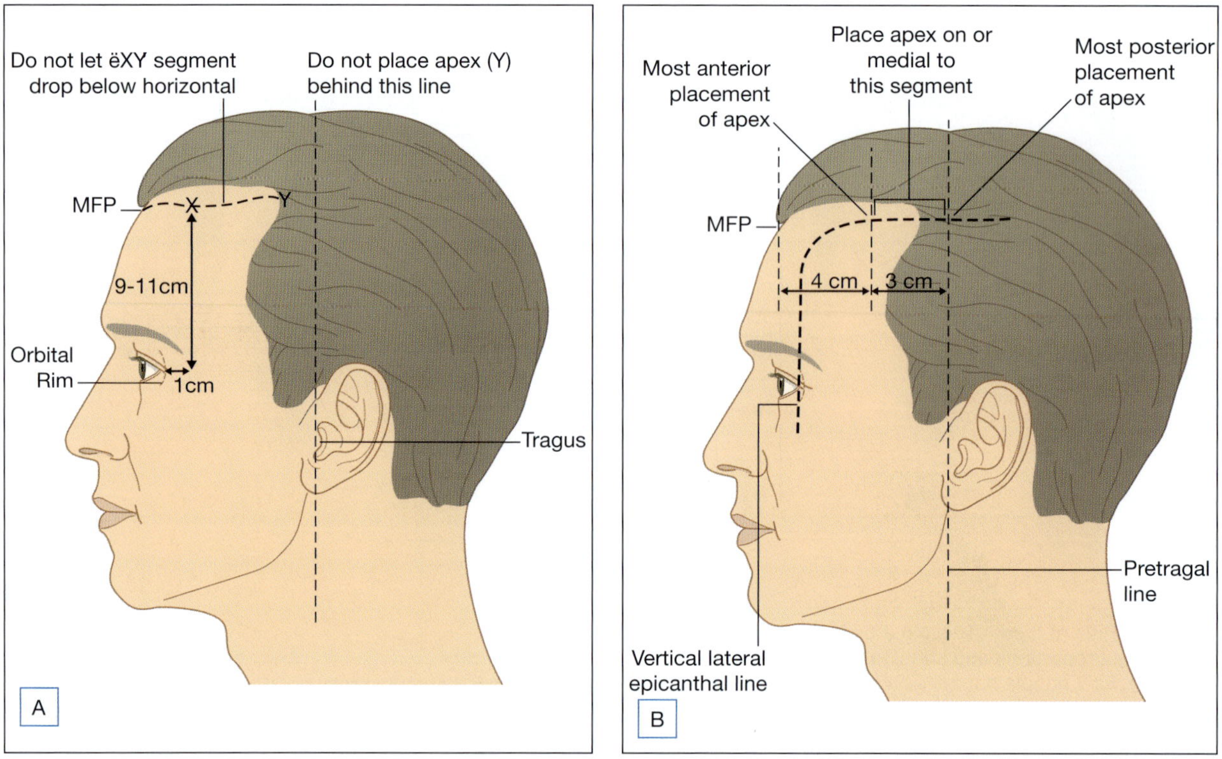


**Fig. 8.12** Location of lateral frontal hairline and apex. (**A**) Location of the lateral portion of the frontal hairline. It is helpful to make a mark (X) 9–11 cm vertical to a point 1 cm lateral to the mid-point of the lateral orbital rim. The line from X to the apex (Y) should not drop below horizontal. The apex (Y) should not be placed posterior to a line drawn vertically from the tragus. (**B**) Anteroposterior boundaries of the apex. The apex should be located anterior to the pretragal line and 4–7 cm behind the MFP

later), along with an increasing density gradient as work moves centrally.

## Creating Irregularity

After spending considerable time to ensure symmetry of the basic pattern, some time needs to be spent creating some natural irregularity, lest the transplant catches the eye as unnatural. A natural hairline has a subtle, and sometimes pronounced, irregularity. Two common techniques are used to create irregularity:

1. *Macro-irregularities*. These are 1–3 naturally occurring **peaks** (mounds, undulations) that occur over the medial aspect of the frontal hairline – a central peak (widow's peak) and two lateral peaks can occur in any combination. Approximately 50% of both men and women have at least one of these peaks. Peaks, as opposed to clusters, can be seen from several feet away and affect the general contour of the hairline. Creating them is useful in giving relief from the often overly round appearance of the mid-portion of the frontal hairline. Lateral peaks are useful in allowing patients to cover lateral troughs when brushing their hair posteriorly, while widow's peaks are helpful in slightly lowering the MFP with minimal use of grafts (Fig. 8.13A–E).
2. *Micro-irregularities*. These are subtle irregularities along the entire length of the frontal design, used to avoid the all-too-commonly seen abrupt transplanted hairline. The favorite technique among transplant doctors is the use of 3–6 mm triangular clusters extending forward at a 45-degree angle irregularly irregular to the hairline. It should be pointed out that these are irregularly irregular with the distance of their protrusion and the spacing between them being irregular. Finally, to mimic nature, these clusters should be surrounded by randomly scattered, or island single-hair grafts (sentinel hairs) (Fig. 8.14). Between the clusters are gaps containing little if any hair. A common

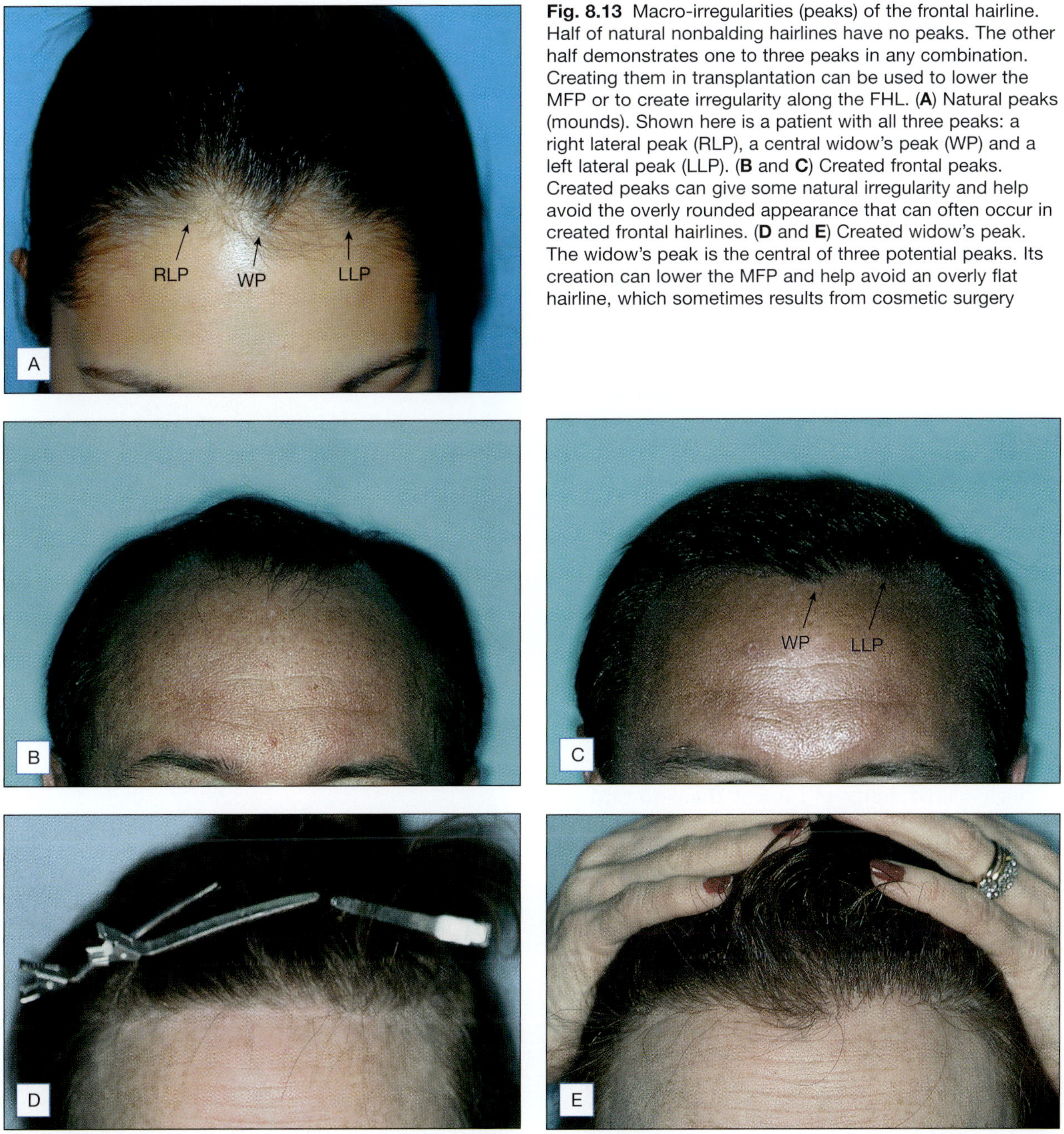


**Fig. 8.13** Macro-irregularities (peaks) of the frontal hairline. Half of natural nonbalding hairlines have no peaks. The other half demonstrates one to three peaks in any combination. Creating them in transplantation can be used to lower the MFP or to create irregularity along the FHL. (**A**) Natural peaks (mounds). Shown here is a patient with all three peaks: a right lateral peak (RLP), a central widow's peak (WP) and a left lateral peak (LLP). (**B** and **C**) Created frontal peaks. Created peaks can give some natural irregularity and help avoid the overly rounded appearance that can often occur in created frontal hairlines. (**D** and **E**) Created widow's peak. The widow's peak is the central of three potential peaks. Its creation can lower the MFP and help avoid an overly flat hairline, which sometimes results from cosmetic surgery

mistake in subsequent transplants is to fill in these gaps. If anything, the clusters should be made denser and the gaps left alone.

## Helpful pointers

1. Never chase receding parietal borders (lateral fringes) with the hairline. Raise the borders by transplanting the parietal humps (see Fig. 8.16).
2. Measure as much as possible, but then stand back and make sure it visually looks proper. Also consider having assistants provide feedback. Some faces are asymmetrical and measurements alone may not be adequate.
3. As the designed frontal hair line (FHL) moves posteriorly, from the side view it should be horizontal or move superiorly, never inferiorly (see Fig. 8.12A.)

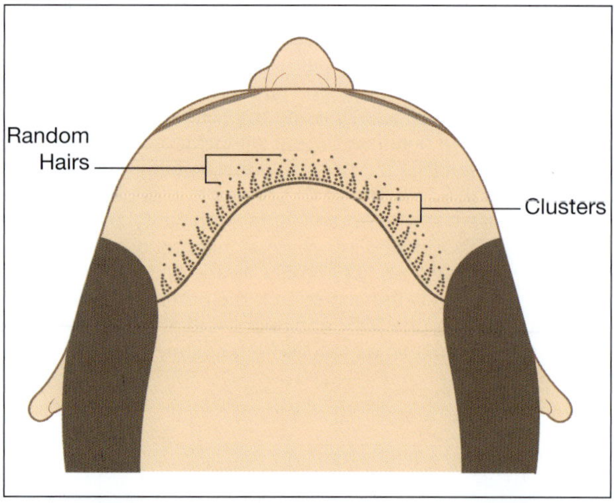


**Fig. 8.14** Micro-irregularities of frontal hairline. Clusters, gaps and random single hairs are the most commonly used designs for the transition zone, allowing the hairline to have a soft appearance yet avoiding an abrupt hairline. Triangular clusters forming a roughly 45-degree angle to the hairline are the favorite design of many doctors

4. Use the function of the mostly horizontal superior scalp with the mostly vertical forehead and temple as the outer most regions of the safe zone for transplanting. Do not transplant onto the vertical walls surrounding the frontal scalp.
5. Create widow's peaks with densely packed single-haired grafts and orient them toward the temple or ear on the nonpart side. This is not only the most common natural orientation of widow's peak hairs, but also gives the appearance of greater density.
6. If an error is to be made, make the hairline slightly too high. This is an easily correctable error. A hairline that is too low can be a difficult problem.
7. The default direction of the transplanted grafts is the direction of the existing hair unless there is some over-riding reason to change.

### Temple hairline

Transplanting the temples should only be attempted if there is confidence that the donor supply will support the present and future demand for grafts; in a properly selected patient, the results can be very pleasing. Absence of temporal points or severely recessed upper temples can restrict the amount of advancement of the frontal hairline. Overly advancing the frontal hairline without grafting the temples can give the frontal hairline the appearance of a 'lid.'

## Patterns

### Overview of patterns

Transplanting the temples can take three forms:

1. Restoring only the temporal points.
2. Restoring only the upper temporal border.
3. Restoring both.

#### *Restoring only the temporal points*

Occasionally the temporal points are weak or missing, yet the upper temporal border is acceptable. In this case, consider only transplanting the temporal points, making sure to blend into the surrounding temple.

#### *Restoring only the upper temporal border*

If the upper temporal borders are quite concave or inferiorly recessed but the temporal points are adequate, this technique can be performed, again remembering to blend.

#### *Restoring both*

Usually if the temporal points are weak or missing, the upper temporal borders are recessed (both inferiorly and posteriorly), creating a vertical line. In this case, both the temporal points and the upper temporal borders need to be restored.

#### *Locating the temporal points*

The most desirable method is to locate the patient's natural temporal points by looking for residual terminal or vellus hair. Often, oblique lighting will help. If the original temporal points cannot be located, Mayer and Perez-Meza give excellent advice for locating the temporal point. Draw two lines:

1. Tip of the ear lobe → Projected mid-point of the frontal hairline
2. Tip of the nose → Pupil of the eye – and extend it until it crosses line '1'

This intersection works well for creating a cosmetically acceptable temporal point (Fig. 8.15).

### *Helpful pointers*

1. Observe the **direction** of the patient's natural temple hair before creating sites. The direction of temporal hair can vary considerably from person to person.
2. Temple hair exits the skin at an **acute angle**, so make sure that sites are created with a small-diameter instrument (it holds the angle better) inserted at a very acute angle of less than 20 degrees. Consider lateral (coronal) grafting here.
3. Only use one- or two-haired grafts for the temples, and only one-haired grafts for the most peripheral 8–10 mm.

## Parietal Hairline (Lateral Fringe)

If the lateral fringe has dropped to the point that a desirable frontal hairline cannot connect to it, the lateral fringe needs to be raised by grafting, creating new parietal 'humps.' This is a valuable tool in creating a natural overall design.

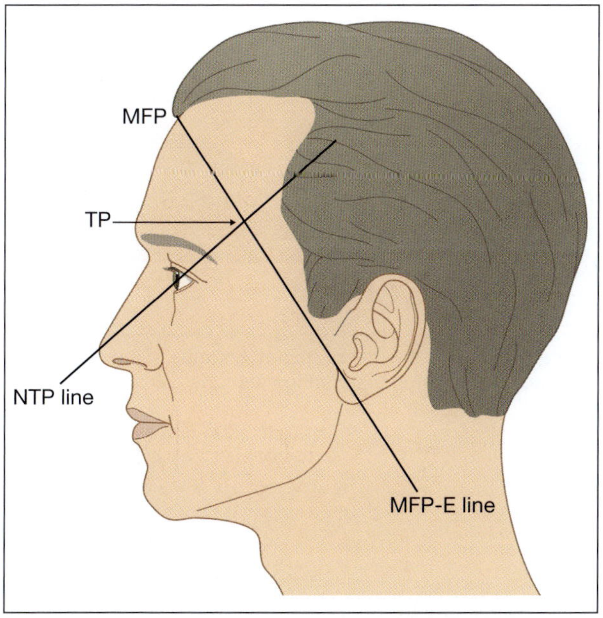


**Fig. 8.15** Temporal point location. The optimal temporal point (TP) can be found by locating the intersection of two lines: the nasal tip–pupil (NTP) line and the mid-frontal point–tip of ear lobe (MFP-E) line

### Patterns

Parietal humps are created by extending the lateral fringes superiorly to connect with the desired frontal hairline or slightly above it, making sure to follow the natural hair direction in that area (Fig. 8.16A–D).

### Helpful pointers

1. The direction of hair grafts at the upper border of the parietal hump should be more forward than inferior, with the direction gradually sweeping to be more inferior as work moves lower. This allows for a transition from the forward direction of the frontal and mid-scalp to the naturally inferior direction of the mid- to lower parietal zone. The patient's natural hair direction, if visible, is always followed.
2. The anterior portion of the parietal hump should always blend into the upper temporal line. For example, if the temple is concave, the anterior portion of the created parietal hump should follow this line and gradually form a convex superior segment.

### Vertex

The vertex (crown) is the posterior zone that lies between the mid-scalp and occipital zones. Even though hair loss in this zone has less impact on a patient's appearance than in the frontal and mid-scalp regions, baldness in this zone still concerns many patients. Because the zone can become quite large with time, it can require a significant percentage of the donor reserves, if transplanted. One problem in transplanting the entire vertex is that there is no permanent border, as the peripheral border keeps migrating and can leave an 'island' of central hair. Many doctors will delay the decision to transplant this zone until a patient is at least 35–45 years old, but this is a loose rule and the decision must be made on an individual basis. To influence patients to delay the decision to transplant the vertex, it is helpful to tell them 'hair loss in the front hurts one's appearance while hair loss in the crown just hurts one's feelings.' Even so, transplanting the vertex when appropriate can please many patients. If the decision is made not to transplant the vertex, an anterolateral border must be created at the junction of the mid-scalp and vertex, unless there is a retained mid-scalp.

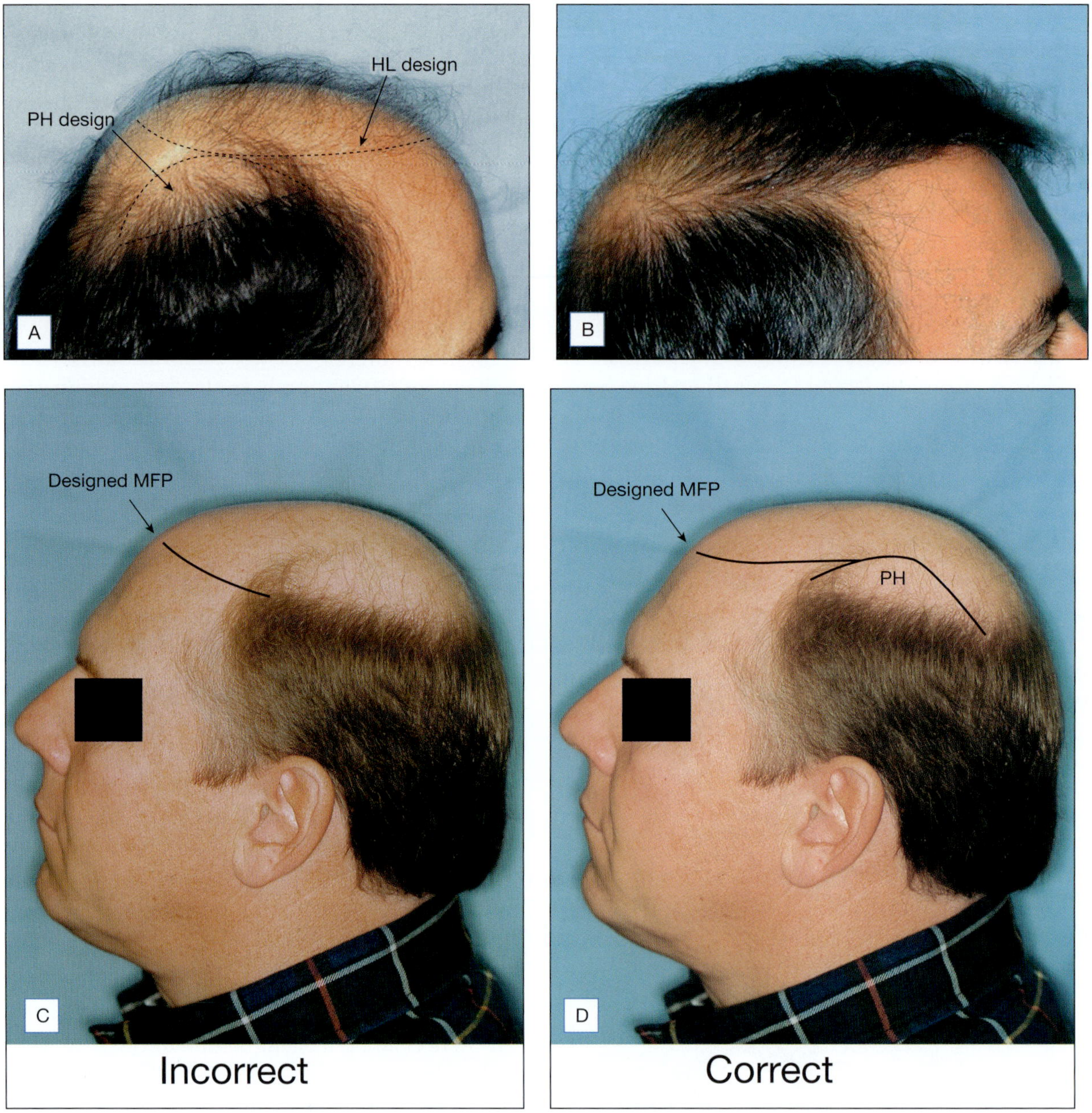


**Fig. 8.16** Created parietal humps. (**A** and **B**) Lifting the temporoparietal fringe with the use of 'parietal humps' allows the frontal hairline to remain in its proper position. (**C**) Never chase the receding temporoparietal fringe with the hairline. (**D**) Instead, build up the 'parietal humps'

## Patterns

### *Overview of patterns*

1. Transplant the entire vertex: (1) with graded density; or (2) with uniform density.
2. The vertex is not transplanted, creating a need to create an anterior-lateral border: (1) creating an oval/round bald vertex; or (2) creating a kidney-shaped bald vertex.

#### Transplant the entire vertex.

In transplanting the entire vertex, the first step is to find the center of the whorl(s) and follow the natural hair direction as it radiates peripherally, which it usually does in a radial curvilinear pattern (Fig. 8.17A–C). Some will plant the vertex with a graded density (denser at the periphery and less dense centrally) and some will transplant with uniform density (Fig. 8.18A and B). Both designs occur naturally. Care should be taken to not make the vertex too dense, as further hair loss can create a troublesome peripheral halo. The larger the size of the vertex baldness, the more it should be considered to use a gradient density pattern.

#### Vertex is not transplanted, creating need to create an anterolateral border.

If it is decided not to transplant the vertex, an anterolateral border (hairline) needs to be created unless the patient has a retained mid-scalp. It is advised that the design not be posterior to the vertex transition zone (see Fig. 3.5), the curved line

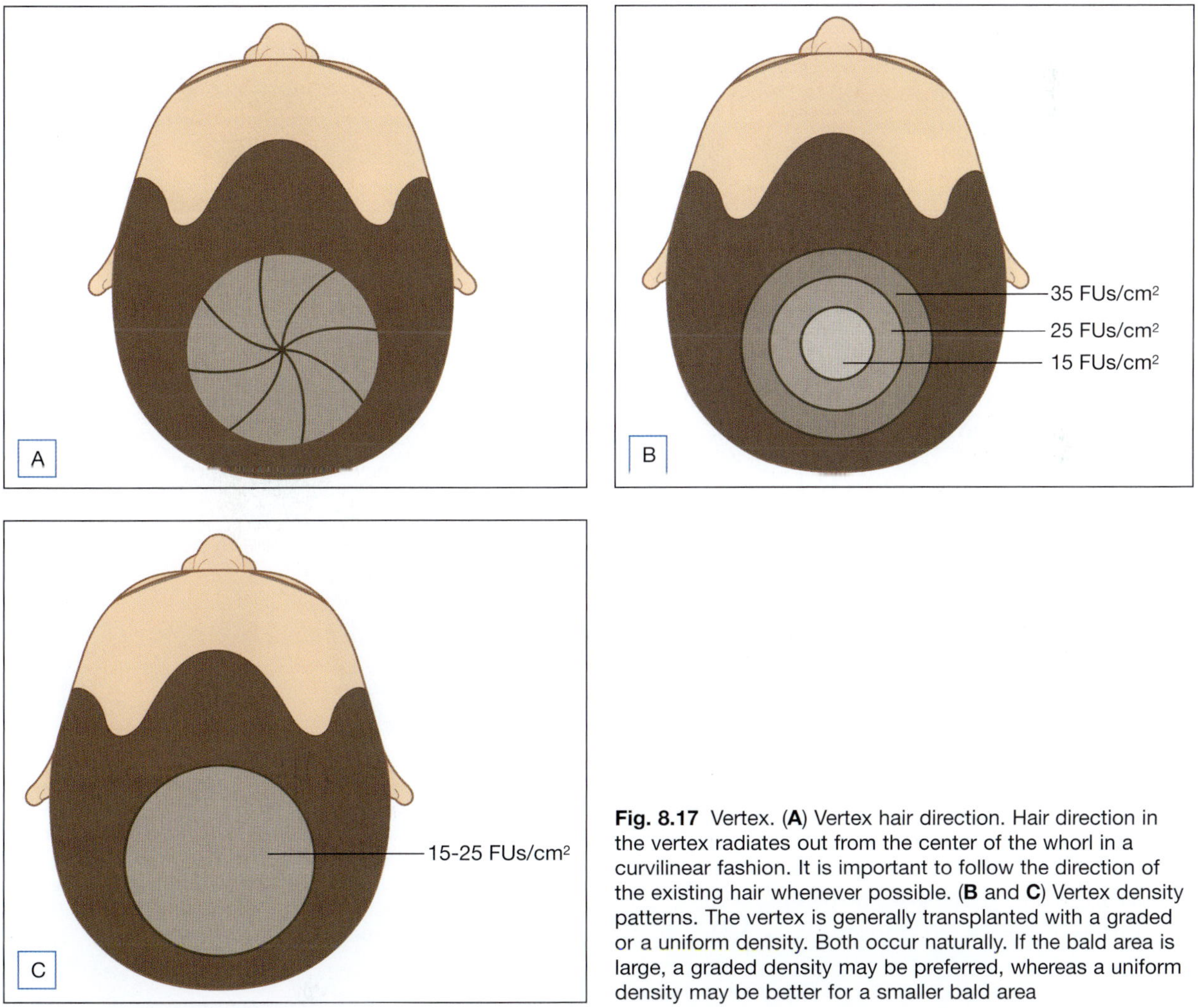


**Fig. 8.17** Vertex. (**A**) Vertex hair direction. Hair direction in the vertex radiates out from the center of the whorl in a curvilinear fashion. It is important to follow the direction of the existing hair whenever possible. (**B** and **C**) Vertex density patterns. The vertex is generally transplanted with a graded or a uniform density. Both occur naturally. If the bald area is large, a graded density may be preferred, whereas a uniform density may be better for a smaller bald area

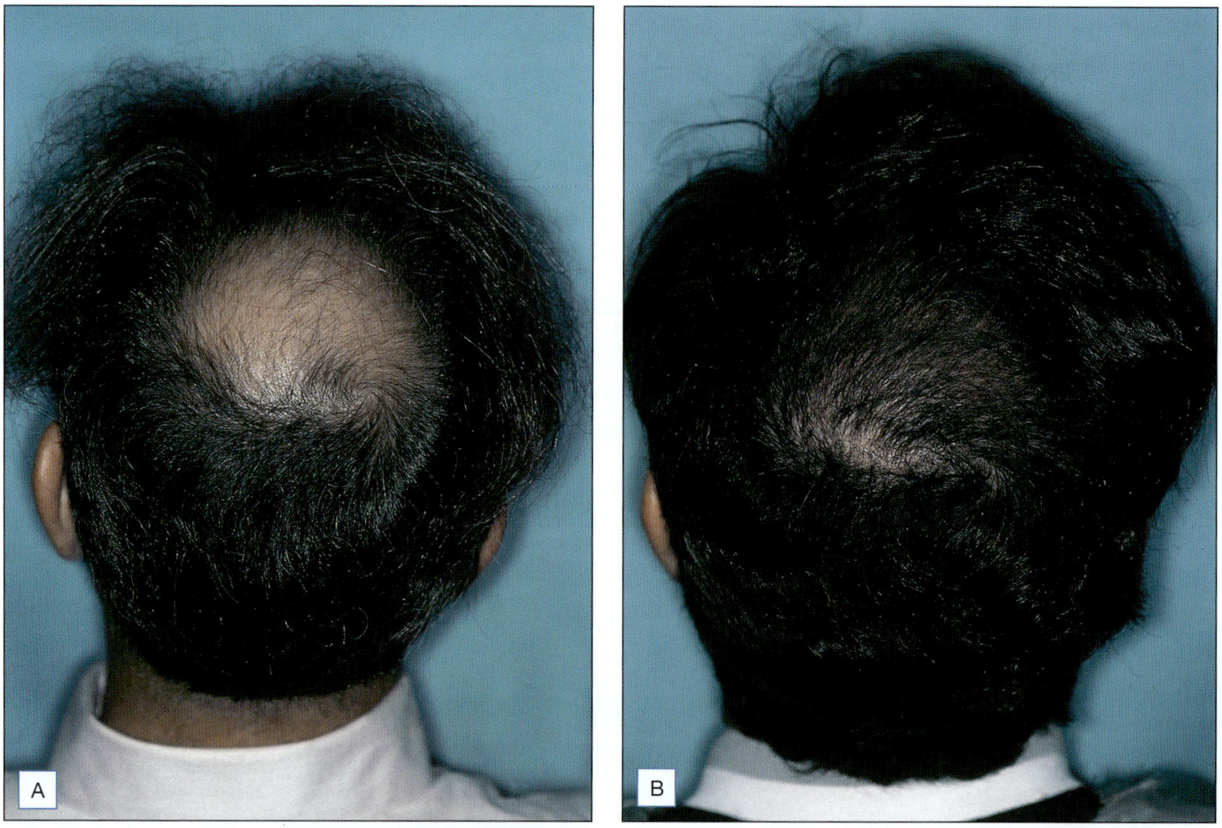


**Fig. 8.18** Vertex transplantation with uniform density. (**A**) Before surgery. (**B**) After one session. If the vertex loss is very large, a graded density will have a better cosmetic appearance

demarcating the point at which the posterior scalp transitions from horizontal to vertical. A round/oval and a kidney-shaped pattern are the most popular designs (Fig. 8.19).

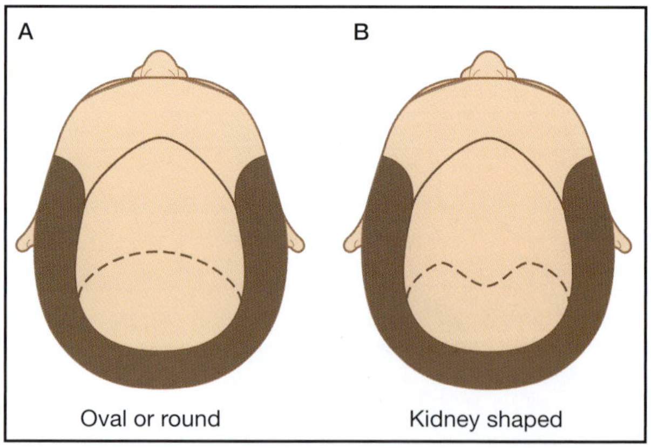


**Fig. 8.19** Anterior vertex hairline design. If the vertex is not transplanted and if the mid-scalp is bald, an anterior vertex hairline needs to be designed. The most commonly created patterns are to leave the vertex round (or oval) or kidney shaped. Do not go posterior the vertex transition zone, where the scalp transitions from horizontal to vertical

## Helpful pointers

1. To help locate the center of the whorl, there is occasionally a retained cluster of hair, given the slang term 'funch', or residual anatomic plug (RAP) (see Fig. 4.8).
2. A kidney-shaped vertex design can help lessen the 'flat head' appearance of a bald crown when viewed from the side.

## Conclusion

There are many choices when picking a design for the different zones. To be safe, it is better to be somewhat conservative, particularly in young patients, in the vertex, or in patients programmed to have advanced baldness. The anticipated designs of the different zones must be coordinated before starting surgery and should not be created later as an afterthought. Finally, it is strongly advisable to become a student of natural hair patterns, and only create designs that are both natural and pleasing. Selecting an appropriate naturally occurring pattern on the proper patient can be one of the most rewarding facets in the field of hair transplantation.

## Further Reading


Basto F 2005 Irregular and sinuous anterior hairline: Prior technique refinement and male and female trace parameters. HT Forum International 15:15–16

Beehner M 1998 Where is thy crown, Your Majesty? HT Forum International 8:18–19

Beehner ML 1998 The Vertex Transition Zone Revisited. HT Forum International 8:33

Mayer M, Perez-Meza D 2003 Temporal points classification and surgical techniques. ESHRS Journal 3:6–7

Parsley WM 2004 Natural hair patterns. Facial Plastic Clinics of North America 12:167–180

Rose PT 1988 Considerations in establishing the hairline. International Journal of Aesthetic and Restorative Surgery 1:24–26

Rose PT 2002 Hairline design. Hair Transplant Forum International 12:180

Shapiro R 2001 Creating a natural hairline in one session using a systemic approach and modern principles of hairline design. International Journal of Cosmetic Surgery and Aesthetic Dermatology 3:89–99

Shapiro R 2004 Principles and techniques used to create a natural hairline in surgical hair restoration. Facial Plastic Clinics of North America 12:201–217

Simmons C 2004 Five old lines and three new lines that can help when designing a male temporal hairline or when transplanting the frontotemporal apex. Hair Transplant Forum International 14:201–203

Unger WP, Shapiro R 2004 Planning the Hairline Zone. Hair Transplantation. 4th edn. Marcel Dekker, New York, p 107–164

Unger WP, Shapiro R 2005 Transplantation of temporal points. Hair transplantation. 4th edn. Marcel Dekker, New York, pp 584–590

# 9 Nerve Block and Local Anesthesia

*Sajjad H. Khan, Shagufta Khan*

## Introduction

### Sensory supply of scalp

The trigeminal and upper cervical nerves are the principal sensory nerves of the scalp. These nerves enter the scalp as main nerve trunks, permitting successful nerve blocks for most of the scalp. The scalp can be divided by a line drawn from ear to ear and passing up through the middle of the vertex. Sixty percent of the scalp is anterior to this line and is innervated by the trigeminal nerve, while 40% of the scalp is posterior to this line, and innervated by the cervical nerves.

#### *Trigeminal nerve*

The trigeminal nerve has three main sensory divisions: the ophthalmic, maxillary and mandibular nerves. All three divisions contribute in providing sensory innervation to the scalp. The ophthalmic division contributes mainly through the supraorbital and supratrochlear nerves. The maxillary division contributes through the zygomaticotemporal nerve and the mandibular division contributes through the auriculotemporal nerve (Fig. 9.1).

#### *Ophthalmic nerve*

The ophthalmic nerve is the smallest of the trigeminal divisions. The ophthalmic nerve divides into three main internal branches: the frontal, lacrimal and nasociliary branches. These branches enter the orbit through the superior orbital fissure (Fig. 9.1).

#### *Frontal nerve*

The frontal nerve is the largest division of the ophthalmic nerve. It divides into two main sensory nerve branches: the supraorbital and supratrochlear.

#### *Supraorbital nerve*

The supraorbital nerve exits the orbit usually through the supraorbital notch and sometimes through the supraorbital foramen. After exiting through the foramen or notch, the supraorbital nerve branches out into two to five main branches. The medial branch pierces the frontalis muscle just above the superciliary arch to reach the connective tissue plane, while the lateral branches pierce the muscle at the mid-forehead to trichion level to reach the connective tissue plane. The lateral branches are the longest and can extend to the vertex. The supra-orbital nerve supplies the sensory innervation to the forehead up to the vertex; it also sends retrograde fibers to innervate the upper lid (Fig. 9.2).

#### *Supratrochlear nerve*

The supratrochlear nerve exits the orbit mostly through the supratrochlear notch almost 1 cm medial to the supraorbital nerve. Occasionally it exits through the foramen or along with the supraorbital nerve. It reaches the connective tissue plane after piercing the corrugator supercilii muscle. The supra-trochlear nerve supplies the medial upper eyelid and medial part of the forehead up to the trichion (Fig. 9.1).

The earlier discussion depicts the classical anatomy as detailed in most textbooks, however, dissections

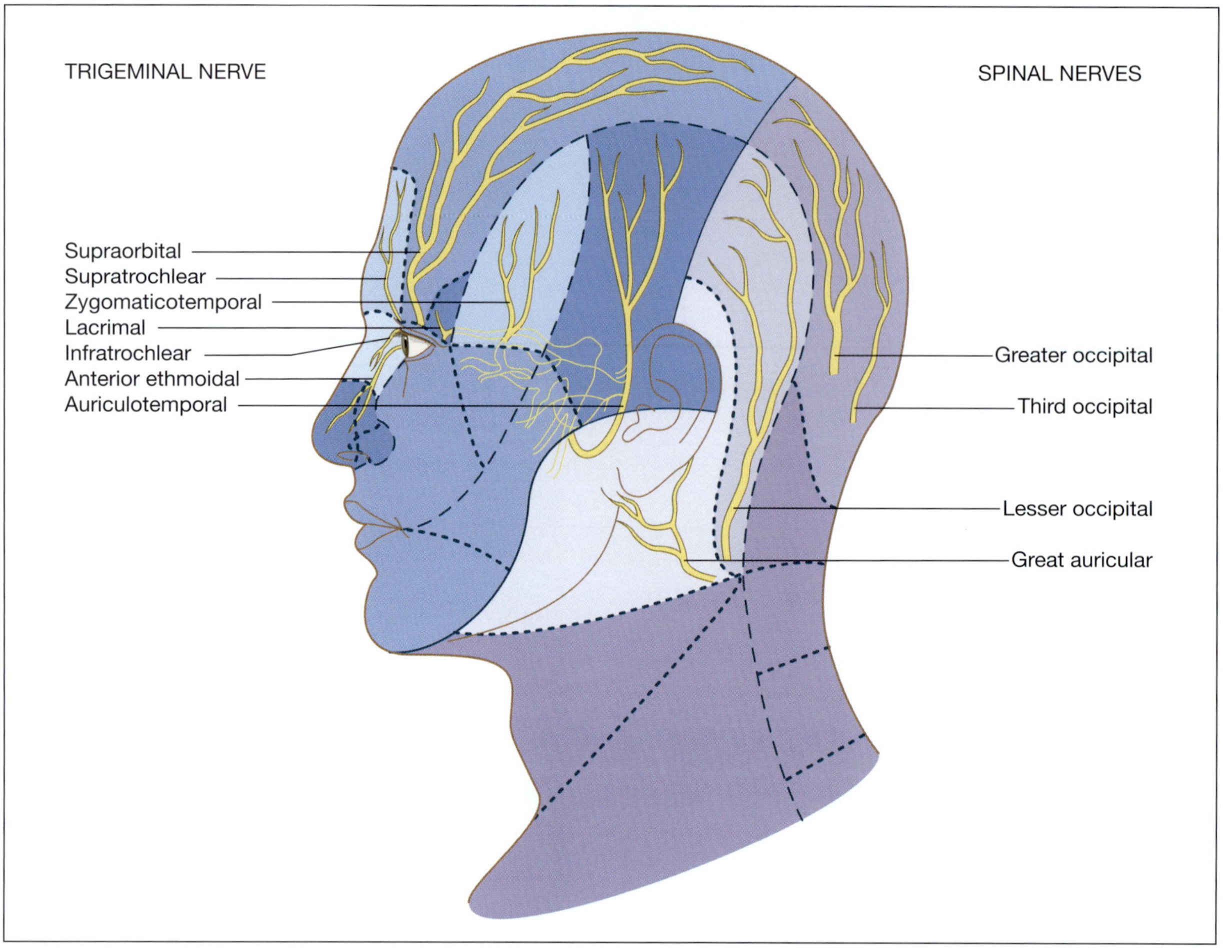


**Fig. 9.1** Sensory supply of the scalp. The trigeminal nerve and its branches are shown in purple color shades. Cervical nerves are shown in different shades of blue

by Fatay show that in only one of 20 cadavers where the traditional supraorbital and supratrochlear nerves are seen. The most medial branch always becomes superficial within a short distance from the orbit, whereas the most lateral branches always remain in a very deep plane below the frontalis muscle until reaching the hairline. It should be kept in mind that the classical, anatomical branching pattern may only rarely be encountered (Fig. 9.3).

### *Maxillary nerve*

The maxillary nerve has three main branches: the infraorbital, zygomaticofacial and zygomaticotemporal.

The zygomaticotemporal is the only branch of the maxillary nerve that innervates the scalp (Fig. 9.1).

### *Zygomaticotemporal nerve*

The zygomaticotemporal nerve emerges from a small foramen on the frontal process of the zygomatic arch near the lateral orbital margin and innervates the temple.

### *Mandibular nerve*

There are three cutaneous branches of the mandibular nerve: the auriculotemporal, buccal and mental nerves.

### *Auriculotemporal nerve*

The auriculotemporal nerve is the only branch of the mandibular nerve that innervates the scalp. The main trunk of the auriculotemporal nerve passes in

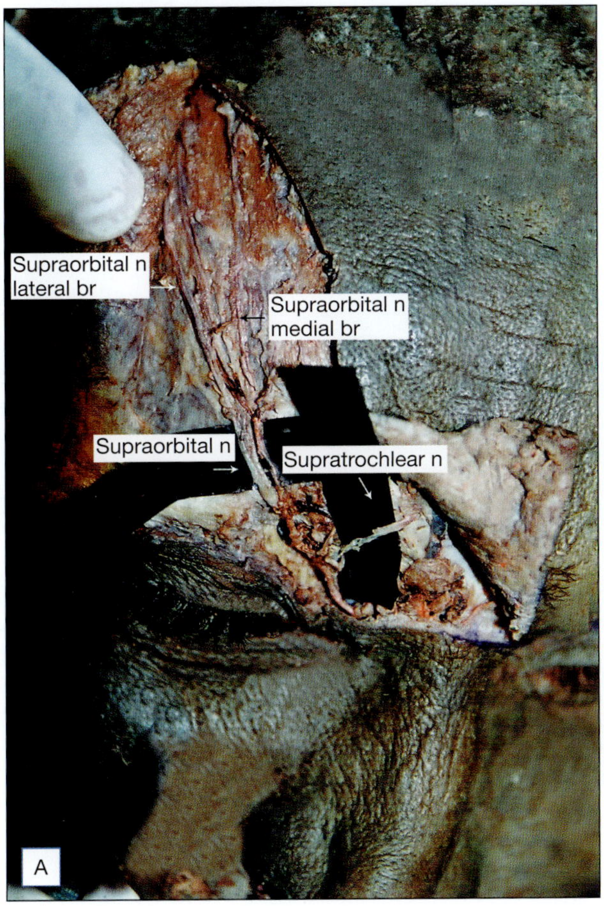


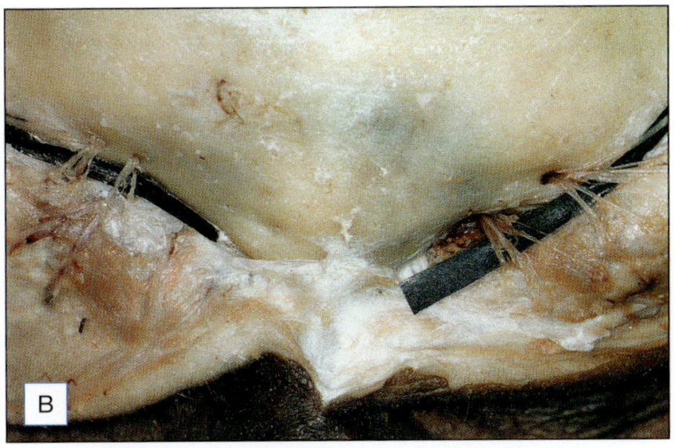


**Fig. 9.2** (**A**) Cadaver dissection demonstrating the emergence of the supraorbital and supratrochlear branches of the frontal nerve. Medial branches of the supraorbital nerve pierce the frontalis muscle proximally, while the lateral branches pierce the frontalis more distally. (**B**) Cadaver dissection demonstrating the emergence and course of the supraorbital and supratrochlear branches of the frontal nerve innervating the forehead and frontal scalp (Reproduced from Stough D, Haber RS 1996 Hair replacement: Surgical and medical. Mosby Year Book Publishing Company, St Louis. Fig 3.9A, p 91, with permission)

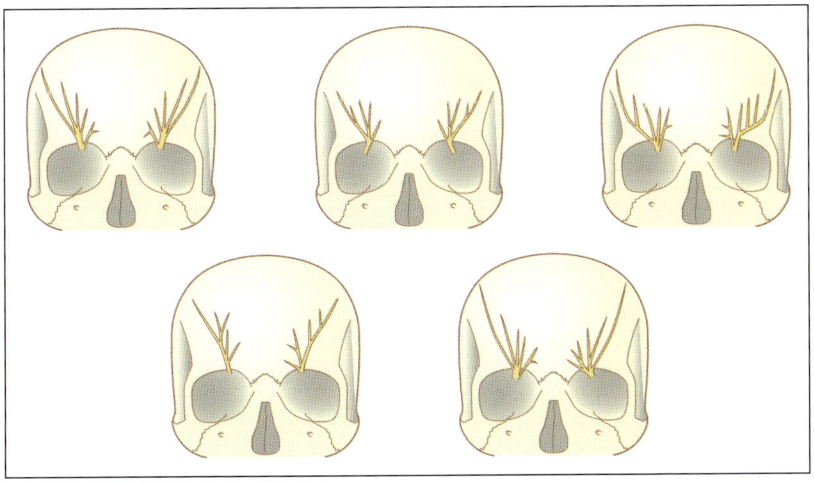

**Fig. 9.3** Variations in the pattern of division of frontal nerve outside the orbit (Modified from Stough D, Haber RS 1996 Hair replacement: Surgical and medical. Mosby Year Book Publishing Company, St Louis. Fig 3.7, p 89, with permission)

front of the tragus and supplies part of the auricle, the temple and temporoparietal scalp (Fig. 9.1).

### *Cervical nerves*

The upper ventral rami through the great auricular and lesser occipital nerves, and the dorsal rami through the greater occipital and third occipital nerves provide the sensory innervation of the scalp behind the ear to the ear line, which passes through the vertex (Fig. 9.4A–D).

### *Ventral rami*

The ventral rami of the upper four cervical nerves form the cervical plexus. There are four sensory

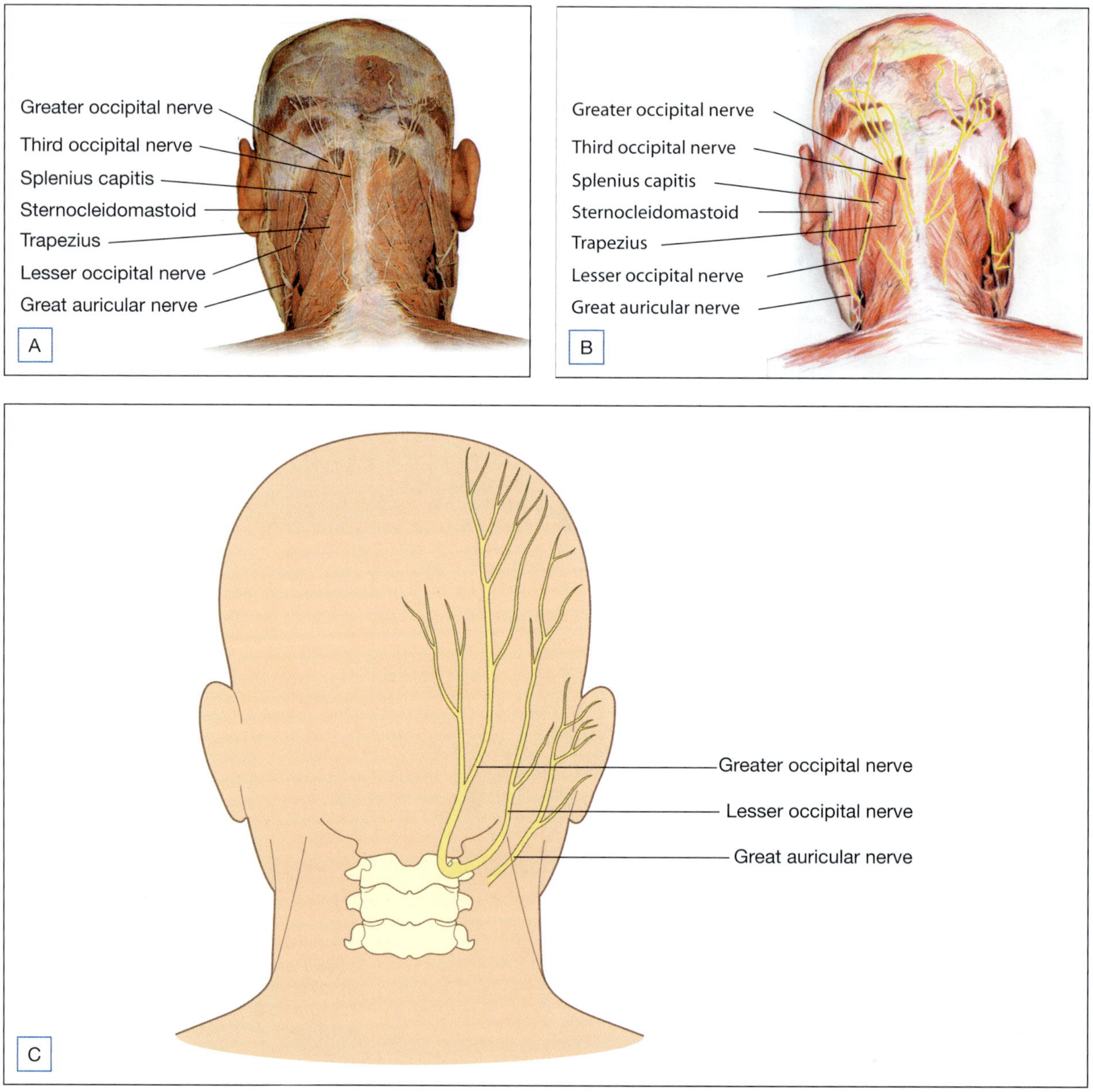


**Fig. 9.4** (**A**) Cadaver dissection showing the emergence of ventral rami nerves and dorsal rami nerves of the scalp. (**B**) Ventral and dorsal rami nerves are highlighted on original cadaver dissection. (**C**) Nerve supply to the posterior scalp (Reproduced from Stough D, Haber RS 1996 Hair replacement: Surgical and medical. Mosby Year Book Publishing Company, St Louis. Fig 3.12, p 93, with permission).

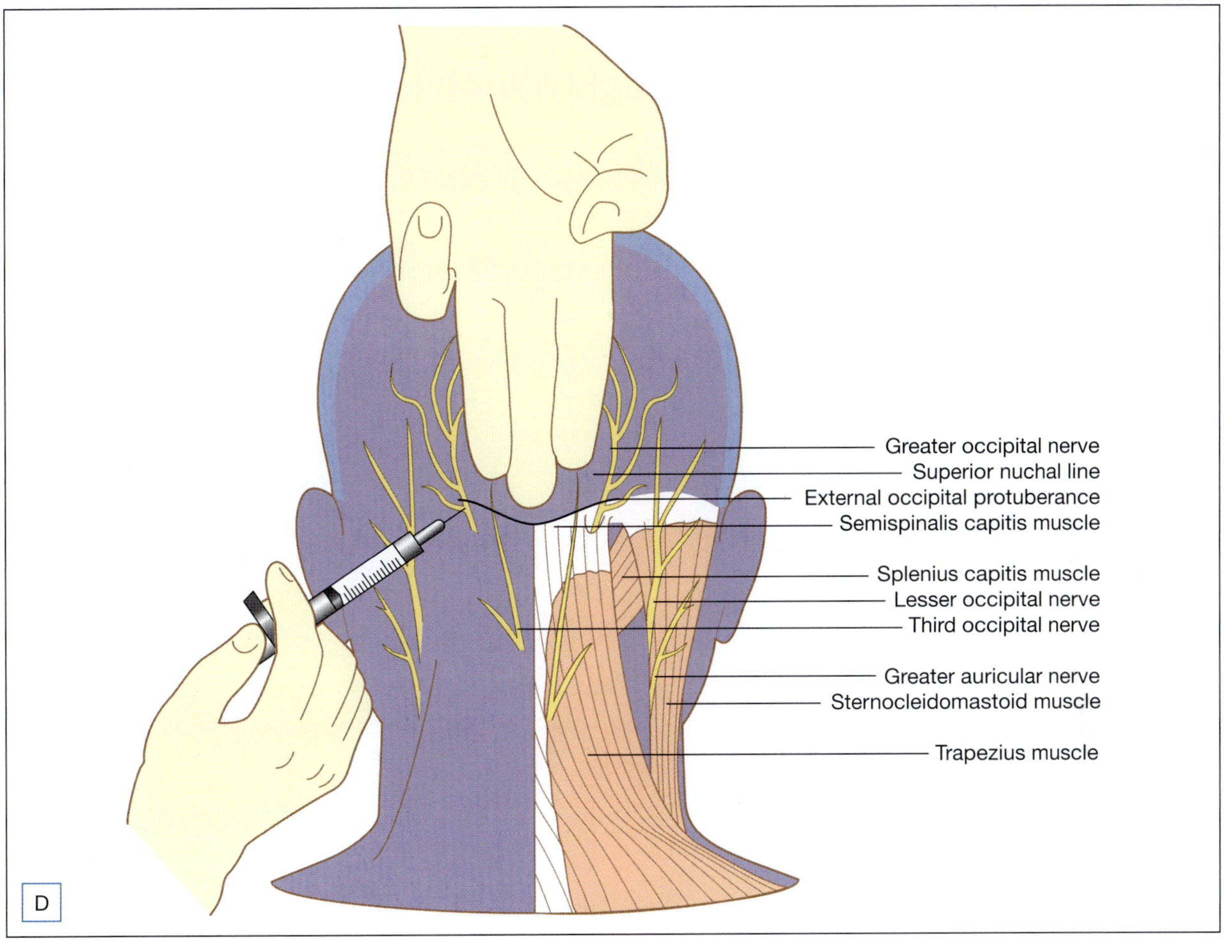


**Fig. 9.4** *Continued,* (**D**) Illustration of original cervical nerve pattern from cadaver dissection. M = muscle

nerves that arise from the cervical plexus: the great auricular, lesser occipital, transverse cervical and supraclavicular. Only the great auricular and lesser occipital nerves innervate the scalp.

### *Great auricular nerve*

The great auricular nerve emerges from behind the posterior border of the sternocleidomastoid muscle and courses upward and toward the lobule of the ear accompanied by the external jugular vein. It innervates the skin of the lateral neck and divides into anterior and posterior branches to innervate the skin at the angle of the jaw as well as posterior portion of the auricle and posterior auricular scalp (Fig. 9.4A)

### *Lesser occipital nerve*

The lesser occipital nerve emerges from behind and runs parallel to the posterior border of the sternocleidomastoid. It innervates the neck and scalp skin posterior to the ear (Fig. 9.4A).

## Dorsal rami

### *Greater occipital nerve*

The second cervical dorsal ramus is the largest of the dorsal rami. It pierces the semispinalis capitis close to the midline, and running superolaterally between it and the trapezius, pierces the tendinous origin of the trapezius and the deep fascia approximately 2.5 cm lateral to the external occipital protuberance as the greater occipital nerve to supply the posterior part of the scalp as far as the vertex. It communicates in the scalp with the great auricular, lesser occipital, posterior auricular, supraorbital and third occipital nerves (Fig. 9.4D).

### *Third occipital nerve*

The third dorsal cervical ramus divides into medial and lateral branches. The medial branch passes posteriomedially, and pierces the semispinalis capitis and trapezius close to the median plane as the third occipital nerve. It supplies the skin and fascia of the upper part of the back of the neck and small adjacent areas of the scalp between the two greater occipital nerves (Fig. 9.4A).

All the sensory nerves of the scalp run along with their respective arteries and veins. These nerve trunks branch out in a linear axial pattern with each nerve innervating a specific vertical zone of the scalp. The terminal branches reach the dermis by the fibrous septa connecting the galea and the dermis.

## Nerve Blocks and Scalp Anesthesia

### Supraorbital nerve block and recipient area anesthesia

Nerve blocks are useful because they can substitute a single injection for a large number of injections and anesthetize a large area with a small amount of anesthetic. A nerve block involves the infiltration of a small volume of anesthetic around a nerve trunk. Diazepam 10 mg is given orally 30 minutes before the procedure. A topical anesthetic such as EMLA or LMX may be applied at the site of injection under occlusion for 60 minutes and will lessen the pain of the block (Fig. 9.5A). While waiting for the topical anesthetic to exert its effect, donor area anesthesia may be performed and the donor area may be harvested.

### *Technique*

The supraorbital nerve block is administered below the eyebrow due to the wide separation of the branches of the supraorbital and supratrochlear nerves above the orbital rim. Place the three middle fingers centered vertically over the glabella. The major nerve branches of the supraorbital nerve emerge just lateral to the outer fingers (Fig. 9.5B, C and E). A 30 gauge half-inch needle is inserted just under the eyebrow until it touches the superior orbital margin. Special attention is paid not to enter into the notch or foramen or elicit paresthesias. Attempt aspiration to ensure that a vessel has not been entered, then inject 2 ml of 0.5% Lidocaine with epinephrine 1:100,000 at this location. The anesthetic will diffuse around the main trunk of the nerve. The needle is then partially withdrawn and redirected medially without exiting the skin and an additional 0.5 ml of anesthetic is injected at the periosteum level (Fig. 9.6). The patient will often note within a few seconds a sensation of heaviness of the upper eyelid due to anesthesia of the retrograde branch of the supraorbital nerve that innervates the upper eyelid. This indicates a successful nerve block. This procedure is followed on the contralateral side as well and both sides are then massaged briefly to help distribute the anesthetic. A complete nerve block is achieved within 30 seconds of the injection in more than 95% of patients.

After achieving the supraorbital nerve block, infiltration block of the recipient area is performed. These injections are extremely painful without the preceding nerve blocks. For infiltration block 0.5% Lidocaine with epinephrine 1:100,000 is injected into the superficial dermal plane. Injection in the dermal plane increases the distance from the base of the hair follicle to the nerves, so during site preparation there is no damage to the main nerves and vessels, and postoperative hypoesthesia is minimal.

### Auriculotemporal nerve block

The auriculotemporal nerve block can be achieved by passing the needle deep into the dermis, just in front of the tragus. Attempt aspiration to ensure that a vessel has not been entered, then inject 2 ml of 0.5% Lidocaine with epinephrine 1:100,000. The block is 95% effective.

### Zygomaticotemporal nerve block

The zygomaticotemporal nerve block can be achieved by injecting 1.5 cm lateral from the outer canthus on the zygomatic arch. A quantity of 2 ml of Lidocaine with epinephrine 1:100,000 is injected deep at the periosteum level to achieve this block. The zygomaticotemporal nerve block can also block the temporal branch of the facial nerve. It can lead to temporary ipsilateral inability to wrinkle the forehead or raise the eyebrow.

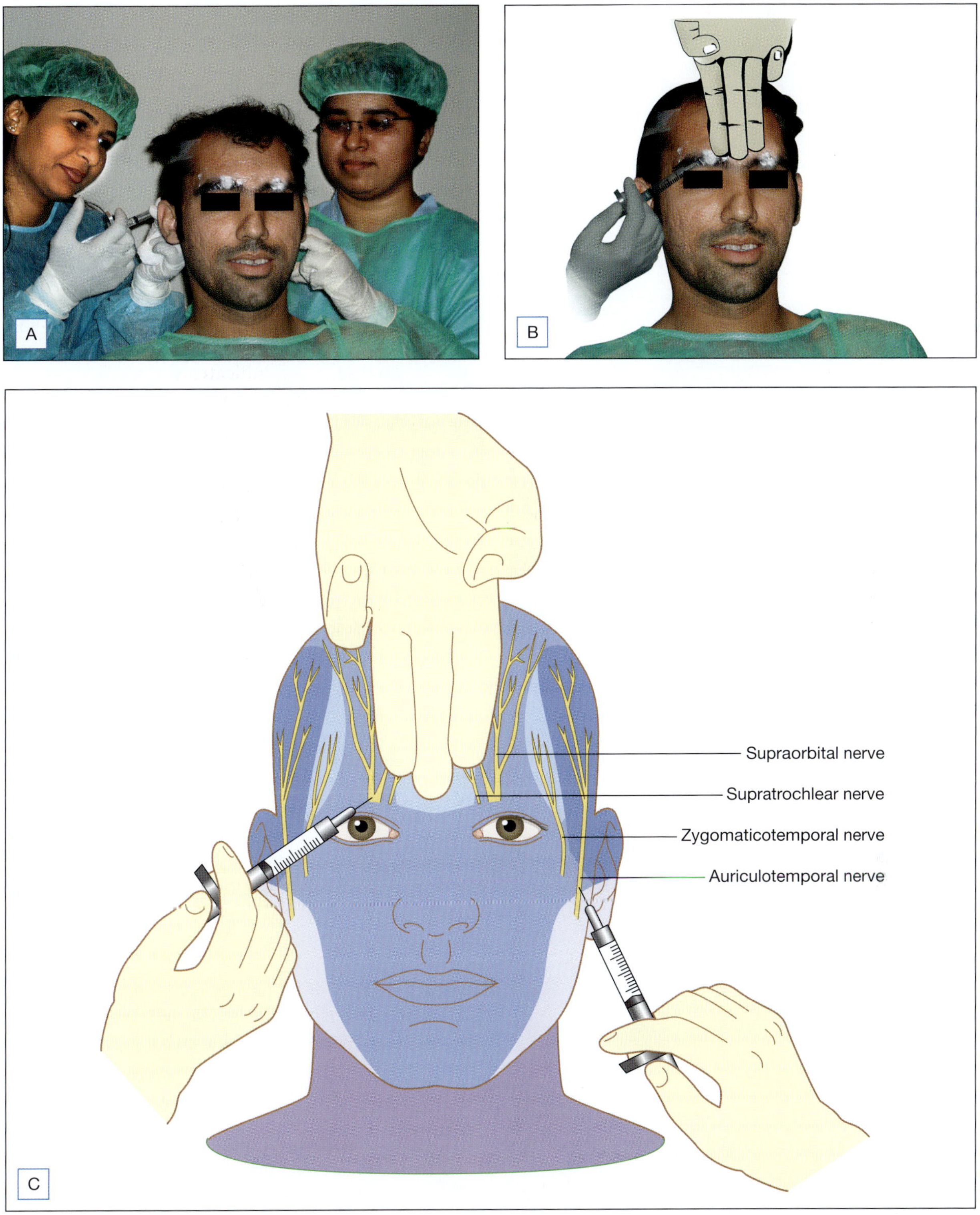


**Fig. 9.5** (**A**) Occlusive application of EMLA before supraorbital nerve block. (**B**) Supraorbital block is achieved by using three-finger rule. (**C**) Original cadaver nerve work is drawn on an illustration.

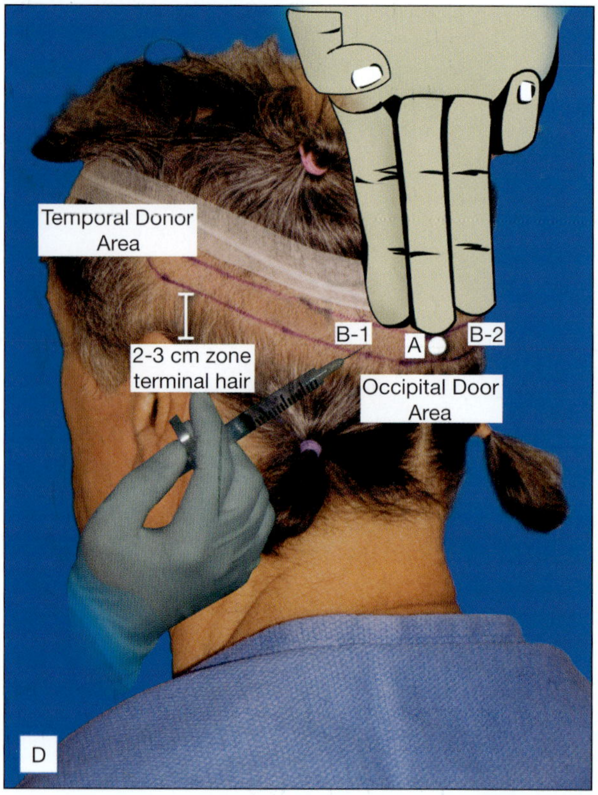


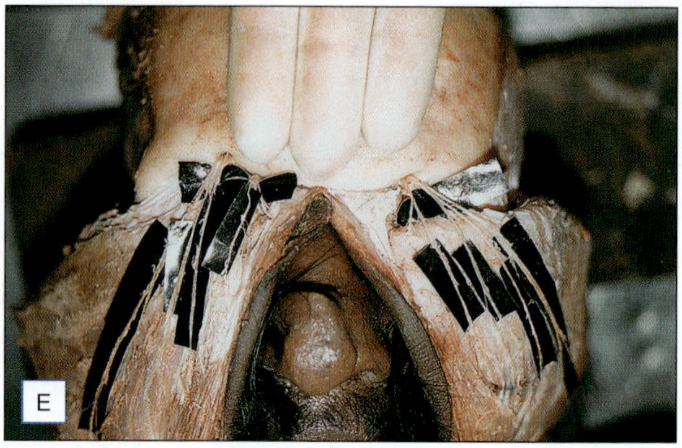


**Fig. 9.5** *Continued,* (**D**) Occipital nerve block technique using three-finger rule. (**E**) Three finger rule. Note the position of the fingers and the emergence of the major nerve branches just lateral to the outer fingers (Reproduced from Stough D, Haber RS 1996 Hair replacement: Surgical and medical. Mosby Year Book Publishing Company, St Louis. Fig 3.10, p 91, with permission)

## Donor Area Nerve Blocks

### Greater occipital nerve block

Three fingers are placed vertically at the level of superior nuchal line with the middle finger over the external occipital protuberance. A 30 gauge half-inch needle is inserted just lateral to the fingers (Fig. 9.5D). When the needle touches the periosteum, 2 ml of Lidocaine with epinephrine 1:100,000 is injected on each side. The occipital nerve block is effective in 90% of the patients. Topical anesthetics can be applied prior to the occipital nerve block as well.

## Donor Area Field Block

A wheal is initially raised at the midline by injecting anesthetic in the superficial dermis. Two other wheals are also raised, one on each side, 4 cm apart from the midline. A needle is then inserted dermally through the previously anesthetized wheal and the anesthetic is injected slightly to the right and then to the left until a solid line of anesthetic is created. Finally the whole donor area is infiltrated at the superficial dermal level, which raises the base of the follicles away from the neurovascular plane (Fig. 9.7). Further dermal supertumescence can be achieved with saline. There is no damage to the neurovascular plane during harvesting with this approach. After harvesting, 0.25% bupivacaine is injected dermally into the dermal area for prolonged anesthetic effect. If the procedure is prolonged, at the first sign of pain, the donor area is injected again in the same manner. Buffering the Lidocaine by adding 1 ml of sodium bicarbonate 8.4% to 10 ml of Lidocaine neutralizes the acidic pH and decreases the pain of injection. Warming the solution to body temperature lessens discomfort as well.

## Summary

Providing a high standard of comfort to the patient is important before, during and after the procedure. Comfort can only be increased by having a thorough knowledge of the sensory nerves of the scalp and knowing the proper techniques of blocks.

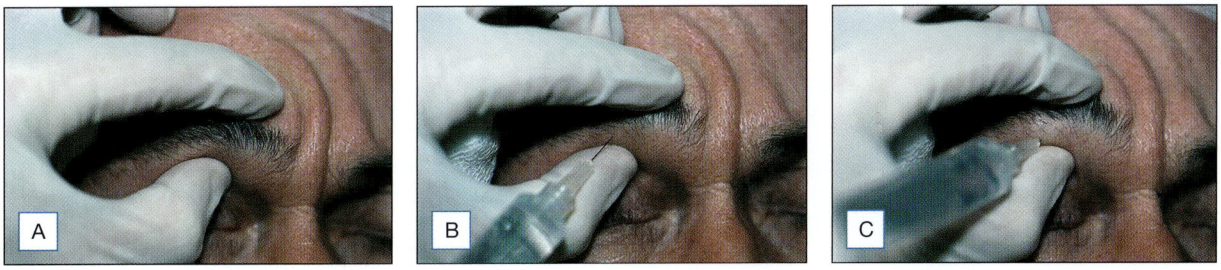


**Fig. 9.6** (**A**) Technique for locating the supraorbital notch. (**B**) Proper position and direction of needle during infiltration of anesthetic for nerve block. (**C**) Needle redirected medially to block supratrochlear nerve (Reproduced from Stough D, Haber RS 1996 Hair replacement: Surgical and medical. Mosby Year Book Publishing Company, St Louis. Fig 3.11, p 92, with permission)

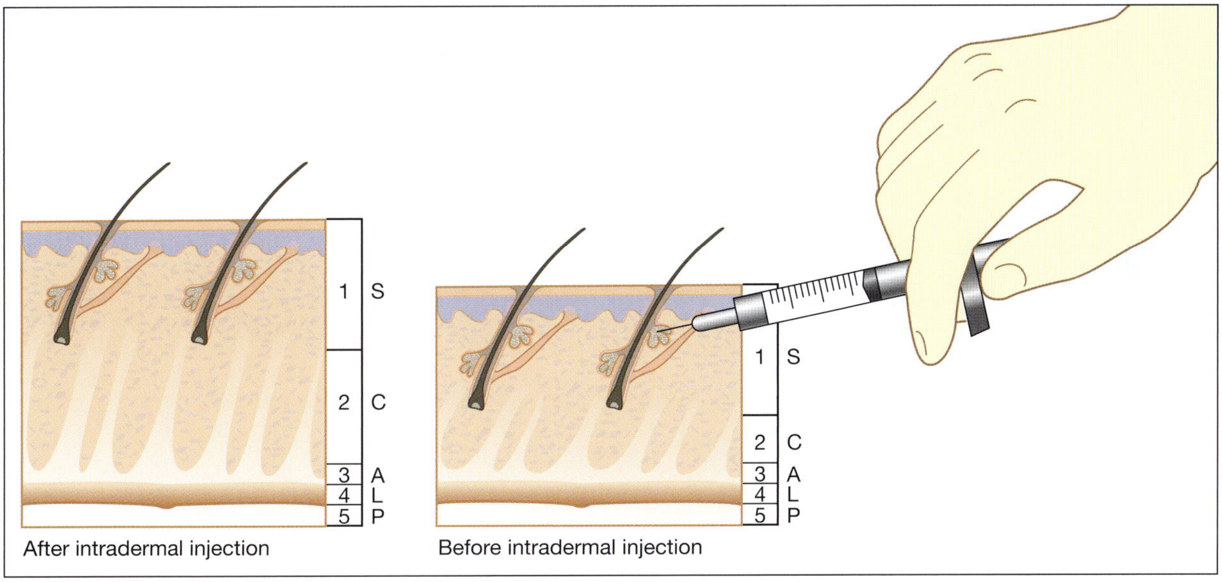


**Fig. 9.7** Superficial dermal infiltration increases the distance between the lower part of the follicle and the neurovascular plane

## Further Reading

Colaric KB, Overton DT, Moore K 1998 Pain reduction in lidocaine administration through buffering and warming. American Journal of Emergency Medicine 16:353

de Jong RH, Heavner J 1971 Diazepam prevents and aborts lidocaine convulsions in monkeys. Anesthesiology 41:226–230

Frankel EB 1981 Nerve block anesthesia for hair transplantation. Journal of Dermatologic Surgery and Oncology 7:73

Haber RS, Khan S, Stough DB 1996 Nerve block anesthesia of the scalp. In: Stough DB, Haber RS (eds) Hair Replacement, Surgical and Medical. Mosby-Year Book, St Louis, pp 89–93

Markham A, Fauld D 1996 Ropivacaine. A review of its pharmacology and therapeutic use in regional anesthesia. Drugs 52:429

Palmon SC, Lloyd AT, Kirsch JR 1998 The effect of needle gauge and Lidocaine pH on pain during intradermal injection. Anesthesia and Analgesia 86:379–381

Roberge CW, McEwen M 1998 The effects of local anesthetics on postoperative pain. AORN Journal 68:1003

Scarfone RJ, Jasani M, Dracely EJ 1998 Pain of local anesthetics: rate of administration and buffering. Annals of Emergency Medicine 31:36

Seager DJ, Simmons C 2002 Local anesthesia in hair transplantation. Dermatologic Surgery 28:320–328

Skidmore RA, Patterson JD, Tomsick RS 1996 Local anesthetics. Dermatologic Surgery 22:511–522

Wahlgren CF, Quiding H 2000 Depth of cutaneous analgesia after application of A eutectic mixture of the local anesthetics Lidocaine and prilocaine (EMLA Cream). Journal of the American Academy of Dermatology 42:548

Williams PL, Warwich R, Dyson M, Bannister LH 1989 Gray's anatomy. 37th edn. Edinburgh: Churchill Livingstone, p 1100

# 10 Single-scar Harvesting Technique

*Mario Marzola*

## Introduction

Assessing the quality of the patient's hair at the back and sides of his scalp and visualizing what will still be there when he's about 60 years old can be loosely called the 'permanent hair fringe' or 'available donor hair.' The best hair and certainly the safest for long-term survival of the transplant is usually located in the center of this hair fringe. The upper part could be susceptible to pattern hair loss if the future loss is underestimated and the lowest part of it may be lost through neck baldness advancing from below.

Once these parameters have been established mentally, mark the middle of this donor hair from ear to ear. Preferably this should be marked with a ruler to ensure that the correct plane is achieved. When marking freehand, there is a tendency for the lines to 'drift.' The strip will be harvested along the pre-drawn lines in this location. It should be remembered that each patient is different and it is important to follow the curves of the pattern displayed in front of the practitioner rather than some preconceived idea that may be held about where the donor area should be. In a patient with normal healing ability, when strip harvesting is correctly preformed the scar will be nearly invisible. The patient should be warned that this very high standard may not be achievable in subsequent surgeries. Like the available donor hair, the scalp's elasticity is finite and each excision reduces the elasticity as it reduces the remaining donor hair. Increasing tension on closure of the donor defect after strip harvesting will result in increasing the size of the donor scar. However there are techniques of minimizing this phenomenon so that the resulting scar after three, four or five surgeries will still only be 1 or 2 mm wide (Box 10.1).

## First Procedure

Make the strip as long and thin as possible, even for small number graft sessions. The one immutable law on best scar outcome is: **no tension on closure**. Make the incision clean and parallel to the hair follicles, tapered at each end and only deep enough to remove the hair follicles, no deeper. By limiting follicular unit graft numbers below 2000 in one session the strip is rarely more than 8 or 9 mm wide. Sometimes the patients prefer larger sessions such as 3000, 4000 or even 5000 grafts per session. This takes some gearing up to do but if it is offered, then the patient must be told that the wider strip of 10–20 mm will result in an easily identifiable scar, even though it will still be well hidden by the fall of hair. There is no escaping this reality. The invisible scar mentioned earlier is only achievable with follicular unit graft procedures somewhere near 2000 or less.

**Techniques for imperceptible donor scars**

1. The strips should be as long and thin as possible
2. There should be limited tension on closure
3. Make the incision as clean as possible and parallel to the hair follicles
4. Recognize that strips greater than 1 cm wide will have a tendency for wider, more cosmetically noticeable scars
5. For sessions requiring wider strips, and more than 2000 follicular unit grafts, expect wider scars
6. Trim off 1–2 mm of the top edge of the donor defect utilizing the trychophytic closure
7. Use single-layered 4/0 nylon closure with removal in 7 days
8. Wait six months between procedures.

**Box 10.1** Techniques for imperceptible donor scars

Before closing the donor defect, trim off 1–2 mm of the top edge, which is an acute angle and often 'lips over' anyway (Figs 10.1 and 10.2). This technique is called trichophytic closure. The de-epithelialization of one or two follicular units in this way allows them to grow up through the eventual scar, thereby dispersing its linearity. It is a technique with origins in transposition flap hairline surgery, where the front hairline scar was a problem without this dispersal.

The use of tumescence described elsewhere in this text will have kept the scalpel away from significant vessels and if enough time is given for the tumescence to work efficiently, there will be almost no bleeding from smaller vessels. If use of a cautery to control bleeding is necessary, then the protocol needs another look.

Because the strip is so long and thin, the donor defect is not wide, so closure should be possible with very little tension. Minor loosening of the edges (undermining) just under the hair follicles but still superficial to the neurovascular bundles may be useful in tight scalps to allow the edges to move together easily. Closure may involve a two-layered closure with buried dissolvable sutures or single-layer closure only. Single-layered closure with continuous 4.0 nylon sutures is easy and produces great results. Remove all sutures at postoperative days 7–10. At all times approximate the edges accurately so that dermis meets dermis and the de-epithelialized upper edge sits neatly next to the non-de-epithelialized lower edge. It is not necessary to bury all the de-epithelialized follicles into the wound to achieve dispersal of the resulting scar.

Follow these rules and nearly all scars will be of excellent quality. There is a small subset of patients however who do not heal well, producing a scar measuring 3 mm or wider regardless of which system is used. These people may have Ehlers–Danlos syndrome or a similar connective tissue disorder, so it is important to stop and discuss further management before the patient is given wider scars (Box 10.2).

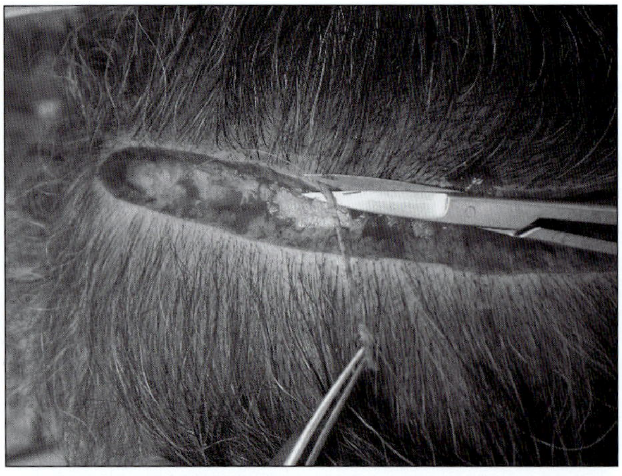

**Fig. 10.1** Trichophytic closure. A thin strip of skin is removed from the upper wound border. When closed, the lower border will overlap the upper border

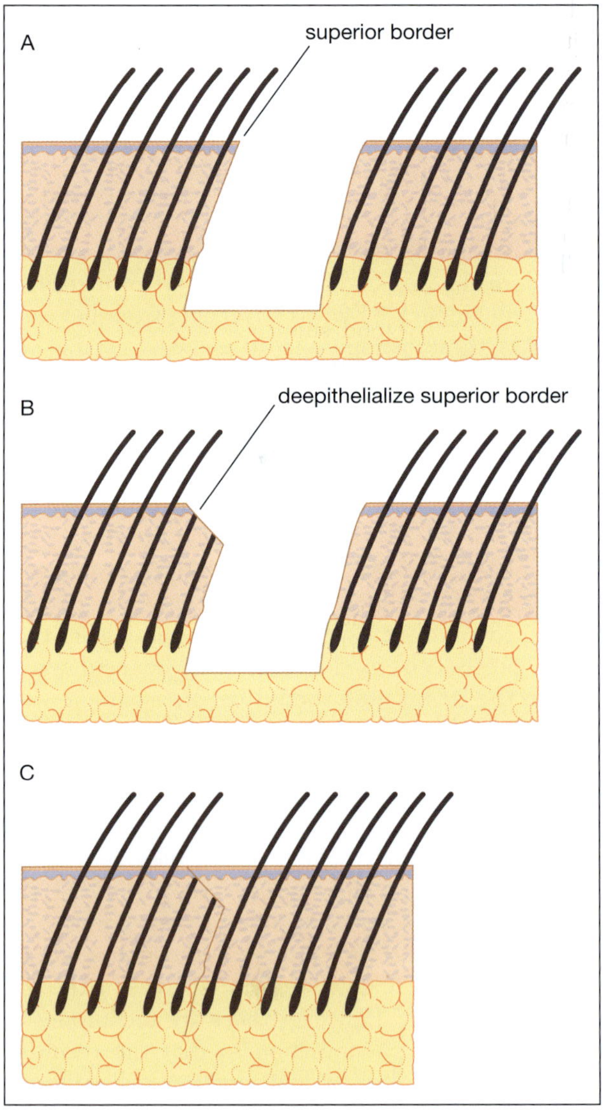


**Fig. 10.2** Diagram illustrating the trichophytic closure procedure. (**A**) Step 1. (**B**) Step 2. (**C**) Step 3

**Problem patients**

- Those with scars 3 mm width or wider
- Those with Ehlers–Danlos syndrome
- Blacks
- High contrast between hair and skin color (individuals with dark hair and very light scalps)

**Box 10.2** Problem patients

## Subsequent Procedures

Most experienced transplant surgeons today practice the removal of the existing scar in subsequent procedures, leaving the patient always with just one scar. The patients certainly like this idea, however there are some practical considerations in doing so. Because there is often a temporary shock loss along the suture line, be it ever so small, it is important to wait for these hairs to regrow so they can be seen and harvested the next time. Without this regrowth the dormant follicles will be invisible and discarded with the waste tissue. To be safe, 6 months must elapse between procedures. It is good surgical practice anyway to space out the operations but it may not suit the patient's program if he's in a hurry.

It is best to place the existing scar in the middle of the new strip. In this way the surgical assistants with their better view using microscopes can safely dissect the follicular units distorted by the scar. This distortion may extend a few millimeters either side of the scar and can result in transection if near the new incision line. There is much more control of angle and depth with single-blade scalpels than when using two or more blades together. Multiple-blade scalpels should therefore be left in the hands of very experienced surgeons and in virgin scalps where there is no scar distortion of growth.

Because the previous closure will have slightly decreased the density of growth near the scar by stretching, the yield per square centimeter will be decreased in second and subsequent harvests. To keep producing the best scar possible, the graft numbers will have to be gradually reduced with each procedure, e.g. 2000, 1500, 1000, 750, 500 and taking the longest and narrowest strip possible each time. For example, the fifth procedure of 500 follicular unit transplants may have a strip from ear to ear that is only 3–4 mm wide. In this way the gradually increasing tension with each closure can be kept at bay and the scar after the fifth procedure will not be much worse than the first scar. A single-layered trichophytic closure as described earlier is recommended at all times.

## Conclusion

Many practitioners today produce very fine scars that are almost invisible yet use different techniques. In one way or another, however, all these practitioners will treat the tissues with respect and close the wound accurately, with little or no tension. Single-scar harvesting leaves the scalp with minimal injury and minimal scarring, the current authors' patient treatment goal.

### Further Reading

Frechet P 2005 Donor harvesting with invisible scars. Hair Transplant Forum Int 15:119–20

Marzola M 2005 Trichophytic closure of the donor area. Hair Transplant Forum Int 15:113–16

Rose P 2005 Ledge closure. Hair Transplant Form Int 15:120

# 11 Donor Strip Slivering and Microscopic Dissection

*Bobby L. Limmer, Bradley Limmer*

## Introduction

Hair grows in the human scalp mostly in groupings of one to four terminal hair follicles, which may also include one or two vellus follicles (Fig. 11.1). These groupings are called follicular units (FUs). In individuals having great hair density such FUs rarely may contain five or six terminal follicles. Headington described the histologic anatomy of such FUs in 1984 to include the associated sebaceous lobules, arrector pili muscle insertions, vascular plexus, and neural network.

From 1959–1988 hair transplantation surgery was performed exclusively by the use of random groupings of multiple FUs into 'plugs,' 'minigrafts,' and 'micrografts.' On October 21, 1988 the author performed the first transplant procedure exclusively using individual FUs as the basic graft. Between 1988 and 1991 the procedure was modified to include the basic principles of single-blade elliptical donor harvest followed by microscopic dissection of individual FU grafts and implantation of such grafts into small needle tunnel recipient sites (the 'stick and place' method of implantation).

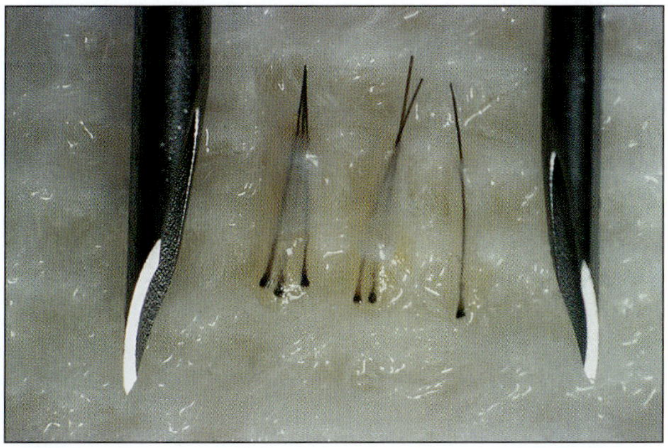

**Fig. 11.1** Follicular unit grafts containing one, two and three hairs

## Method

Donor hair must be taken from an area not genetically susceptible to future loss. The most common donor zone lies in the occipital scalp extending as a horizontal band of approximately 5 cm in width defined by the superior and inferior attachments of the cartilaginous pinna. This band may be carried superiorly into the supra-auricular parietal scalp and forward into the posterior temporal scalp if necessary; however, the preferred donor remains the occipital zone. A single-blade elliptical excision is preferred over multi-bladed knives to minimize marginal transection of follicles. The average density of FUs in the occipital scalp is approximately 100 units per square centimeter; however, the range of such densities is approximately 50–160, making it imperative that the density be measured preoperatively to determine the donor surface area needed to harvest the number of FU grafts desired. Donor site closure with minimal tension is critical to achieving a narrow surgical scar. Double-layer suture closure may offer some advantage, especially on subsequent re-harvest. The donor tissue and grafts generated must be kept well hydrated by immersion in chilled normal saline or lactated Ringer's solution. Other media are under investigation.

## Microscopic Dissection of Donor Tissue

To avoid unnecessary follicular transection, all graft production is accomplished under binocular stereomicroscopic dissection characteristically at approximately 10-power magnification. The initial step of slivering the donor tissue into smaller units is the most critical and technically exacting step. The use of a single assistant who is very precise and capable of this step assures minimal transection of follicles. An excellent assistant can sliver the donor tissue into thin sections with less than 1% transaction. The remaining individual FU graft production and careful trimming can be accomplished with virtually no follicular transection when done by experienced assistants. Grafts are separated by numbers of hair in each graft and kept immersed in chilled holding solution at all times.

## Graft Implantation

FU grafts may be implanted in pre-made incision sites created by small blades, or into needle tunnel incisions using the 'stick and place' method. Punch recipients sites, once the most popular method, are seldom used today because of the greater vascular injury produced. Graft densities of 20–60 grafts per square centimeter are commonly performed to achieve suitable cosmetic densities in a single pass over the recipient zone. Most authors feel that graft densities of 30–40 grafts per $cm^2$ accomplish adequate cosmetic densities with a single pass. Obviously, the single-hair grafts are used to produce a soft transition zone along the frontal hairline with the multi-hair grafts placed to produce greater density, especially in the central frontal core zone. Selective distribution is used to accomplish desired density in each scalp region. Recent emphasis on the angulation of the recipient incision site using very small blades has led some surgeons to change the direction of the incision from anterior/posterior (sagittal) to a more lateral (coronal) incision direction. This coronal angle incision has been proposed as a means to take advantage of the somewhat linear native distribution among many two- to four-hair FUs.

## Postoperative Care

The vascularity of the scalp promotes rapid healing, therefore dressing applications to the grafted area are not essential since healing will occur with shedding of the tiny crusts in 7–9 days with or without special care. However, healing can be expedited by a moist environment of saline or water misting onto the scalp, or routine occlusive wound dressings.

## Disadvantages and Advantages of FU Transplantation

### Disadvantages

The process is time consuming and labor intensive. Special training is necessary to produce skilled assistants who understand the precision needed to generate and place high-quality grafts. The physician must understand and be proficient with each step in order to train assistants and to supervise quality control. Special equipment includes binocular stereomicroscopes, loupes for implantation, and a custom blade cutter if it is desired to produce cut-to-size blades for implantation site creation. Most important of all are skilled and well-trained assistants dedicated to excellence. Without such a staff, this procedure cannot be properly executed.

### Advantages

The greatest advantage of FU transplantation is the naturalness of the final cosmetic result. The tufting seen with plugs and multi-follicular unit grafts does not occur with follicular unit grafts. Grafts may be placed among pre-existing hair in zones of thinning without the loss of such pre-existing hair in most cases. If such pre-existing hair should partially shed due to the procedure, in most instances it will regrow synchronously with the newly placed grafts. Healing of both donor and recipient areas is rapid. Scarring of cosmetic significance is uncommon in both donor and recipient areas if known surgical principles are followed. The most important of these principles is donor closure without significant tension. While no rules are absolute, a good rule of thumb is not to exceed 1.3 cm in width on the initial donor strip and not more than 1 cm on subsequent re-harvest in the donor area. Manual checking of mobility prior to marking the donor width may change such general rules.

FU transplantation has greatly expanded the number of candidates for transplantation because of its careful use of the donor area. Rarely is the donor area depleted before the recipient area is completed to realistic expectations established before the outset. Cases done by 'plug' and 'minigraft' methods may be greatly improved by elimination of tufting, usually with a single session of FU transplantation. Scars involving the scalp, beard, and mustache are acceptable for grafting and the rate of graft survival in such scars is high. Cases of inactive cicatricial alopecia including lupus, scleroderma, lichen planopilaris, and pseudopelade of Brocq as well as traumatic surgical and radiation alopecia, accept grafting in the author's experience as well as normal, nonscarred alopecic scalps. Eyebrows can be suitably restored as can eyelashes, but methods in these critical areas are more complex than routine grafting elsewhere.

## Summary

FU hair transplantation in this author's opinion represents the end refinement of surgical hair transplantation. Other methods of donor harvest or graft implantation may alter in some ways the methodology evolved some 16 years ago, but the use of the naturally occurring FU will likely remain as the basic graft due to naturalness and density consistently and predictably produced.

## Editor's Comment

Dr Norman Orentreich is known as the father of the standard punch autograft technique. Dr Bobby Limmer is recognized as the innovator of modern transplant techniques. This preceding chapter is elegant and succinct. Despite its brevity, readers should note the impact of his findings as described earlier. It is highly recommended that all readers view the accompanying DVD illustrating the technique that has been produced in his office.

## Further Reading

Headington JT 1984 Transverse microscopic anatomy of the human scalp. A basis for a morphometric approach to disorders of the hair follicle. Archives of Dermatology 120:449–456

Limmer BL 1994 Elliptical donor stereoscopically assisted micrografting as an approach to further refinement in hair transplantation. Journal Dermatologic Surgery and Onocology 20:789–793

Limmer BL 2004 The history of follicular unit micrografting technique: A personal view. In: Unger W, Shapiro R (eds) Hair transplantation. Marcel Dekker Publishers, New York, p 383–388

Norwood O, Limmer BL 1999 Advances in hair transplantation. Advances in Dermatology 14:89–113 [discussion 114]

Shapiro R 2004 Principles and techniques used to create a natural hairline in hair restoration. Facial Plastic Surgery Clinics of North America 12:201–217

# 12 Follicular Unit Transplantation

*Robert M. Bernstein, William R. Rassman*

## Introduction

The underlying concept of follicular unit transplantation (FUT) is that, in order to maximize the cosmetic benefit of the hair transplantation, only naturally occurring, individual follicular units (FUs) should be transplanted. In the purest form of FUT, FUs are neither divided into smaller units, nor combined into larger ones.

FUT had its origins in the microscopic dissection techniques of Limmer, developed in 1988. The conceptual framework for FUT was introduced in the hair transplant literature by the authors in their 1995 publication *Follicular Transplantation* and further detailed in 1997. The name **follicular unit transplantation** was formalized by a group of hair transplantation surgeons in a 1998 publication in *Dermatologic Surgery*. In that article, an attempt was made to precisely define FUT and included the two basic techniques of Limmer, single-strip harvesting and stereomicroscopic dissection, as integral parts of the procedure. Since FUs can now be harvested directly from the donor area without the necessity of a strip excision (using follicular unit extraction or FUE), the original definition of FUT has become obsolete. FUT is simply the transplantation of FUs by any means.

Other surgeons previously regarded FUT as the transplantation of FUs by any means, thus a strict definition of this involving strip harvesting and stereomicroscopic dissection was never accepted by all. FUs can be produced by many methods, one of which is FUE. Transplantation of grafts obtained by FUE is still regarded as a form of FUT.

In order to transplant grafts in very high densities or in very large numbers per session, some practitioners have limited FUs to those containing a maximum of three hairs, particularly in those patients with coarse hair. This would necessitate dividing a naturally occurring four-hair FU into smaller grafts, essentially creating micrografts. Other practitioners of FUT occasionally combine two FUs with the intention of creating more density in the frontal core area, particularly in patients with fine or light-colored hair. Other physicians may combine one-hair FUs into 'twos' simply to minimize the number of recipient sites needed. Finally, unlike strip harvesting with stereomicroscopes, where intact naturally occurring FUs are generated, for the vast majority of the time with FUE techniques the physician is not always able to harvest intact units and therefore must work with partial groups or groups devoid of some of the connective tissue support structures.

Considering these relatively common variations on FUT and the often imperfect FUs that are generated in the increasingly popular technique of FUE, FUT should be considered as any procedure in which the goal is to restore a person's hair using predominantly naturally occurring individual FUs. It is important that where significant exceptions or deviations are made from the pure FUT procedure these modifications are clearly explained.

FUE may be considered a specific harvesting method in FUT in which FUs are obtained directly through small circular incisions rather than through a microscopically dissected donor strip. However, the nature of the technique itself can have a significant impact on other aspects of the surgery, including the quality of the grafts, their number, the organizational aspects of the surgery, and possibly its design.

## Transplanting Individual FUs

There are two central arguments for transplanting individual FUs. The first is that using individual FUs will produce the most natural results. The second is that it allows the practitioner to transplant the maximum amount of hair into the smallest possible wound.

## Natural results

Since hair naturally grows as individual FUs, it is logical to conclude that transplanting hair exactly the way it grows would produce the most natural results. This apparently obvious conclusion however may not always be true. The normal density of FUs is approximately $100/cm^2$. If an average FU contains 2.3 hairs, there will be $230$ $hairs/cm^2$. In the context of this density, FUs of any size will look natural. However, if 2400 FUs are transplanted evenly over the front and top of a bald scalp (excluding the crown), an area that generally measures 150 $cm^2$, the new transplanted density is 16 follicular $units/cm^2$ or 16% of the original density. A second procedure of 2000 grafts, evenly distributed, will increase the average density to just under 30% of the original density. However, most physicians transplant greater densities toward the front part of the scalp (40–50%), leaving the area toward back of the scalp thinner. Therefore, even with two sessions totaling 4400 grafts, there may be as little as 20% of the original density on the top of the scalp and as little as 10% towards the back. If the crown is transplanted, these numbers will be even lower.

At low densities, there may not be enough hair to 'visually support' the larger FUs and four-hair grafts may have a slightly unnatural look. This may present a particular problem in patients with coarse, dark hair and light skin. One solution is to try and bury the larger units in areas of greater density, such as in the frontal core area, and use the smaller grafts towards the periphery, but in patients with extreme skin/hair color contrast this may not be enough and it may be appropriate to split some of the four-hair units into two, two-hair grafts.

A second issue is that merely using individual FUs will not insure that the grafts look natural. The right-sized units must be placed in the right place. Since the normal hairline consists mainly of single-hair FUs, so must the transplant. This, however, is not always easy to do. Transplanting the naturally occurring FU implies keeping the support structures intact, which is best accomplished using a 'chubby' graft. Chubby grafts, however, increase the chance that empty telogen follicles are included in the dissection. Although this is beneficial to achieve maximum fullness for most of the scalp, at the hairline this may result in two-hair grafts. To avoid this problem, FUs at the hairline should be trimmed 'thin,' which may expose the graft to mechanical injury and desiccation.

Another problem occurs when small transplant sessions are performed. This may be due to a demand issue (i.e. if the patient is a Norwood Class III and only requires 800 grafts) or a supply issue (i.e. if the patient can only afford a small number of grafts or FUE is planned and a limited number of grafts is a constraint due to the capabilities of the surgical team).

Since the normal donor scalp contains only around 10–15% one-hair FUs, a donor strip of 800 grafts would only yield 80–120 single-hair FUs, far short of the 250–300 generally needed for the frontal hairline.

Therefore, with strip harvesting, if the surgeon desires to restore a hairline in one session then he or she must resort to splitting larger FUs into one-hair grafts. FUE presents another problem since harvesting single-hair FUs with this technique greatly increases the number of the recipient wounds. In FUE, in order to minimize injury to the donor area, it may be beneficial to harvest the largest FUs and then divide them into one-hair grafts for the hairline. This has been a common practice for over a decade among transplant surgeons and is a minor departure from "pure" follicular unit transplantation.

## Small wounds

Observing hairs growing in FUs, rather than individually, is most easily done through densitometry, a simple technique where scalp hair is clipped to approximately 1 mm in length and examined through a high-magnification instrument (Fig. 12.1). From this vantage point, it can also be appreciated that follicular units are relatively compact, but are surrounded by substantial amounts of nonhair-bearing skin. The actual proportion of nonhair-bearing skin is probably about 50%, so that its inclusion in the dissection can have a substantial effect upon the outcome of the surgery. When multiple follicular units are used, and the skin is included, these effects are magnified.

The advantage of FUT over mini-micrografting and other grafting techniques is that in the former

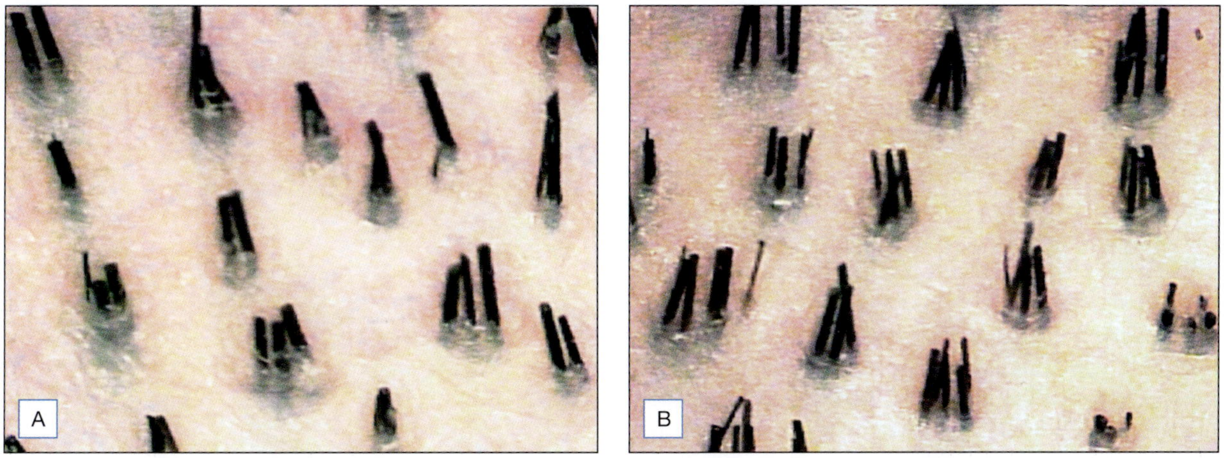


**Fig. 12.1** Densitometry showing discrete natural groups as the hair emerges from the scalp. These groups are the clinical correlate of the FU. (**A**) Slightly low donor hair density at 2.0 hairs per FU. (**B**) High donor hair density at 3.2 hairs/FU. Both patients have the same FU density of 1 FU/mm$^2$

procedure the excess skin between FUs is trimmed away rather than transplanted. Therefore, a two-hair FU will consist of two closely spaced follicles and a single sheath of circumferential connective tissue. In contrast, a two-hair micrograft comprised of two distinct one-hair FUs will contain both the circumferential sheaths of each unit and the connective tissue between them, significantly increasing the bulk of the graft and the subsequent wound that must accommodate it (Fig. 12.2). The same argument can be made for grafts containing three or more hairs that are not pure FUs.

A great benefit then, of using individual FUs, is that the wound size can be kept to a minimum, while the amount of hair that can be placed into it is maximized. Having the flexibility to place up to four hairs in a tiny recipient site has important implications for density, the design, and the overall cosmetic impact of the surgery.

The importance of minimizing the wound size cannot be overemphasized, particularly in larger hair transplant sessions or when grafts are densely packed. Larger wounds risk damage to the larger blood vessels in the scalp as well as disrupting the microcirculation. Poor recipient circulation increases the risk of postoperative infection, skin necrosis and poor or no hair growth. This is of particular concern when the blood supply to the scalp is already compromised from severe solar degeneration or chronic smoking, or if it is diminished from longstanding baldness.

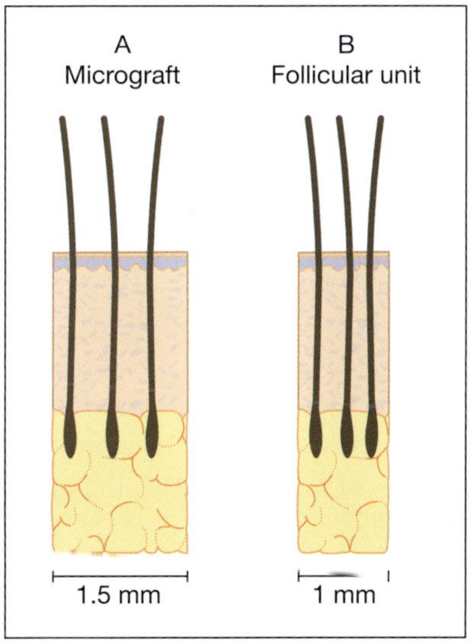


**Fig. 12.2** (**A**) A three-hair micrograft. (**B**) A three-hair FU. Note the much smaller volume of the follicular unit compared to the corresponding micrograft

The compact FU is of course, ideal, permitting the use of the smallest possible recipient wounds, and has made the transplantation of large numbers of grafts technically feasible. At times, however, when dense packing is taken to the extreme, such as when the goal is 50 or more grafts per cm$^2$ in one session, even four-hair naturally occurring FUs may be too large for the surgeon's needs. In this case, the largest FUs must be split in order to fit them into smaller sites. Although these authors prefer to make the recipient sites slightly larger to accommodate the larger grafts, some surgeons performing very large sessions of densely packed grafts prefer to split the units to keeps the sites uniformly small.

Another important advantage of the small wound is a factor that can be referred to as the 'snug fit.' Unlike a punch, which removes recipient connective tissue, a small incision, made with a needle or similar fine instrument, retains the basic elasticity of the recipient site wall. When a properly fitted graft is inserted, the recipient site will then hold it snugly in place. For example, two- to three-hair FUs will fit snugly into 20 or 21 gauge needle sites, while single-hair FUs will fit nicely into 21 or 22 gauge needle sites, or into sites made with 0.6–0.7 mm rectangular blades. This 'snug fit' has several advantages. During surgery, it minimizes popping, and the need for the potentially damaging re-insertion of grafts. After the procedure, it ensures maximum contact of the implant with the surrounding tissue, so that oxygenation can be quickly re-established. In addition, by eliminating dead space, there is less coagulum formed and wound healing is facilitated. The time it takes after a transplant for grafts to be securely fixed in place can be shortened by as much as 4 days if a coagulum is not allowed to form.

## Transplanting in Large Sessions

A main advantage of using FUs is that the small sites permit the transplantation of large numbers of grafts with minimal wounding. The advantage of transplanting in large sessions include: (1) social issues; (2) planning for surgical effluvium; (3) economizing the donor supply; and (4) flexibility in using different-sized FUs.

### Social issues

An obvious advantage of transplanting in large sessions is to achieve the patient's objectives as quickly as possible with as little interference with their lifestyle. For patients who have hair loss through Norwood Class VI, the transplantation of 2400 FU grafts will provide coverage, albeit thin, from the frontal hairline to the vertex transition point (Fig. 12.3). It will give the patient a natural look after one session and if distributed properly will allow one procedure to stand on its own. A second session can be used to add density, but should not be required for the procedure to look natural, a goal that should be accomplished in the first session.

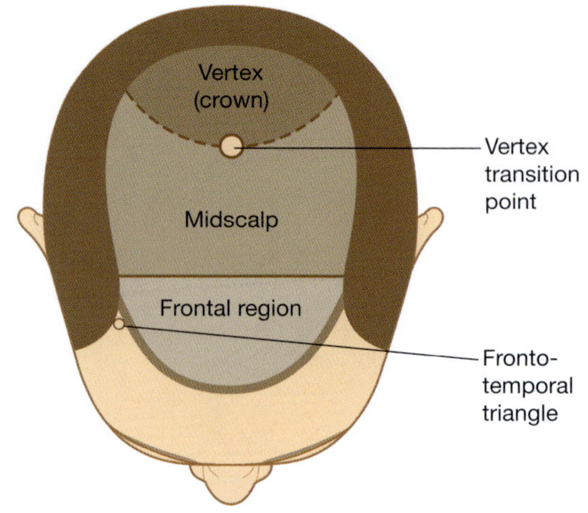


**Fig. 12.3** Regions of the scalp anterior to the vertex transition point

Some physicians advocate a 'one-pass' procedure to achieve the final density. It is felt by proponents of the one-pass session that graft growth is maximum in a virgin area and, therefore, as much density as possible should be achieved in the first session. It is these authors' opinion that if this approach leaves the patient with areas uncovered anterior to the vertex transition point, then it would be better to distribute the same number of grafts more broadly to produce a more natural distribution in the first session. It will also decrease the risks associated with very dense packing, namely graft popping and desiccation, insertion injury, and possible vascular compromise that may lead to poor growth. Poor growth associated with dense packing is of particular concern in longstanding baldness and in areas of significant solar damage, which alters the cutaneous vasculature.

### Surgical effluvium

Regardless of the technique, an inevitable aspect of hair transplant surgery is that the patient's existing hair in and around the transplanted area has a chance of being shed as a result of the procedure. The hair that is at greatest risk of being lost is the hair that has already begun the process of miniaturization and if this hair is near the end of its lifespan, it may not return.

Often this shedding is mild and insignificant, but at times it can leave the patient with a thinner look after the procedure. Identifying those patients especially at risk by assessing increased levels of miniaturization, educating all patients that this process can occur, and planning for effluvium surgically are important aspects of the hair transplantation process.

Performing large-transplant sessions are particularly useful if there are large areas of miniaturization that produce insufficient coverage and have not been responsive to finasteride and/or minoxidil. In these cases transplanting through (rather than around) an area that is highly miniaturized should be considered, since it is likely that this area will be lost by the time the transplant has grown in. An example would be to transplant through the 'bridge' of Norwood Class V patients who are beginning to show signs of thinning in that zone.

The surgeon should plan to use enough FUs so that, if possible, the volume of transplanted hair is greater than the volume of hair that will likely be lost from surgical effluvium. In areas of extensive miniaturization, it may be appropriate to transplant FUs in the same density as if the area was totally bald.

## Economizing Donor Supply

Regardless of how impeccable the surgical technique is, each time an incision is made in the donor area, and each time sutures are placed, hair follicles are damaged or destroyed. This damage can be minimized (but not eliminated), by keeping the sutures very close to the wound edges (so that they don't encompass much hair), removing them early, and using nontension closures.

In addition, the healing distorts the direction of the hair follicles and increases the risk of transection in subsequent procedures. In subsequent procedures the damage can be reduced by using the previous scar as the upper or lower border of the new excision. In this way the amount of distortion and possible damage to existing hair is limited to only one free edge.

Another problem is that the fibrosis from the healed linear scar makes the scalp less mobile for subsequent surgeries, thus decreasing the amount of additional donor tissue that can be harvested. Each time there is surgery these factors come into play, therefore transplanting in large sessions, which minimizes the total number of individual procedures, will conserve total donor hair.

FUE techniques would seem to circumvent these problems; however, they also cause fibrosis of the donor area, limiting the yield in future surgeries. The extent to which present FUE procedures limit future ones is not yet known, but considering that FUE relies on secondary intention healing, the effects are likely to be significant.

## Follicular Unit Sorting

In FUT the numbers of grafts present in any given size donor strip is determined by nature, since each graft represents one FU. It follows that if only the

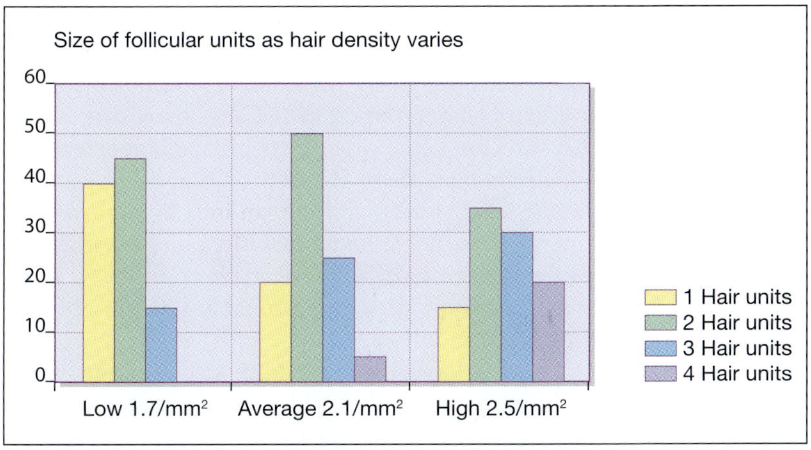


**Fig. 12.4** Distribution of FUs in the scalp in patients with low, average and high hair densities. This would correspond to the graft yield using stereomicroscopic dissection

naturally occurring individual units are to be used, practitioners are limited by their normal distribution in the scalp (Fig. 12.4). Using larger sessions, greater numbers of each type of unit will be generated, adding flexibility to the surgery. This will enhance the cosmetic outcome of the procedure when the surgeon seeks to create soft transition zones using single-hair units or when creating central density with three- and four-hair FU grafts.

## Clinical Characteristics of FUs

### FU constant

One of the interesting aspects of transplanting with FUs is that nature was kind to space them at approximately one per $mm^2$. This has been observed clinically using densitometry and stereomicroscopic dissection and histologically using transverse microscopic sections of the skin (this was first described by Headington in 1984). Not only does a FU constant of 1 unit/$mm^2$ make the math easy, but it makes accurately estimating the donor harvest possible, and gives a logical basis for planning the density and distribution of the grafts.

The constancy of FU density has been studied, but inconsistent study designs prevent accurate conclusions. There is general agreement on the following:

1. FU density generally decreases as work moves laterally from the mid-occiput at the level of the occipital protuberance towards the temples.
2. FU density varies among races such that the darker skinned races tend to have the lowest FU densities and light-skinned races the highest (Table 12.1).
3. Within the same race and same location on the scalp, there is significant person-to-person variation in FU density.
4. Given points 1–3 above, the constancy of the FU density is still rather striking so that patients with high hair density have more hairs per FU rather than FUs spaced closer together and those with low hair density for the most part have fewer hairs per FU rather than units spread further apart (Fig. 12.1).

Racial variations in hair and follicular unit densities

| Factor | Caucasians | Asians | Africans |
|---|---|---|---|
| FUs/$mm^2$ | 1.0 | 1.0 | 0.6 |
| Average density (hairs/$mm^2$) | 2.2 | 1.7 | 1.6 |
| Predominant hair grouping | 2 | 2 | 3 |

**Table 12.1** Racial variations in hair and follicular unit densities

Although the FU density is not exactly 1/$mm^2$, it is close enough to this number that it can be extremely useful in the surgery. Once it is realized that the FU density is relatively constant and that hair density varies, it follows that the number of hairs per follicular unit largely determines hair density. The implications of this in hair transplantation can be summarized as follows:

- Since the FU density is relatively constant, the same number of FUs should generally be used to cover a specific-sized bald area regardless of the hair density of the patient.
- With low hair density, using the same number and spacing of FUs as in a patient with high density will help to ensure that there is proper conservation of donor hair for the long term.
- Hair density is a characteristic of the FU specific to each individual, and together with hair shaft diameter, color and wave, will determine the cosmetic impact of the transplant.

### Hair characteristics

The results of a hair transplantation procedure are determined as much by the characteristics of the individual hairs as the number of hairs per FU. Since hair counts are easily measurable, the more subjective hair characteristics, or the ones more difficult to measure, are often discounted. Many characteristics including hair shaft diameter, hair color, texture (wave, curl, kink) and other factors such as the emergent angle of the hair, static, oiliness, or sheen, all contribute to the appearance of fullness, however, hair shaft diameter probably has the greatest impact.

The total volume of hair determines the visual impact. Doubling the hair density doubles the hair volume, while doubling the hair diameter quadruples the hair volume (remember $\pi r^2$). Hair density varies

| Relative significance of hair density and hair shaft diameter | | |
|---|---|---|
| **Characteristic** | **Range** | **Cosmetic impact of doubling** |
| Hair density | 1.5–3.0 hairs/$mm^2$ | 2× |
| Hair shaft diameter | 0.06–0.14 mm | 4× |

**Table 12.2** Relative significance of hair density and hair shaft diameter

from 1.5–3.0 hairs/$mm^2$, while hair shaft diameter varies from 0.06–0.14 mm. Therefore, hair shaft diameter plays a greater role than absolute hair numbers in determining overall cosmetic impact (Table 12.2).

## Conclusion

The introduction of FUT created a revolution in hair transplantation surgery, with doctors discarding their multi-bladed knives, buying stereomicroscopes, and training their staff in the dissection of individual FUs. However, the belief that in order to get the best results, only naturally occurring individual FUs should be transplanted has not been universally accepted.

With the new harvesting method of extracting FUs directly from the donor area, new technical issues are challenging the wisdom of always keeping FUs intact. In particular, if the object is to minimize the number of recipient wounds when performing FUE, it may be best to split larger units into single hairs to create a soft hairline rather than making separate punch holes to harvest each one-hair graft. This and other technical issues of FUE, where only partial units are removed, require fresh thinking about what should constitute FU transplantation.

## Editors' Note

This chapter succinctly outlines the importance of the FUs. Many of the concerns raised in this chapter over the use of magnification and transplanting only intact FUs pertain to the Caucasian population. Transplant surgeons who operate primarily on Asians and those of middle-eastern descent have not found the requirement for stereomicroscopic magnification absolute. These surgeons have also routinely divided FUs in order to achieve more single-hair grafts in the frontal hairline.

### Further Reading


Bernstein RM, Rassman WR 1997 Follicular transplantation: Patient evaluation and surgical planning. Dermatologic Surgery 23:771–784

Bernstein RM, Rassman WR 1997 The aesthetics of follicular transplantation. Dermatologic Surgery 23:785–799

Bernstein RM, Rassman WR 1999 The logic of follicular unit transplantation. Dermatologic Clinics 17:277–295

Bernstein RM, Rassman WR, Seager D, et al 1998 Standardizing the classification and description of follicular unit transplantation and mini-micrografting techniques. Dermatologic Surgery 24:957–963

Bernstein RM, Rassman WR, Szaniawski W, Halperin A 1995 Follicular transplantation. International Journal of Aesthetic and Restorative Surgery 3:119–132

Limmer BL 1994 Elliptical donor stereoscopically assisted micrografting as an approach to further refinement in hair transplantation. Dermatologic Surgery 20:789–793

Rassman WR, Bernstein RM, McClellan R, Jones R, et al 2002 Follicular unit extraction: Minimally invasive surgery for hair transplantation. Dermatologic Surgery 28:720–727

# 13 Follicular Unit Instrumentation

*William M. Parsley*

## Introduction

As described by Headington in 1984, scalp hair grows in bundles of 1–4 or more individual follicles called follicular units (FUs). By definition, follicular unit grafting (FUG) implies that donor FUs are harvested as they naturally occur, discarding the surrounding hairless skin. The small size of these FUs demands meticulous technique along with the use of good magnification and illumination. A reasonably accurate assessment of the number of grafts needed and the required donor size should be made before harvesting the donor strip. In this chapter, a summary will be given as to the most commonly utilized instruments to accomplish these goals (Box 13.1).

## Calculations to Determine Donor Needs

### Recipient site measurement

A rough estimate must be made of the recipient area and required planting density before starting. Usually the borders of the recipient site are irregular, creating some difficulty in determining the size. Steven Chang developed a useful technique – he recommends placing polyurethane wrap (i.e. Saran wrap) in an **embroidering hoop**, laying it over the recipient site, and tracing the outline of the recipient site. A dry erase pen is helpful. The wrap is then placed over grid paper with 1 $cm^2$ boxes. Counting only the intersections of the boxes within the tracing will relatively accurately give the number of square centimeters in the designed recipient zone – a math principle called 'morphometry.' Using morphometry, the formula for calculating the area inside an asymmetrical field is:

$$A = n \times a$$

where A is the area to be measured, n is the number of intersections within the area to be measured and a is the area of one grid box. Therefore, multiplying the number of intersections by the desired number of grafts/$cm^2$ will give the number of grafts needed to complete the procedure (Fig. 13.1A–D).

**Generally accepted standards for FUG**

- Donor removal
  - Single blade (single strip)
- Graft preparation
  - Stereomicroscopes
  - Preserve natural FUs
  - Discard interfollicular hairless skin
- Recipient sites
  - Incisions (not punches)

**Box 13.1** Generally accepted standards for FUG

### Donor site measurement

Now that the desired number of grafts has been determined, it is necessary to establish the size of the donor strip needed to produce that number of grafts. Donor density should be measured by a device with high magnification and high-quality optics. Hand-held illuminated magnifiers are the most popular, but digital imaging devices may also be used. A small field of view makes counting FUs easier, but requires calculation to convert this measurement into a standard density (FUs/$cm^2$). The Rassman Densitometer was an early device used, but it suffered from poor optics and quality control. The 10× Trichoscope (Welch Allyn) is a relatively accurate instrument, which consists of a standard Episcope head with an accessory plate.

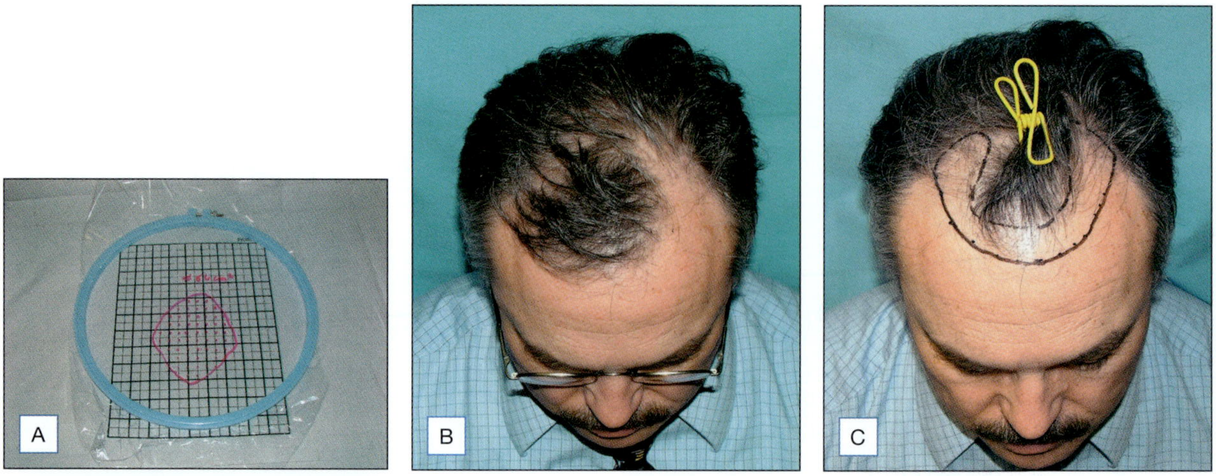

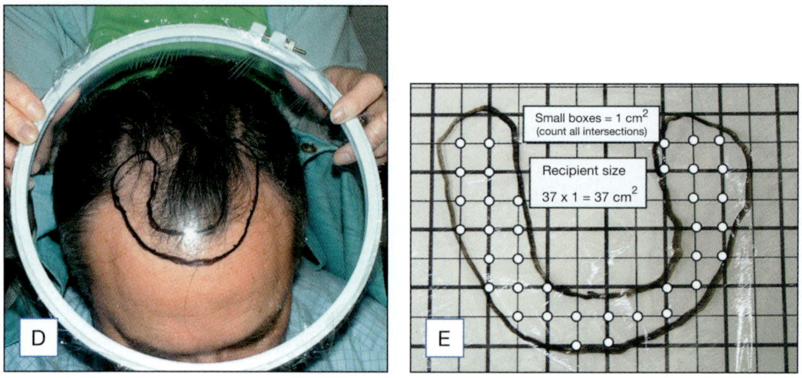


**Fig. 13.1** Chang measuring hoop (**A**). Saran wrap in an embroidery hoop allows the donor area to be traced. The tracing is then placed over a grid to allow measurement of the recipient area. (**B**) Patient before measurement. (**C**) Recipient site traced. (**D**) Recipient site traced onto clear plastic sheet. (**E**) Count intersections in the grid using the principle of 'morphometrics;' the number of intersections × the area of the grid squares will closely approximate the area inside the tracing

This plate comes with either a 4 mm circular or a 5 mm square cutout (special order). The 4 mm circle provides a measuring area of 12.5 mm$^2$, so the counted FUs in this area must be multiplied by 8 to obtain the FUs/cm$^2$. The 5 mm square provides a measuring field of 0.25 cm$^2$, so the counted FUs in this area must be multiplied by 4 to obtain the FUs/cm$^2$. Another method is to make a 5 mm square (0.25 cm$^2$) cutout in a plastic sheet and use loupes to count the FUs within the area, multiplying by 4 to get the FUs/cm$^2$. Fields larger than 0.25 cm$^2$ become difficult to count.

To determine the size of the strip (in cm$^2$) required, the desired number of FUs needs to be divided by the average FUs/cm$^2$ in the donor area, taking several measurements along the strip (Figs 13.2 and Box 13.2).

Another useful tool for assessing donor density is the macro video camera, which projects a clear macro image onto a computer screen. Plastic sheet cutouts or an accessory computer grid can be used

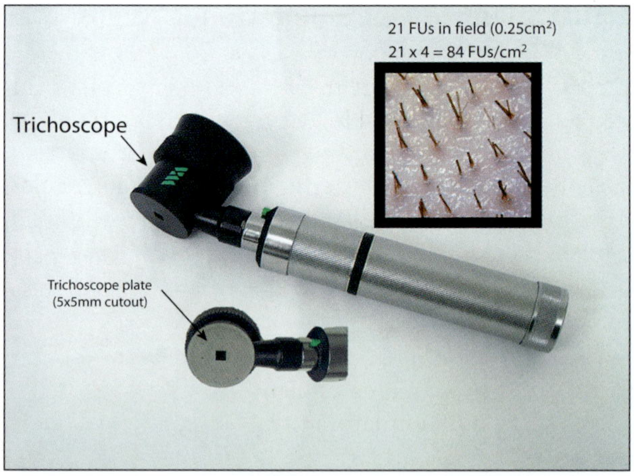


**Fig. 13.2** Trichoscope. The trichoscope (an Episcope with a measuring plate, Welch Allyn, Inc.) is a reasonably accurate instrument for calculating donor FU density. The 5 × 5 mm cutout creates an area of 0.25 cm$^2$. Counting only the visible FU bases, the count in the above example is 21 FUs. Multiplying × 4 gives a count of 84 FUs/cm$^2$. An average of several measurements along the donor strip are needed

**Recipient and Donor Site Calculations**

1. **Determine donor FU density**
   Donor density in FU/cm$^2$ = (FU's in field) × 4
   (with Trichoscope, 0.25cm$^2$ field)
2. **Determine number of FU grafts needed**
   FU's needed = (Recipient size in cm$^2$) × (Desired density in FU/cm$^2$)
3. **Determine size of donor strip needed**
   Strip area (cm$^2$) = (FU's needed) / Donor density (FU/cm$^2$)

**Example:**
Assume the following:
Average donor density = 84 FU/cm$^2$
Donor recipient size = 37 cm$^2$
Desired recipient density = 25 FU/cm$^2$
**Number of grafts needed: 37 × 25 = 925**
**Donor strip needed: 925 / 84 = 11cm$^2$**

**Box 13.2** Recipient and donor site calculations. The recipient needs and the donor size required must be calculated before beginning the procedure.

for density counts. Popular models are the Micro-VID (*http://micro-vid.com*) and Capillicare (*http://www.hansenfontana.com/capillicare.html*).

At present there is no practical method by which the practicing physician can measure hair loss, hair growth, or simply determine how much hair a patient has. The problem has been addressed by Dr Bernard Cohen, who has developed a new device that measures the cross-sectional area of hair growing within a circumscribed area of scalp.

Dr Jim Arnold originated this methodology several years ago by isolating a bundle of hair from a circumscribed area, but measured its circumference with a small thread. He called its value the 'hair mass index'. Cohen suggests that the term 'hair mass' would also reflect the hair's length and has suggested the term density-diameter index (DDI) as a more precise definition. Both methods simultaneously measure the density of surface hairs and their collective diameters.

Evaluations are performed in a simple office setting. A 2 × 2 cm area of the scalp is defined using a skin-marking template and the uncut hair within the area is isolated from the surrounding hair. The bundle is captured in a caliper-like device and compressed with a standardized load. Its cross-sectional area (mm$^2$) is displayed on an LED screen.

If hairs are shed, new hairs emerge, hair diameters increase, or hair diameters decrease, the value of the DDI will increase or decrease accordingly. To quantify hair loss and/or growth, the same 2 × 2 cm area is measured and then re-measured at a later date. To calculate the percent hair loss of a balding area, the DDI of that area would be simply divided by the DDI of a normal area, i.e. the permanent horseshoe-shaped fringe.

The device may be used to identify when stabilization occurs and recovery begins in patients with telogen effluvium. It may also be used to measure the effectiveness of hair growth drugs and devices.

## Strip Removal

### Single blade vs. double blade

Even though a few surgeons remove the donor strip with a two-bladed scalpel, the gold standard for FUG is a single blade, most often with a No. 10 Personna blade due to its sharpness. The goal in strip harvesting is to use the least amount of cutting necessary to get the donor tissue to the stereomicroscopes, where transection rates are very low. Owing to the curvature of the scalp, more transection will occur with a multi-bladed knife because it can't be adjusted for differences in hair angle between the top and the bottom of the strip. Skin hooks to expose the wall of the strip are useful during the excision.

An innovative technique for strip removal was developed by Arturo Sandoval, MD, in which the strip margins are superficially scored with a #10 blade to a depth of 1.5-2.0 mm. The strip walls are then separated by blunt dissection with a curved hemostat. Robert Haber, MD has developed an ergonomic instrument for a more efficient blunt dissection (Fig. 13.3). It consists of 4 staggered aligned sharp prongs, 2 on each end of arms that can be spread apart by gripping the opposite arms of the instrument rather than by pulling the arms apart (as with a hemostat).

### Strip removal

Once the walls of the strip have been cut with the scalpel, the strip must be removed from its subcutaneous attachments. While many use the scalpel for this process, **undermining scissors** are less likely to sever the deeper vessels and nerves, and is this author's instrument of choice. If a scalpel blade is used for removal, it should be done with a pushing (not slicing) motion while lifting the strip.

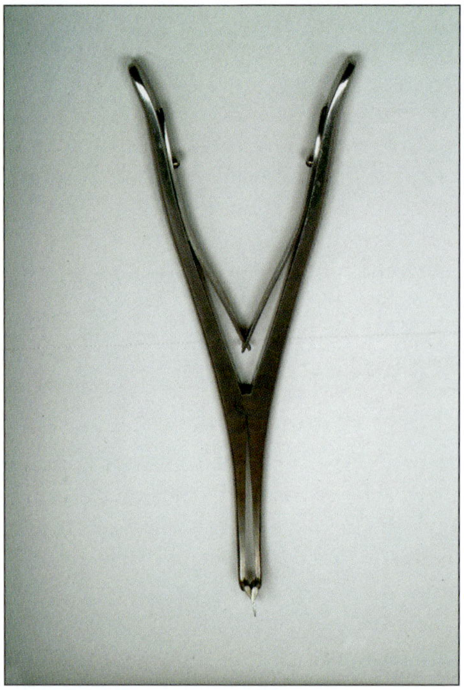

**Fig. 13.3** Ergonomic device designed to permit low transection rates during donor dissection

## Recipient Sites

There are many types of instruments used to create graft sites for FU grafting. The two main groups are needles and flat blades. Site size is important. Most experienced hair surgeons will rarely make sites larger than 1.4 mm in length for FUG (Table 13.1) Round punches and slot punches are generally not part of FUG.

The cutting surface of the needle or blade can be oriented so that the incision is made perpendicular to the intended direction of hair growth. This type grafting is called lateral, perpendicular or coronal-angled grafting (CAG). The cutting surface can also be oriented so that the incision is made parallel to the intended direction of hair growth. This type of grafting is called parallel or sagittal-angled grafting (SAG). Chiseled blades are better for perpendicular grafts, while angled blades are better for parallel grafts. Needles and spearpoints are used for both (see Chapter 15.)

## Needles

Needles have the advantage over flat blades in that they are easily accessible, inexpensive, easy to hold, and are color coordinated to help avoid mistakes in size (Fig. 13.4A and B). In addition, they give a brief but helpful dilatation, which is particularly useful in stick-and-place techniques, where each graft is placed immediately after making the incision. Sharpness and burrs can be a problem. Needles are popular for both perpendicular grafting with the bevel up or down, as well as parallel grafting with the bevel on edge.

| Diameter (length) of various needles and blades | | |
|---|---|---|
| **Needles** | **Spearpoint** | **Chisel blades** |
| 16 g–1.60 mm | SP88–1.00 mm | SM61–1.5 mm |
| 17 g–1.44 mm | SP89–1.25 mm | |
| 18 g–1.26 mm | SP90–1.5 mm | Sharpoint |
| 19 g–1.09 mm | SP91–2.0 mm | 15°–1.59 mm |
| 20 g–0.90 mm | | 22°–1.69 mm |
| 21 g–0.82 mm | NoKor needles | 30°–1.90 mm |
| 22 g–0.73 mm | 16g–2.30 mm | |
| 23 g–0.65 mm | 18g–1.79 mm | Minde |
| 25 g–0.51 mm | | Blue: 1.3 mm |
| | Cutting Edge | Black: 1.5 mm |
| | any size: custom | Green: 1.8 mm |
| | | Beige: 2.0 mm |

**Table 13.1** Diameter (length) of various needles and blades

### Hypodermic needles: regular, bent

Standard hypodermic needles used for hair transplantation are generally 18–22 g, all of which are color coded to the diameter. Their primary use in general medicine is to deliver medicine or draw fluids, so there is a central canal (core). Some planters turn the bevel up to aid in planting the grafts. Dr Mario Marzola developed a variation by bending the needles into a 'shoehorn' shape to allow easier insertion and to aid depth control.

### Solid wire needles

As their name implies, there is no central core; thus they are solid. Also known as solid core needles, they either come with universally color-coded plastic handles (17–20 g) or with no attached handle (16–22 g), requiring a holder. The color coding is identical to that of hypodermic needles. They have the advantage of not picking up debris in a central core and being safer in case of an accidental needle stick. Consistent sharpness and burrs have been problems.

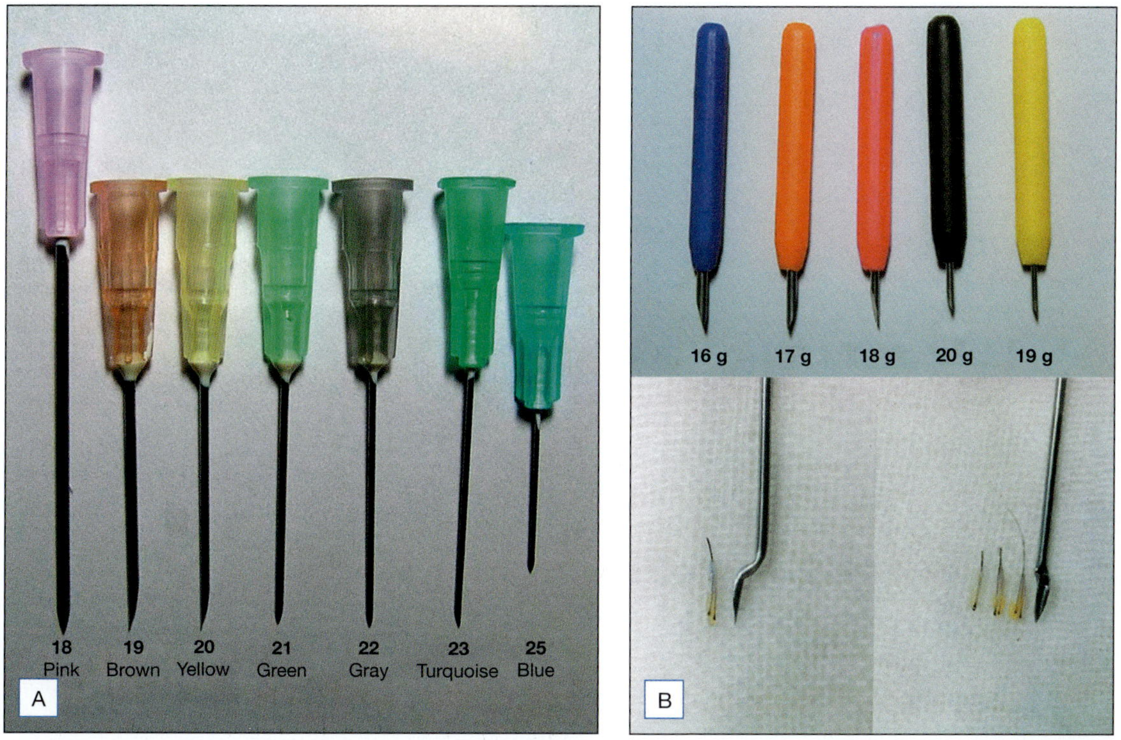


**Fig. 13.4** Needles. (**A**) Hypodermic needles. Hypodermic needles come in a number of sizes (gauges) and are universally color coded. (**B**) Solid wire needles and Shoehorn Modification of hypodermic needles. Solid wire needles, also color coded, are convenient and more durable than hypodermic needles, and reduce blood exposure in case of an accidental stick. Additionally, there is less debris transfer. Sharpness and burrs can be a problem. The Shoehorn Modification allows depth control and greater ease of insertion. The bending must be done by the office staff. (Picture courtesy of Dr Mario Marzola)

## Flat blades

Flat blades tend to be sharper than needles and cause less popping of grafts. Most brands offer multiple sizes (Fig. 13.5). The important measure is the length of the blade edge, which determines the recipient incision size, as the width is normally minimal. Potential disadvantages are that most require a separate holder and that they provide little or no dilatation.

## Chiseled (rectangular) blades

Chiseled blades are primarily used in perpendicular (coronal) grafting. If rotated for parallel (sagittal) grafting, the lower edge may go too deep and create damage to the deeper vessels. They can be purchased from several different companies or can be created by cutting single- or double-edged surgical razor blades (Fig. 13.6A and B).

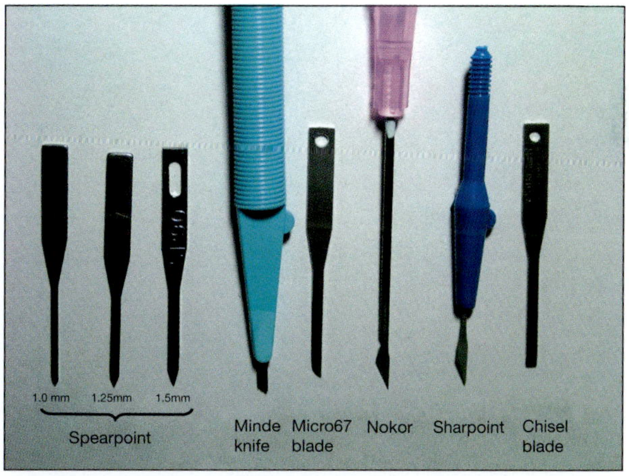


**Fig. 13.5** Flat blades. The basic shapes of flat blades are Spearpoint (two cutting surfaces), angled, scalpel shaped, and chiseled (rectangular)

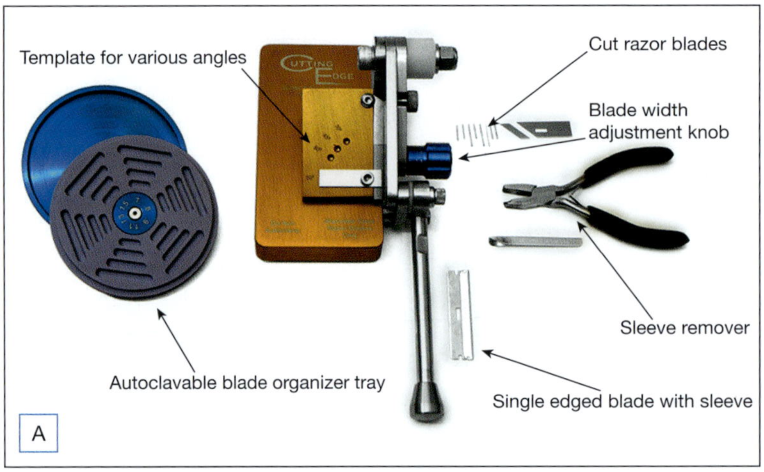


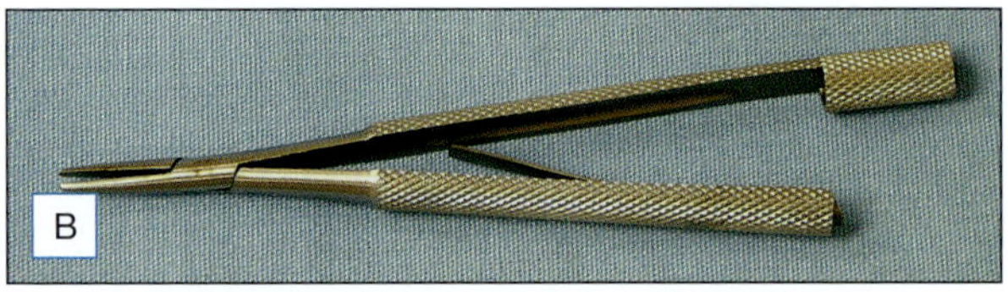


**Fig. 13.6** Custom cutting tool and blade holder. (**A**) Blade cutting tool (www.CuttingEdge-Surgical.ca). This is a convenient tool for making personalized recipient blades from either Personna single-edged razor blades or from Personna double-edged razor blades. Angles of 30, 45, 60 and 90 degrees (chisel) can be created. A separately purchased blade holder or a fine needle holder can be used to hold the blades and control depth. (Courtesy of Cutting Edge Ltd.) (**B**) Blade holder (Ellis Instruments- No. 145-042E). A blade holder should hold the blade firmly, have good ergonomics, allow depth control and allow for quick blade change. The above holder works well in all categories

### Angled (SharpPoint, Minde, cut razor blades)

Angled blades are best for use in parallel (sagittal) grafting. They are generally angled to 15–45 degrees and cut through the skin with minimal resistance, thus causing very little popping of grafts. Generally the angled edge is sharp but the side in line with the shaft is dull to prevent inadvertent extension of the cut through the skin. To minimize the depth of the incision, the cutting surface should be flush or nearly flush with the skin. Sharpoint blades give very little resistance as do Minde ('**Min**imal **de**pth') blades, which are useful for depth control. Minde blades have the advantage of a generous range of sizes and angles, and they are color coded to size. Angled blades can also be created with a blade-cutting device.

### Spearpoint

The spearpoint has two angled edges, coming together to make a point, and both lateral edges are sharp. Having a sharp tip, they give little resistance on incision. These blades can be used reasonably well for both perpendicular and parallel grafting.

## Other Considerations

### Minimal depth

Efforts to cause minimal damage to the vasculature are important. Most doctors feel that the recipient incisions should be through the dermis but not reach the supragaleal plexus. A good technique is to use the provided blade holder or a needle holder clamped onto the blade in order to limit the depth to the length of one of the patient's grafts. A useful technique is to lay a graft containing terminal hairs on the end of the blade to determine the proper depth of the incision. Recipient tumescence also helps by providing separation of the subdermal plexus from the supragaleal plexus.

### Sharpness

The sharper the cutting instrument the less transection of existing hairs, popping of grafts and irregularity of the wound. The sharper the better.

### Multibladed devices

Several devices are available for holding up to six or more flat blades to speed up making recipient incisions. These should be used on totally or near-totally bald recipient areas to avoid damage to existing recipient hair.

## Graft Preparation

### Visualization tools

Owing to their small size, magnification and illumination are necessary in order to prepare FUs. The gold standard for FUG is stereomicroscopes, and many do not consider it true follicular unit transplanting without their use. However, other methods such as magnifiers and digital camera magnification have been utilized, and they are certainly superior to the naked eye. The strip is first cut into segments along the strip (blocking). These segments are then cut like a bread loaf into slivers 1–2 FUs wide (slivering). Finally the slivers are dissected into the individual FUs, and are ready for planting.

### Magnifiers and loupes

Magnifiers consist of a magnification plate mounted on a desk stand, headband or eyeglass frame. The general magnification range used is 1.5–4×, but is short of the ideal range of 6× or above. With the long hours of FU preparation that is often required, the headband and the need to flex the neck can become quite uncomfortable. Illumination must be furnished separately. Binocular loupes are available but due to expense their use is generally limited to planting grafts.

### Digital camera with screen

A relatively new innovation is the use of a digital camera above the specimen to magnify and project it onto an LCD screen. The magnification is adequate but the images are only two dimensional, as opposed to the three-dimensional images of magnifiers, loupes and stereomicroscopes. For this reason, the devices are better for dissecting slivers (which are very thin) into FU grafts than for blocking and slivering the thicker donor strip. Advantages are the 0-degree viewing angle and the ability to visually assess the assistant's performance.

### Stereomicroscopes

Stereomicroscopes are the gold standard for FU graft preparation (Fig. 13.7). Their optics, magnification range and illumination are unsurpassed by other methods. They are actually a combination of two compound microscopes coming into the specimen at roughly a 10-degree angle, allowing stereomicroscopic vision. As opposed to microscopes, stereomicroscopes have erecting prisms to prevent image reversal. Top brands to consider are Meiji, Nikon, Motic, Zeiss and Mantis.

A number of options are available when purchasing a stereomicroscope. The most important considerations are as follows.

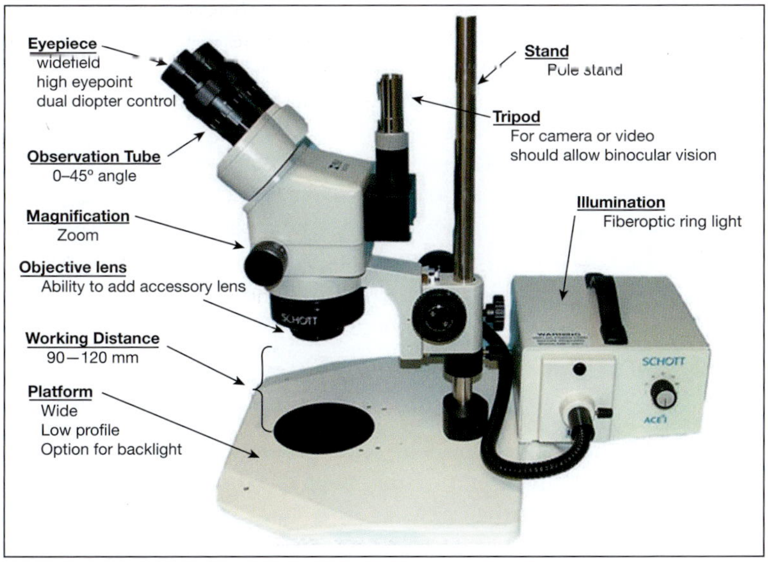


**Fig. 13.7** Stereomicroscope – desirable features. Listed are worthwhile features to look for when purchasing a stereomicroscope. This scope is a Meiji EMZ-8TR on a Diagnostic Instruments TLB1000 pole stand with a fiberoptic ring light

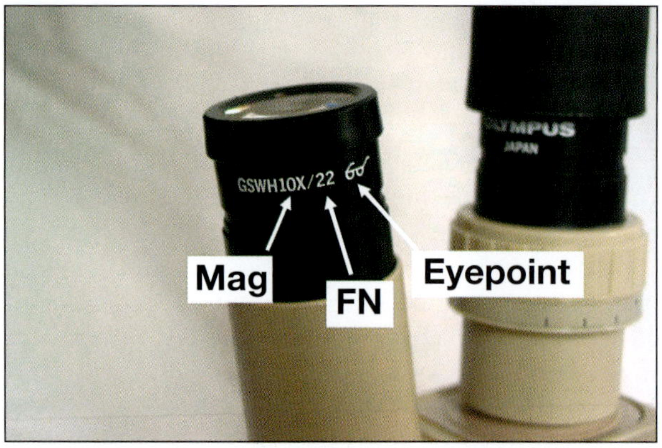


**Fig. 13.8** Stereomicroscope eyepiece. Two desirable qualities of the eyepiece are 'widefield,' represented by a FN of 22 or greater, and 'high eyepoint,' usually represented by a diagram of spectacles. Magnification is normally 10×, but Meiji makes a 12.5× extremely widefield eyepiece, which is popular

## Eyepiece and observation tube

There are five important characteristics of an eyepiece: (1) field number (FN); (2) eyepoint; (3) magnification; (4) diopter control; and (5) tube angle (Fig. 13.8). The FN represents the width in millimeters of a diaphragm directly below the lens – the more millimeters, the bigger the field of vision. It is important to get a **widefield eyepiece** with a FN of 22 or higher; this gives a wider field of view and is much more comfortable for long hours of use. The eyepiece should also be **high eyepoint**, meaning the focal point of the eyepiece is at roughly 20 mm or more above the lens, allowing eyeglass wearers and assistants with long eyelashes to use the scope in comfort. High eyepoint is usually indicated with a diagram of 'spectacles' on the side of the eyepiece. Recommended eyepiece magnification is 10× or 12.5× (the Meiji 12.5× eyepiece has a greater FN for roughly the same price as the 10×). **Diopter control** allows adjustment for the diopter difference between the assistant's eyes; dual-diopter controls are best. **Observation tube angles** are normally either 45 degrees or 60 degrees to the horizon. The lower the better, but 20-degree tube angles and adjustable heads are expensive. Fortunately, 45-degree observation tubes generally work very well.

## Stereomicroscope Magnification

Total magnification is determined by multiplying the magnifications of the eyepiece, intermediate lens and objective/accessory lens. Magnification adjustments are generally made with the intermediate lenses (zoom, turret, and fixed), with most assistants using 6–10× magnification. The best method of magnifiation adjustment is with zoom magnification, allowing seamless magnification adjustments throughout the zoom range, usually 6–40×. Other methods are turret style (click stop with 2–5 magnification levels but no intermediate magnification), and fixed (no magnification adjustment). The objective lens is the lowest standard lens and is the first lens to gather light from the specimen. It is usually 1×, thus not influencing the magnification. It is highly advisable to have an objective lens that allows attachment of an accessory lens to its lower edge. Addition of an accessory lens below the objective lens allows a change of the working distance (WD) (distance between the specimen and the objective/accessory lens, which measures the room for the assistant's hands). While accessory lenses change the overall magnification, their primary use is to alter the WD (WD ÷ accessory lens magnification = new WD). A 0.5× accessory lens, for example, will double the WD.

## Stands and Platforms

Plain stands are those in which the platform and the body of the scope are a unified piece, not allowing rotation of the upper body. Pole stands hold the microscope body and attach to the platform, but allow rotation (a minor advantage). Some pole stands have platforms that are wide and heavy enough to permit the body of the scope to be rotated, allowing assistants to work directly on the counter top. The platform holds the donor tissue that the assistants are dissecting into FUs. A low, wide platform with a sloping edge is better ergonomically for the hands and wrists. The platform should be less than 2 cm in height. An excellent pole stand is the Diagnostic Instruments TBL1000 Stereo Stand, which can accommodate many brands, including Meiji.

## Illumination

All methods of graft preparation require good illumination. The doctor must consider expense, comfort and visual quality when deciding on the type and source.

### Overhead vs. backlighting

Light coming from above the specimen is said to be **episcopic** or **reflected**. This is the most popular type of illumination and can be used for any phase of graft preparation. Backlighting (from underneath the specimen) is called diascopic or transmitted. Diascopic light is best utilized in dealing with thin tissue, as the light must be able to pass through the specimen. This is most advantageous during creation of FUs from slivers. Some feel diascopic lighting helps visualize gray hair.

## Light Sources

### Overheard lighting (episcopic, reflected)

The primary light sources for stereomicroscopes are fiberoptic ring lighting, fluorescent ring lighting, LED ring lighting and incandescent incidental lighting (Fig. 13.9). Fiberoptic lighting is the best and coolest of this group, also allowing the best intensity range. Fluorescent and LED lighting is relatively cool but lacks intensity. While they come with intensity adjustments (dimming only), they are normally not needed as maximum intensity will usually be used.

For cutting without stereomicroscopes, fiberoptic dual-arm lights are best. Standard fluorescent lighting or incandescent lighting can be also be used.

### Backlighting (diascopic, transmitted)

The best lighting is a fiberoptic box light, which comes in different sizes. Not only is it cool but intensity can be varied. A popular and inexpensive light is a photoslide-sorting box (or viewing box). It is thin and relatively cool, but intensity might be a problem (Fig. 13.10).

## Other Considerations

### Mantis scope

The Mantis scope is a stereo-optical viewer with no eyepiece. Even though the optics are mediocre and there is a limitation to two fixed magnifications (choice of 2, 4, 6, 8, or 10×), it has a big advantage with a 0-degree viewing angle and has gained considerable popularity. It is more expensive than most scopes.

### Teaching scope

The most important scope in any office is a teaching scope with dual stereoscopic viewing. The scope can be used for blocking, slivering and final FU preparation, but more importantly is an invaluable tool for training new assistants and monitoring quality. Most have the ability to add a video output to a VCR, computer or TV screen. The Motic DSM500 Dual Viewing teaching scope is a reasonably priced choice (Fig. 13.11).

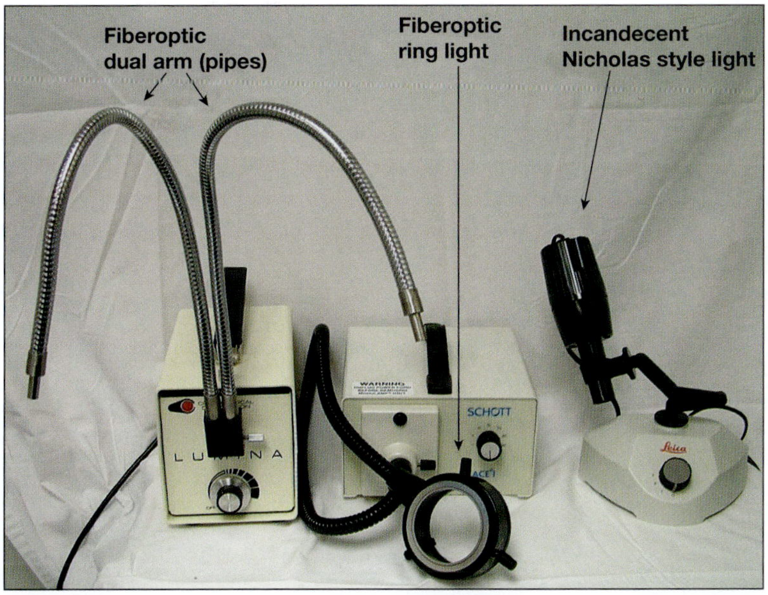


**Fig. 13.9** Episcopic (overhead, reflected) light sources. Fiberoptic is not only the coolest light source but also has the greatest intensity variation

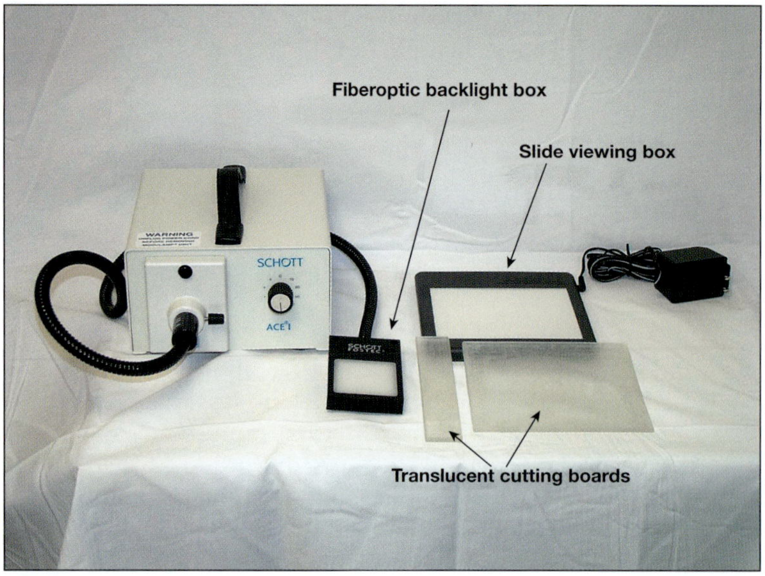


**Fig. 13.10** Diascopic (backlight, transmitted) light sources. Fiberoptic is again the coolest, but great intensity variation may not be necessary. The slide-viewing box is relatively cool and has a very low profile; however, the intensity is fixed. Translucent cutting surfaces are needed

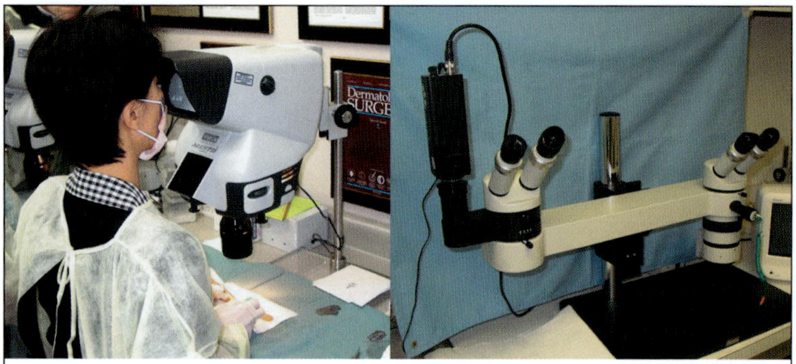


**Fig. 13.11** Mantis and teaching scope. The Mantis scope, despite other shortcomings, has an advantage over other reasonably priced stereomicroscopes with its 0-degree (horizontal) viewing angle, a feature which can reduce neck strain. A teaching scope, right, is an extremely valuable addition to the office for quality control and teaching new assistants

### Cutting board

The cutting board is the surface on which the donor tissue is placed and dissected into grafts. Saline-soaked sterile tongue blades (better traction), saline-soaked gauze without a board, scarified plastic sheets (best for backlighting), and soft silicon pads are all popular cutting surfaces. The choice is based mainly on personal preference.

If overhead lighting is used, any board can work, but if backlighting is used, a translucent board is needed. With overhead lighting, saline-soaked sterile tongue blades have the advantage of giving excellent countertraction during tissue dissection and of being relatively soft and not dulling the blades significantly. With backlighting, silicon pads or plastic scarified (for traction) sheets can be laid over the light source. Problems with counter traction still can be a problem when compared to tongue blades and gauze.

### Cutting instruments

Nontoothed or very fine-toothed forceps are needed to hold the grafts while cutting the tissue; straight and angled forceps are equally popular (Fig. 13.12). To dissect the tissue, No. 10 scalpel blades or sterile razor blades are used. Razor blades can be single edged (no holder required) or double edged (needs a disposable plastic holder) (Fig. 13.13).

## Graft Placement

### Forceps

Grafts are generally placed with fine forceps. They can be nontoothed or fine toothed; nontoothed are the most popular. Teeth, unless very fine, can drag a graft back out of its site after being placed. Forceps can also be straight, curved or angled. If the assistant is pushing the grafts into the site from in front of the

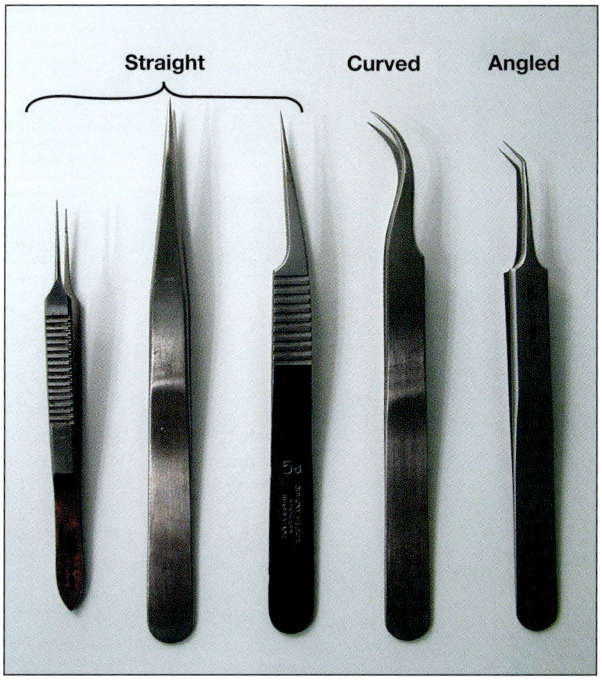


**Fig. 13.12** Planting and graft preparation forceps. A variety of forceps is currently used for planting and graft preparation. Common qualities are fine tips and no (or very fine) teeth

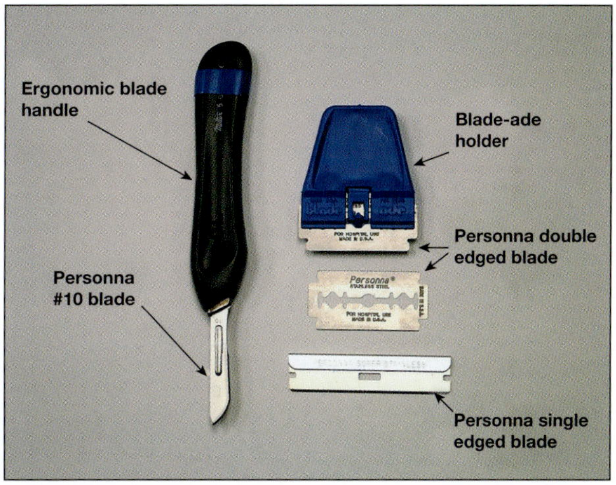


**Fig. 13.13** Graft cutting blades. Extremely sharp cutting blades are a must. The blades must be changed frequently

patient, straight forceps may be favored. If the assistant is behind the patient and pulling the graft into place, 45-degree angled fine-tipped or curved forceps may be best. Personal preference is very prominent in this selection as there seems to be no firm rule. The assistant is encouraged to try them all in order to pick a favorite.

## Miscellaneous Aids

When placing into lateral (coronal) sites, a very fine **skin hook** (Marina Medical No. 190-179) can be helpful. It is used to lift the acute edge, aid graft placement, and also stabilize the skin, reducing popping. Some doctors will dull the tip of a 30 gauge needle, then bend the tip into a hook and place it onto a tuberculin syringe for this purpose. Also, there are **reservoirs** that hook onto a planter's finger for holding grafts to save time in retrieving grafts.

## Magnification

Magnifiers and binocular loupes with fiberoptic illumination are very useful in making recipient sites and also in placing the grafts, particularly in finding the recipient incisions.

## Conclusion

FUG deals with very small units of hair and tissue. Magnification, illumination, fine instruments and sharp blades are critical to a successful outcome. The length of the surgery demands attention to ergonomics and general comfort. The use of less than optimal equipment can lead to eye strain, repetitive motion injuries, and fatigue. The instruments listed earlier have been used successfully in offices over the past 10 years and are highly recommended.

## Further Reading

Keene SA 2003 New cost-effective ergonomic way to magnify donor hair during follicular unit graft dissection: LCD monitor with video magnification. Hair Transplant Forum International 13:470

Nikon Microscopy University. http://www.microscopyu.com/articles/stereomicroscopy/

Parsley WM 2004 Stereomicroscopes for hair transplantation. Hair Transplant Forum International 14:105–106

Unger WP, Shapiro R. Hair Transplantation. 4th edn. Marcel Dekker, New York, p 835–886

# 14 Achieving Optimal Growth

*Jerry E. Cooley*

## Introduction

Achieving optimal growth in hair transplantation is a critical part of obtaining excellent results and high patient satisfaction. Many experienced surgeons quietly acknowledge amongst themselves that graft survival is not consistently as high as is publicly stated, partly because of the natural tendency to avoid publicly admitting to suboptimal results. Furthermore, in the era of follicular unit transplantation (FUT) in which a typical case is 1500 grafts and often more, it can be very difficult to accurately establish the percentage of grafts that survive. Nevertheless, all surgeons should be aware of the factors related to graft survival and develop their surgical technique accordingly.

This chapter will provide a brief overview on the factors related to graft survival. Relatively little is available in the way of valid, controlled scientific studies but important principles can be identified based on existing studies, as well as case reports and the opinions of experienced surgeons. The most important factors determining graft survival are avoiding physical trauma to the grafts (transection, crushing, dehydration) and ensuring the integrity of the recipient area vascular bed. There are other factors that may be important as well (Box 14.1).

## Physical Trauma

### Transection

Hair follicles that are physically intact have a much higher chance of survival than transected ones. This is a major rationale for microscopically controlled FUT, first described by Limmer. By using a single scalpel blade for donor excision, transection is minimized along the wound edge. The strip is then slivered and dissected using stereomicroscopes, where 10× magnification provides for superior visualization of the follicle (Fig. 14.1). A study carried out by the author involving multiple experienced surgeons showed that those who used microscopes had half as many transected hair follicles in random samples of grafts than those who did not use microscopes.

Without the use of microscopes, follicular transection is very likely to occur to varying degrees in all cases (Fig. 14.2). Some have claimed that this is not that important because transected follicles 'sometimes grow anyway.' The probability of follicle regeneration is directly related to the level of transection. If less than half of the follicle is present, regeneration rarely occurs. The author believes that follicle regeneration is an unpredictable process and that the best way to ensure good growth is to transplant physically intact follicles. In the author's practice, the change to follicular unit grafting

**Overview of factors related to graft survival**

Physical trauma
- Transection
- Dehydration
- Crushing
- Vascular factors

Pre-operative factors
- Prior surgery/scarring
- Actinic damage
- Tobacco usage

Operative factors
- Incision size
- Incision depth
- Incision density
- Biochemical factors
- Storage injury
- Ischemia-reperfusion injury

**Box 14.1** Overview of factors related to graft survival

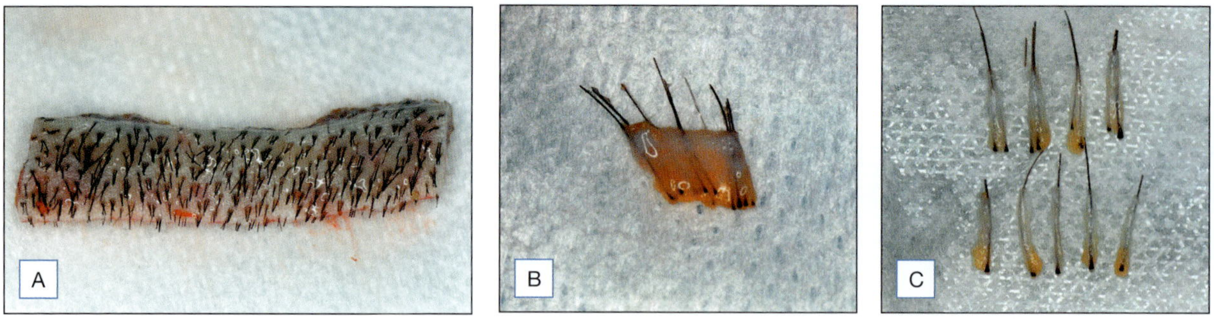


**Fig. 14.1** FU hair transplantation consists of removing the donor strip with a single-bladed scalpel and creating slivers and well-trimmed follicular grafts

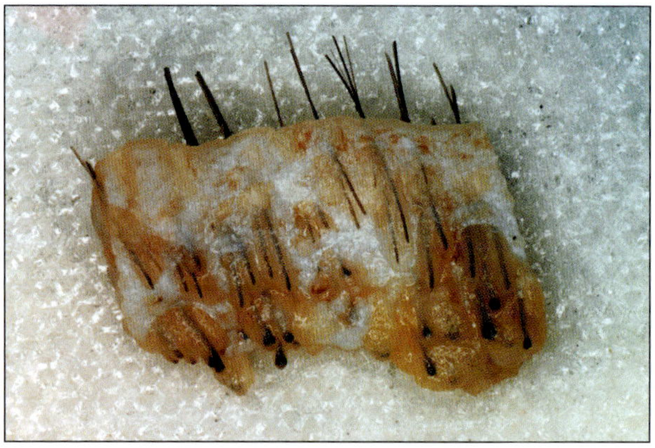

**Fig. 14.2** Without the aid of the stereomicroscope, there is a high probability of follicle transection during dissection of the grafts

(FUG) and all microscopic dissection has been the single most important factor in producing consistently high graft survival.

There are situations in which microscopic dissection is especially critical. In patients with extremely curly hair (e.g. Black people) and in those with extensive scarring in the donor tissue from prior procedures, many of the follicles will be transected if they are not carefully dissected under the stereomicroscope. The patient with gray or white hair is also challenging. Even with the use of the microscope, visualization can be difficult. Some have found that injecting or soaking the donor strip with methylene blue can be helpful in increasing the contrast between follicles and the surrounding tissue. Other have found that dying the donor hair prior to harvesting with over-the-counter brown mustache dye is a useful aid. The author favors the latter approach as well as the use of backlighting.

However, it should be noted that there are situations in which the patients' hair characteristics allow for easier dissection and may not require stereomicroscopes. For example, Asians generally have dark, straight hair, which allows for easy visualization. Furthermore, many surgeons believe that they can have consistently low transection rates with simple loupes and backlighting for all cases. The current author does not concur with this opinion and recommends that beginning surgeons consider microscopic dissection for all cases, to consistently produce the best growth.

## Dehydration

Loss of intracellular water is very damaging to the cells of the hair follicle. There is a high risk of graft dehydration because these small grafts are exposed to the air during dissection and while awaiting placement. There is widespread consensus for the need to keep grafts well hydrated. Achieving this requires constant monitoring of the staff performing the dissection and placement of grafts. One factor that can affect graft drying is the ambient humidity in the operatory environment. This can especially be a factor when forced air conditioning or heat is in use. In the author's experience, having a bacterio-static humidifier running constantly during the surgery helps add moisture to the air and reduces graft drying (Fig. 14.3).

There is some controversy as to whether grafts should be submerged in graft-holding solution or placed at the air–liquid interface on moistened gauze pads. Some strongly advocate the former while other successful surgeons utilize the latter, both with excellent results.

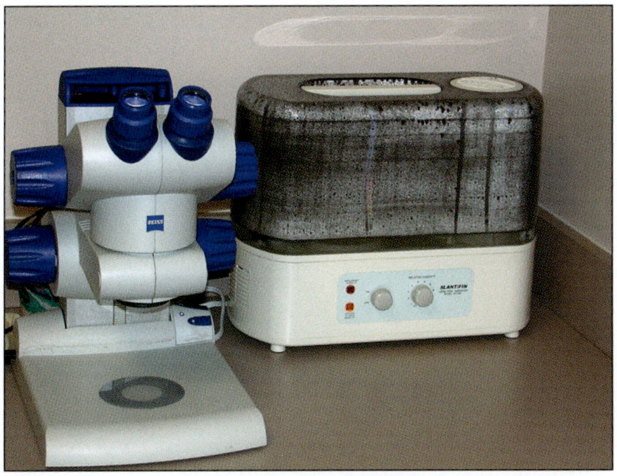

**Fig. 14.3** A bacteriostatic humidifier operates continuously during the transplant to increase ambient humidity and reduce graft dehydration

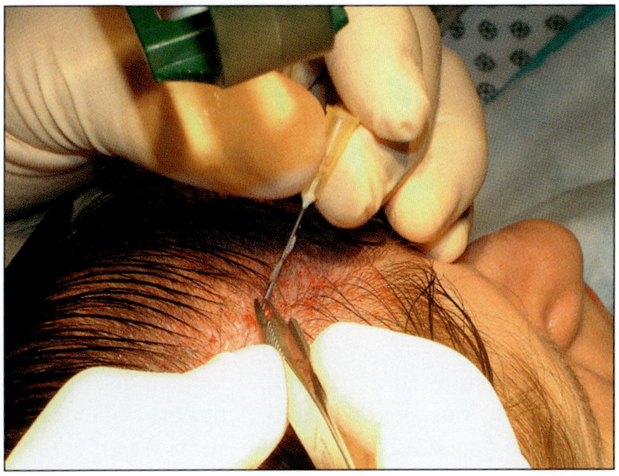

**Fig. 14.4** Modified 'stick and plant' technique. The incisions are made prior to placement. The placer then holds a dull needle in their nondominant hand and dilates the incision opening as the dominant hand uses the forceps to gently place the graft in the site

## Crushing

Given the small size of today's grafts, it is not surprising they may be crushed during placement into small recipient sites, such as 20 or 21 gauge needle incisions. Grafts that have been roughly handled and crushed by forceps have a significantly lower growth rate than grafts that have been handled gently.

Techniques to minimize crush injury during placement include: implantation devices, special forceps, the two-forcep technique, and the 'stick and place' technique. The latter technique, developed by Dr Bobby Limmer, consists of placing the graft immediately after each site is made by a hypodermic needle. Dr David Seager is also a strong advocate of this approach. The author employs a modified 'stick and place' technique where all incisions are pre-made. Then the placers will have their forceps in their dominant hand and a dull hypodermic needle (e.g. 20 gauge) in their non-dominant hand. The dull needle can be used to re-open the incision as the graft is gently placed into the site, nudging the graft downwards using less force and trauma than a one-handed technique (Fig. 14.4).

## Vascular Factors

Grafts must become revascularized to survive after being transplanted. This process takes several days however, and until completed the graft must get its nourishment from 'plasmatic imbibition.' The graft imbibes wound exudate by capillary action through the sponge-like structure of the graft tissue and through the follicular blood vessels. This process determines graft survival until circulation is re-established. Revascularization of the graft occurs by a poorly understood mechanism. Some think that vessels in the recipient area anastomose with the vessels of the grafted tissue while others think that there is an ingrowth of an entirely new network of vessels into the graft. It may be a combination of both. Regardless of how it occurs, full circulation to the graft should be restored by 7 days post grafting. To survive, the graft must adhere within the site, 'imbibe' sufficient nutrients, and then be successfully revascularized.

Grafts may fail to survive because of a failure in the revascularization process. Recipient areas that have scar tissue, whether from previous transplants, scalp reductions, or other trauma, may have an inadequate vascular network to oxygenate the graft during imbibition and revascularization. Likewise, patients who smoke tobacco may have inadequate baseline oxygenation of the skin and are more likely to have poor growth than nonsmokers. Although there are anecdotal reports of lower growth in smokers, there are no convincing studies to prove this.

In addition to pre-existing vascular compromise, the blood supply in the recipient bed can be overstressed by excessive size, depth, and density of incision sites. Some believe that placing grafts at high density (over 35 FUs/cm$^2$) with anything larger than a 19 gauge needle overstresses the vascular network and results in poor growth. Others believe that growth rate drops off at densities over 35 FUs/cm$^2$, regardless of incision size. More recently, this has been challenged by some who have claimed excellent growth at densities over 60 grafts/cm$^2$ but no studies have been offered to support these claims.

In the author's opinion, beginning surgeons should focus on achieving consistently excellent growth with well-trimmed grafts and smaller incision sites (19 gauge needle size and smaller) placed at moderate densities (20–35 FUs/cm$^2$). When consistently high growth is achieved, the surgeon can attempt denser packing of grafts (over 35 FUs/cm$^2$).

Besides size and density, the incision depth into the skin may have an effect on the revascularization and survival of the grafts. Most surgeons feel that ideally the incision should be just deep enough into the subdermal space to allow the graft to sit in its normal anatomical location without injuring deeper blood vessels. Incisions that are too superficial (i.e. within the dermis) or too deep (i.e. in the deeper subcutaneous layer) may result in poor growth. Injecting adequate tumescent solution helps avoid making incisions that are too deep.

Recently, there has been greater use of incisions placed perpendicular to the direction of natural hair growth (i.e. the 'lateral slit' or 'coronal angle grafting'). Some who have tried this technique have experienced decreased or delayed growth. Others claim growth is as good as or better than standard parallel incisions ('sagittal slits'). Theoretically, lateral slits may create greater compromise of the vascularity. The author makes most incisions using the lateral slit but believes there is a greater chance for poor growth if careful technique is not followed. Specifically, when using the lateral slit, the author uses greater tumescence and avoids overly deep incisions. Also, to avoid poor growth, the density of lateral slit incisions should be lower for more acute incisions (e.g. the frontal and temporal hairlines).

## Biochemical Factors

In the field of organ transplantation (e.g. livers and kidneys), surgeons consider biochemical factors to be critical in predicting graft survival, assuming immunologic rejection has not occurred. A tremendous amount of research has been carried out to identify and overcome biochemical injury to transplanted tissue and organs, research which has direct implications for hair transplantation. This biochemical injury may occur to the tissue while it is outside the body ('storage injury') or after it has been transplanted (ischemia-reperfusion injury [IRI]).

Once the donor strip is removed, the cells within the tissue are immediately cut off from their supply of oxygen, glucose, and other necessary nutrients. Oxygen is required for the production of adenosine triphosphatase (ATP), the cell's primary fuel, through aerobic metabolism. When tissue is removed, it switches from aerobic to anaerobic metabolism, which does not produce enough ATP to meet the cell's energy requirements. Lack of energy supplies and absence of other necessary ingredients leads to apoptosis, or programmed cell death, resulting in 'storage injury' of the tissue. If enough cells within the follicle undergo apoptosis, the follicle as a whole might not survive to produce hair.

IRI is the biochemical injury to the grafts that occurs after they have undergone a period of low oxygen (ischemia) after harvesting and during preparation, and are then implanted in the recipient sites where they are exposed to oxygen (reperfusion) (Fig. 14.5). It is an automatic reaction that is only partially understood. What is known is that IRI results from the formation of free radicals, sometimes called reactive oxygen species. This occurs in both the transplanted cells as well as the neutrophils present in the recipient tissue. These free radicals can be thought of as 'molecular poison' that injures the cell (Fig. 14.5). Damaged cells within the hair follicle may result in suboptimal growth. IRI has been demonstrated to occur in transplanted hair follicles.

Efforts to reduce storage and IRI have led to experimenting with different storage solutions. Many have tried using standard cell culture media (e.g. Dulbecco's Modified Eagle's Medium) instead of the commonly used normal saline. Others have found that autologous platelet-rich gel is an ideal environment to protect and nourish grafts prior to transplanting. IRI may be reduced by including antioxidants in the graft-holding solution and by treating the patient with corticosteroids perioperatively.

Another approach to preventing storage injury is by lowering the temperature of the storage solution.

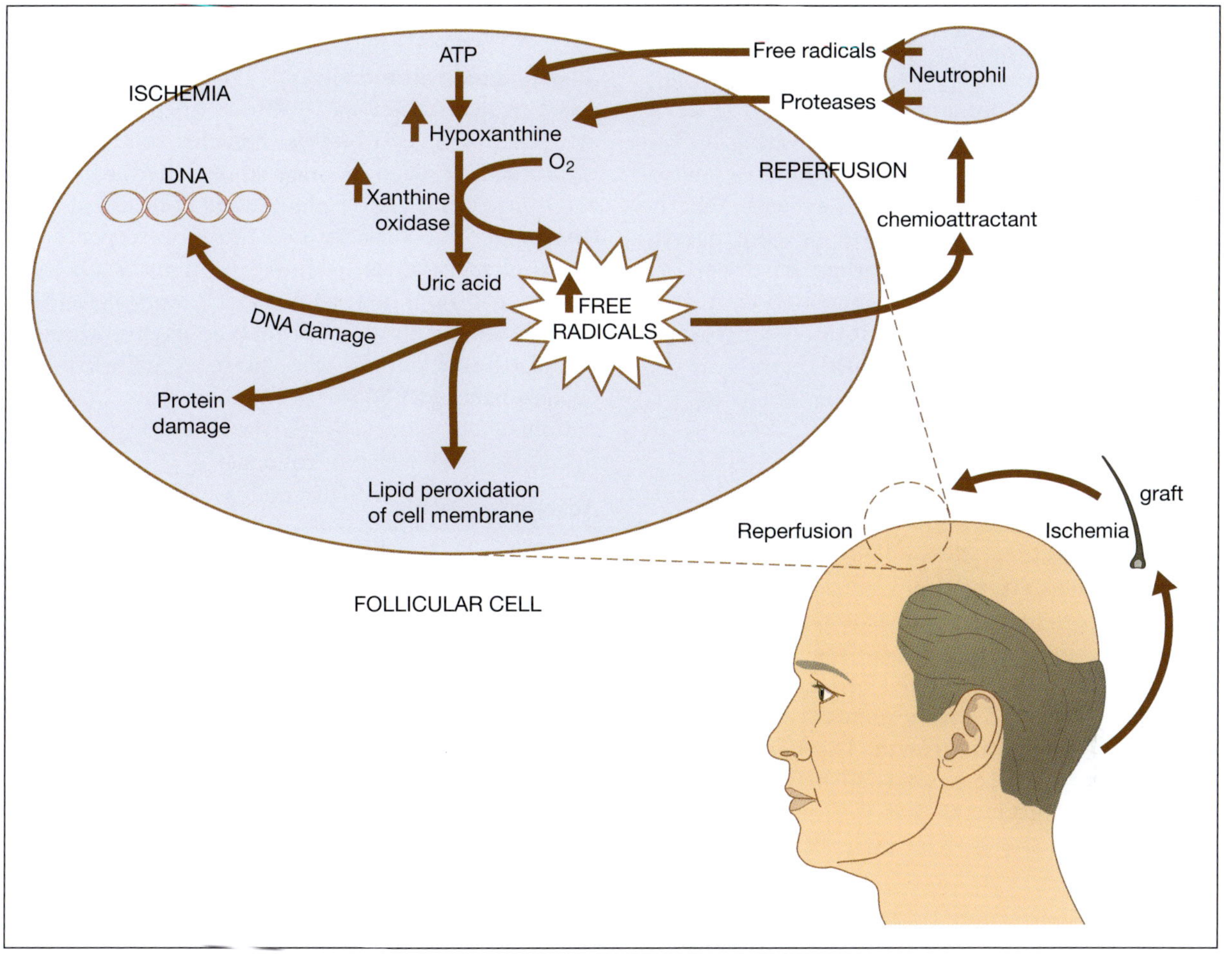


**Fig. 14.5** Ischemia-reperfusion injury. While the hair follicles are outside the body, they are in low oxygen (ischemia). After the grafts are implanted, they are exposed to more oxygen

Cooling has been used for millennia by man to preserve food, and seems like a logical technique to preserve tissue outside the body. However, at lower temperatures, membrane pumps do not function properly, resulting in intracellular edema, a lower pH, and an elevated intracellular calcium concentration, all of which are damaging to cells. It is for this reason that **hypothermic storage solutions** have been specifically designed to support and protect tissue that is being kept at low temperatures prior to transplantation. These solutions prevent the pathophysiologic changes that occur with cooling but it is important to note that they may actually be harmful to tissue at room temperature. In addition, these commercially available solutions (e.g. HypoThermosol, BioLife Solutions, Inc.) contain antioxidants such as vitamin E and glutathione. The author performed a study showing less IRI for grafts kept in HypoThermosol compared to saline.

A hypothermic storage solution such as HypoThermosol may appear to be the ideal choice for keeping hair follicles outside the body before transplantation. However, no comparative studies exist for various storage solutions. Furthermore, recent studies have shown that hair follicles stored in simple lactated Ringer's solution at very cold temperatures (0°C) have excellent survival. Hopefully future research will clarify current confusion over which solution provides the best balance of high graft survival and cost effectiveness. Until that time, chilled saline remains the gold standard as a holding solution for hair transplantation.

## Miscellaneous Issues

### Infection

Fortunately infections are rare. If they do occur, they will usually be due to gram-positive bacteria such as *Staphylococcus*. But other strains of bacteria may infect the transplanted hairs as well. Whether or not infections affect growth is controversial. Some claim less growth while others have seen even better growth, perhaps due to increased circulation. The issue of perioperative antibiotics is controversial but many surgeons continue to use them.

### Patient disruption

When evaluating a patient who claims poor growth, it is important to consider something as simple as the patient accidentally pulling several grafts out during the week after the procedure. The author has had a few patients over the years who confessed to bumping their heads and losing grafts in the postoperative period. If they had not admitted to this, the cases would have presented as unexplained examples of poor graft growth. There may be other things patients do (e.g. unusual diets, supplement usage, topical products) that may adversely affect wound healing and graft growth. Patients may not admit to such events.

### Idiopathic factors ('X factor')

If a patient has poor growth from a transplant and all the other factors discussed earlier have been ruled out, this can be labeled as an unexplained or **X factor**. This phenomenon was described by Richard Shiell in 1984, who estimated that it occurred in 0.5–1% of his patients. By definition, this phenomenon would be expected to occur again in future procedures despite careful surgical technique. Fortunately, the X factor is quite rare.

## Conclusion

Transplanted hair follicle grafts generally survive and grow well. Achieving optimal growth requires attention to several factors. Follicles should not be transected, crushed, or allowed to dehydrate during the dissection and placement phase of the transplant. The vascular bed must be respected in terms of incision size, depth, and density. Ongoing studies will hopefully show which storage solution for hair follicle grafts is optimal. By paying attention to all these factors, the surgeon will produce consistently excellent results and have satisfied patients.

### Acknowledgments

The author has no financial interest in the products mentioned.

### Further Reading

Bernstein RM, Rassman WR 1999 The logic of follicular unit transplantation. Dermatology Clinics 17:277–295, viii; discussion 296 [Review]

Cooley JE, Vogel JE 1999 Follicle trauma and the role of the dissecting microscope in hair transplantation. A multicenter study. Dermatology Clinics 17:307–312, viii; discussion 312–133

Cooley JE 2004 Ischemia-reperfusion injury and graft storage solutions. Hair Transplant Forum 14(4)

Gandelman M, Mota AL, Abrahamsohn PA, De Oliveira SF 2000 Light and electron microscopic analysis of controlled injury to follicular unit grafts. Dermatologic Surgery 26:25–30

Jiange Q, Wenzhong L, Guocheng Z, Liangbin Y, Wei S 2005 How long can hair follicle units be preserved at 0 and 4 degrees C for delayed transplant? Dermatologic Surgery 31:23–26

Krugluger W, Moser K, Moser C, Laciak K, Hugeneck J 2004 Enhancement of in vitro hair shaft elongation in follicles stored in buffers that prevent follicle cell apoptosis. Dermatologic Surgery 30:1–5 [discussion 5]

Limmer BL 1994 Elliptical donor stereoscopically assisted micrografting as an approach to further refinement in hair transplantation. Journal of Dermatologic Surgery and Oncology 20:789–793

Seager DJ 2002 The 'One-Pass Hair Transplant' – A six-year perspective. Hair Transplant Forum 12(5)

Shiell RC, Norwood OT 1984 Hair transplant surgery. Charles C. Thomas, Springfield, IL

Uebel C 2005 A new advance in baldness surgery with the platelet-derived growth factor. Hair Transplant Forum 15(3)

# 15 Perpendicular Angle Grafting

*Victor Hasson*

## Introduction

The establishment of the follicular unit (FU) as the basic building block of the modern hair transplant by Dr Limmer in 1988 marked a turning point in the science of hair transplantation surgery. Later work by Drs Rassman and Bernstein provided a mathematical model relating available donor hair to recipient site area. Creative planning and various distribution patterns of transplanted hair were the only suggested techniques by which the 'cosmetic impact' of what was a finite amount of donor hair could be maximized.

Little or no attention has been paid to the actual FU as a three-dimensional structure and how manipulation of the FU can optimize the cosmetic result of a given surgery.

By studying the distribution, orientation and structure of the FUs in the virgin scalp, several patterns can by recognized. Certain configurations of FUs are seen to cover underlying scalp better than others. Reproducing these configurations in the recipient scalp can significantly improve the final cosmetic result achieved with any finite number of FUs.

The endpoint or cosmetic result of the hair transplant procedure can generally be described in terms of three parameters:

1. **Naturalness**: largely a subjective assessment but will be influenced by a number of technical (e.g. hair angle and direction) and artistic (e.g. hairline design) factors.
2. **Coverage**: largely objective and relatively easily quantified. Used to describe the amount of bald scalp hidden by the transplanted hair.
3. **Density**: largely objective and relatively easily quantified. Divided into two separate components:
    1. **Mathematical density**, i.e. number of hairs/FUs per $cm^2$ of scalp
    2. **Optical density** – the amount of hair between the viewer's eyes and the patient's scalp. This measurement is more subjective and can be influenced by such factors as curl, wave, highlights, hair color, and scalp pigmentation.

In general, patients with less donor hair and a greater degree of final hair loss will need coverage more than density. Patients with relatively more donor hair and a lesser degree of final hair loss will usually desire greater density.

## Anatomic Considerations

In Caucasians the average FU contains approximately 2.3 follicles with a density of 80–100 FUs/$cm^2$. The terminal hair shaft has a diameter usually of between 50–80 μ and extends into the subcutaneous fat to a depth of 3.5–5.0 mm. The important anatomic features are:

1. The anatomic FU
2. FU/FU relationships
3. Hair direction
4. Hair angulation.

### Anatomic FU

The follicles within the FU have specific spatial relationships to one another (Fig. 15.1A). These relationships can be recognized at three specific levels:

1. **In the dermis**. The relationship of the follicles may be random or linear. Regardless of the degree

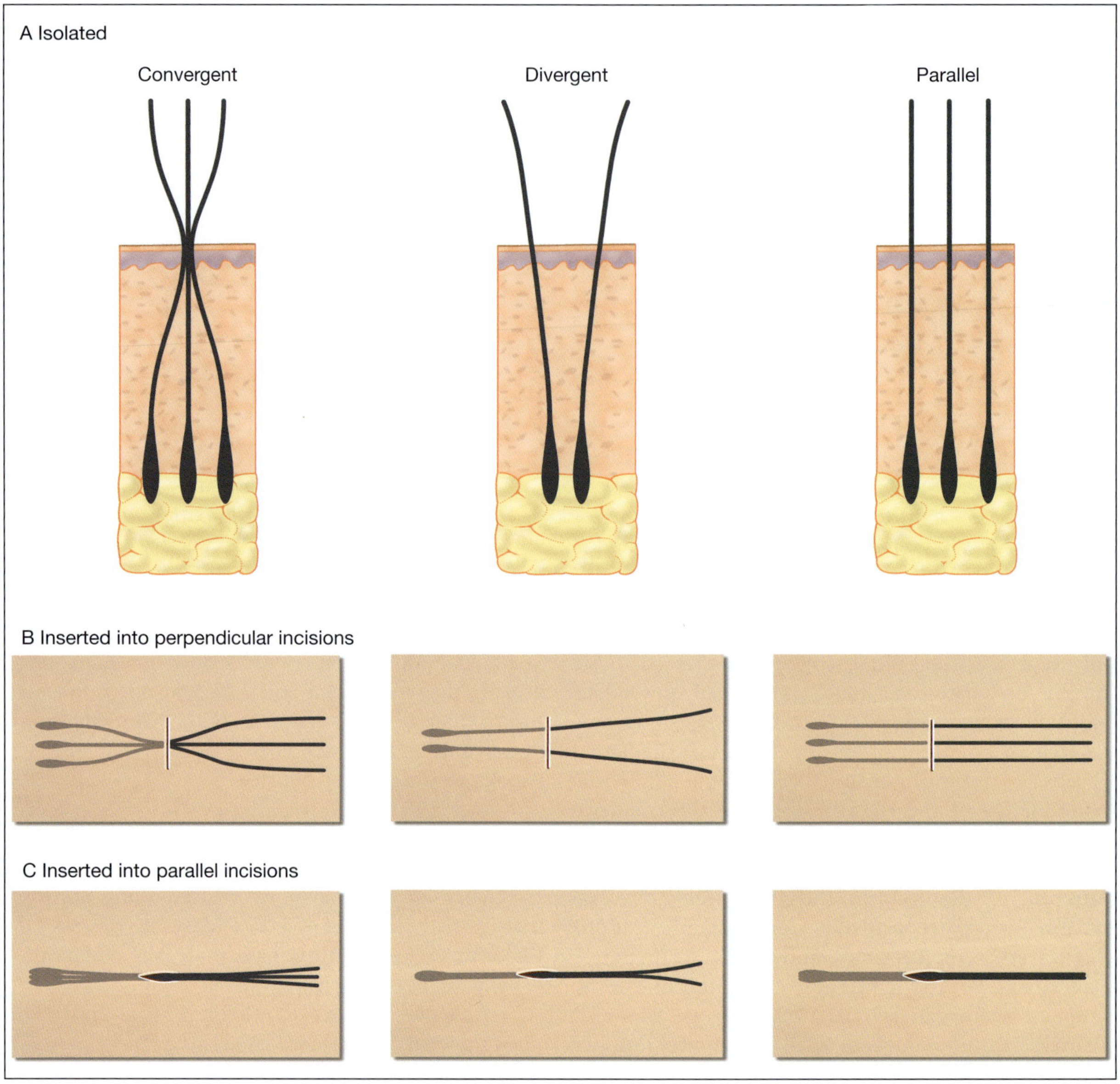


**Fig. 15.1** FU configurations. (**A**) After dissection. (**B**) Viewed from above in perpendicular incision. (**C**) Viewed from above in parallel incision

of natural curve, the follicles may be divergent, convergent, or parallel (Fig. 15.1A).

2. **At the point of exit from the epidermis**. Multi-hair FUs may exit through a single or multiple follicular canals in close association to one another.
3. **The hair shaft extending beyond the epidermis** The immediate orientation of hair above the skin correlates with and reflects the orientation in the dermis (Fig. 15.1B and C).

Regardless of the interfollicular relationships the orientation of the FU tends to be such that its longest axis is arranged at right angles to the direction of hair growth. Follicles of the individual FU tend to arise from the skin in a side-by-side rather than anteroposterior pattern (Fig. 15.2).

This concept is critical to understanding how FU orientation can affect underlying scalp coverage.

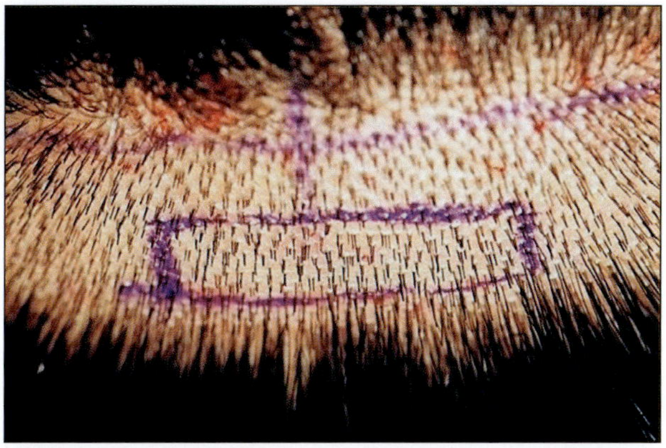

**Fig. 15.2** Orientation of FUs at right angle (perpendicular) to direction of hair growth

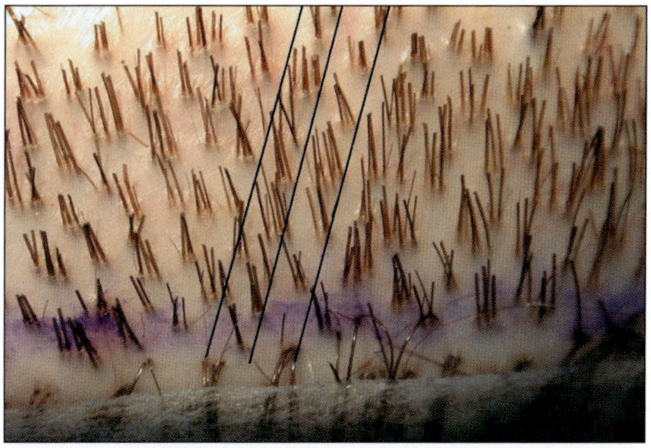

**Fig. 15.3** Linear arrangement of FUs in scalp

### FU/FU relationships

In different areas of the scalp the FU inter-relationships may be random or patterned. In the areas of the scalp where hair angulation is acute the FUs are frequently arranged in a linear fashion. Here the long axis of the FUs are arranged in a line parallel to the skin surface and at right angles to the direction of hair growth (Fig. 15.3).

### Hair direction

On the superior and frontal scalp the hair direction is predominately forward. At the sides and posterior scalp the hair direction is downward. The change in direction from forward to downward occurs most rapidly in the anterior scalp and is more gradual more posteriorly.

In the center of the crown the FUs are arranged in a spiral or concentric pattern. The rotational direction is clockwise in the majority of patients.

### Hair angulation

Hair shaft angulation with respect to the underlying scalp changes from about 90 degrees in the crown to around 30 degrees at the frontal hairline, but varies widely. In the posterior scalp and sides the hair angulation is very acute and may emerge almost flat against the scalp.

Precise control of hair distribution, direction, and degree of angulation will affect coverage. Transition points of both hair direction and angulation should be accurately reproduced to provide a 'seamless' transition between different areas.

### Local Scalp Circulation

The local circulation of the scalp occurs at two main levels: the subdermal vascular plexus and more importantly the vessels that run along the surface of the galea. Although the vascularization is extensive, it is not invulnerable to trauma.

Factors that may affect scalp circulation during hair transplantation include the following:

- Trauma to the vasculature, especially from multiple incisions during megasessions
- Extensive pressure due to dense packing. Hemorrhage into the scalp tissue and changes in tissue osmotic pressure that result should also be considered.
- Epinephrine use.

## Surgical Approach to Perpendicular Angle Grafting

### Preparation of FU grafts

The FU grafts used in perpendicular angle grafting are prepared from a fusiform donor strip, followed by two-stage microscopic dissection (Fig. 15.4A, B and C).

It is the preference of this author to use 'skinny' rather than 'chubby' FU grafts. The reasons for this are several:

1. The 'skinny FUs' are much smaller, allowing for smaller incisions in the scalp. This results in less scalp trauma, less vascular damage, and closer placing of the recipient site incisions.

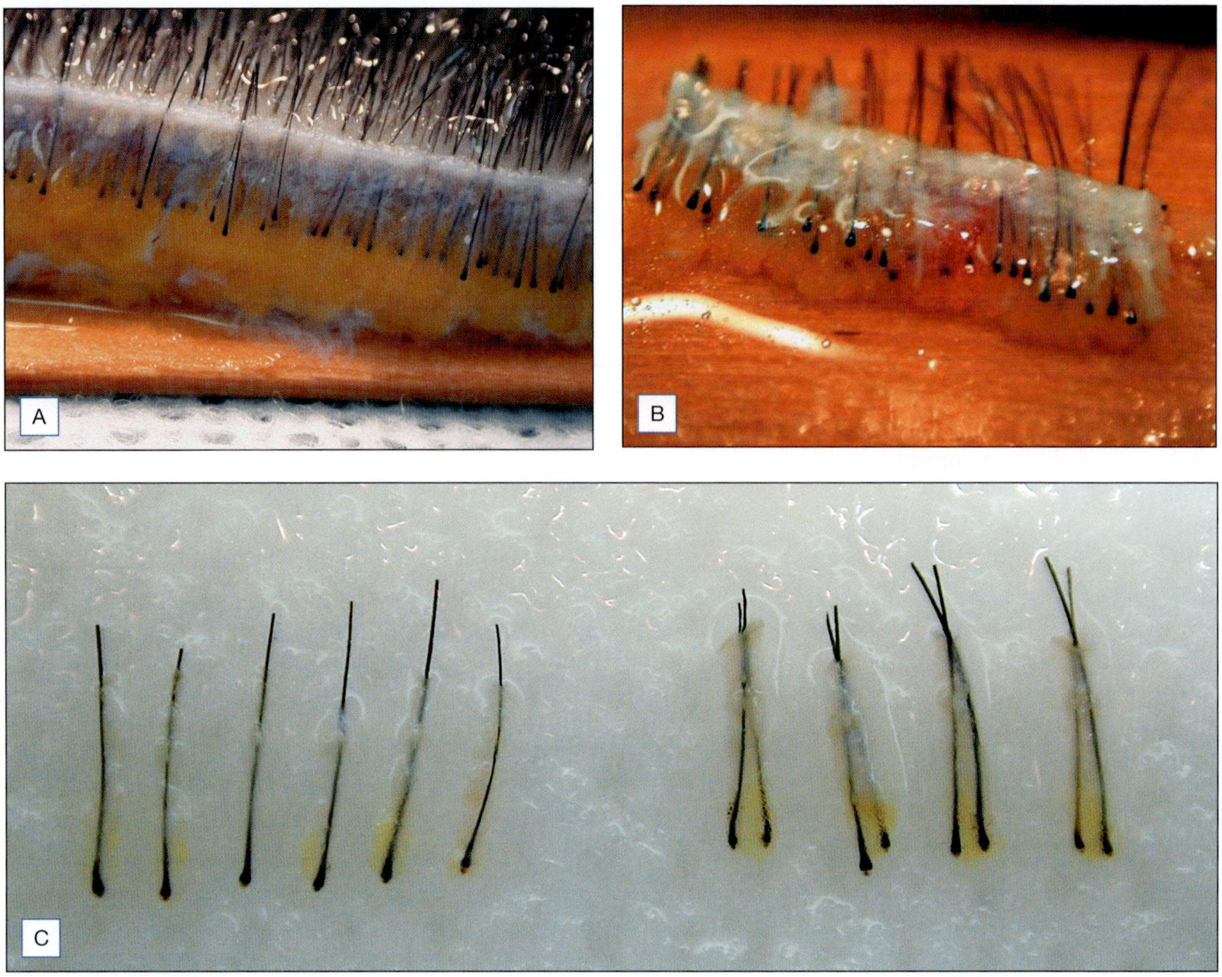

**Fig. 15.4** (**A–C**) Two-stage microscopic dissection of FU. (**A**) Excised donor strip. (**B**) Partially divided strip. (**C**) Trimmed 1 and 2-haired follicular units

2. The less bulky grafts occupy a smaller volume when placed into the incisions. There is less tendency for the grafts to 'pop' and less pressure exerted on the walls of the scalp excision.
3. The reduced dermal and connective tissue surrounding the follicles of the graft allows for easier diffusion of substances between the follicles and the tissue surrounding the recipient site.
4. Removal of tissue between and surrounding the graft follicles 'weakens' the bonds between the follicles, allowing the three-dimensional graft to flatten out and more easily conform to the shape of the recipient site. In addition, follicles exiting the epidermis through a single follicular canal may separate such that when placed into a recipient site, they appear to be exiting at separate points. This is of advantage esthetically as transplanted follicles always appear more natural if they exit the skin separately.

## Preparation of recipient sites

### *Choice of blade*

A chisel-tipped blade is used (Fig. 15.5); this type of blade will produce a perfectly linear incision (at right angles to the direction of hair growth) at the skin surface and a rectangular-shaped space cut into the dermis and subdermal fat. The perpendicular orientation of the incision will be more superficial than the same length parallel incision, with less damage to the underlying circulation (Fig. 15.6).

Needles produce nonlinear crescentric incisions, and spear point and angled blades as well as needles will penetrate the skin more deeply and damage important vasculature. In addition the rectangular shape best matches the shape of the inserted skinny FU.

A blade cutter can be used to produce custom chisel-tipped blades (Fig. 15.7). The back of a single-edged prep blade is removed and the blades are cut accurately to size. The author uses blade sizes ranging from 0.6–1.2 mm in width. The blades are held in a handle, which will allow varying lengths of blade to protrude (and giving a limited depth incision). This is measured to equal the depth of the follicle in the skin. In this manner the blades can be custom sized to the size of each individual's FU. The author uses the smallest size incision that will comfortably accommodate the grafts.

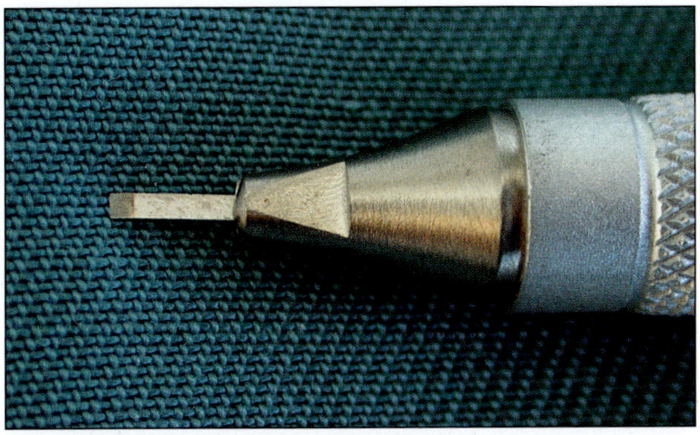

Fig. 15.5 Chisel-tipped blade

## Tumescence of recipient site

The recipient site is tumesced with a solution of normal saline and 1:1,000,000 epinephrine. This tumescence accomplishes several goals:

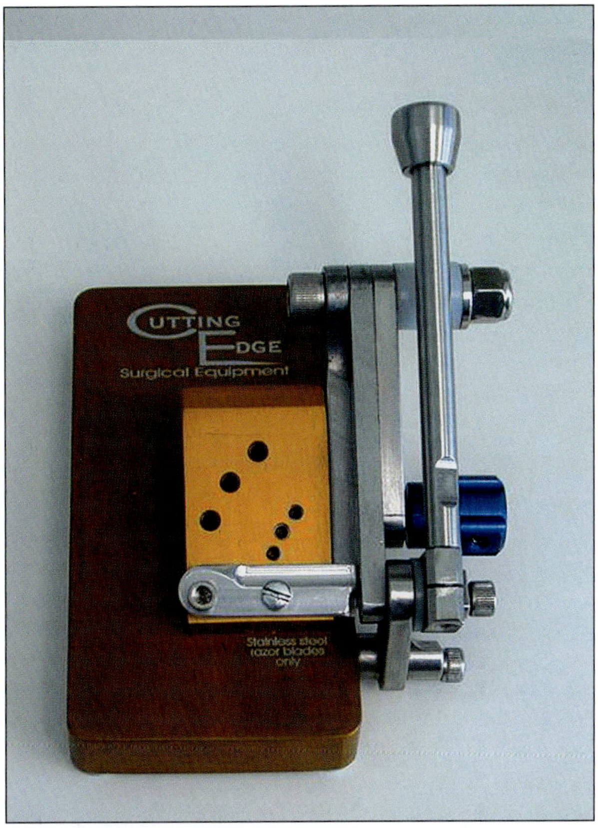


Fig. 15.7 Blade cutter

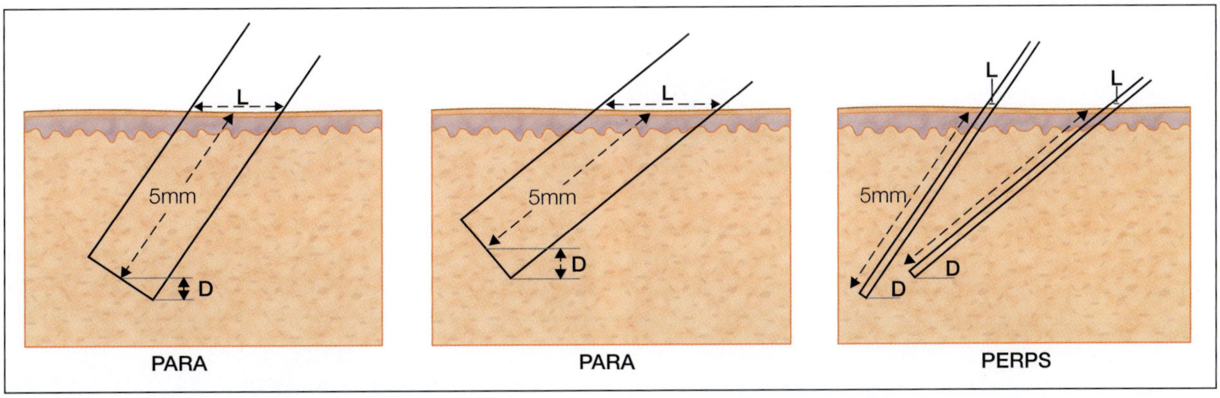


Fig. 15.6 Comparison between parallel and perpendicular incisions. L: length of skin incision. Note that as incision angle becomes more acute, L increases for parallel incisions, but remains the same for perpendicular incisions

1. Vasoconstriction of the scalp, reducing the likelihood of vascular trauma and hemorrhage into the scalp tissue
2. Lifting the skin surface away from the subdermal/supragaleal vasculature and thereby reducing vessel trauma
3. Increasing the surface area of the scalp, allowing for a greater number of recipient site incisions in any given area.

### Placement of incisions

The incisions are made in a linear arrangement and a staggered pattern is created with reference to the lines of incisions in front and behind. This staggered pattern reduces the possibility of redundant skin coverage by adjacent FUs.

The direction of the incisions is perpendicular to the direction of hair flow at any given point in the scalp (Fig. 15.8).

The angulation of the incisions varies according to position on the scalp. It is most acute on the sides and back of the head. On the superior and frontal aspects of the scalp, the angulation is approximately 45 degrees. The angle becomes more acute towards the anterior hairline.

On a bald scalp where improved coverage is required, the angulation may be made more acutely so as to provide greater coverage and a shingling effect of underlying scalp.

On the sides and back of the scalp the perpendicular incision is the only type of incision that can be used to reproduce the very acute angulation of the hair as it lies virtually flat against the scalp.

### FU placement

Custom-sized chisel-tipped blades produce an ideal match for the FUs obtained by microscopic dissection. These FUs will be placed easily (after practice) in the recipient sites.

Owing to the graft shape, the orientation of the FUs (so that the long axis of the graft is perpendicular to the direction of hair growth) will occur automatically or with minimal manipulation. The author believes that placement will be performed with less popping and bleeding than with parallel (sagittal) incisions.

## Summary of Advantages of Perpendicular Angle Grafting

### Coverage

This refers to the amount of bald skin covered by the inserted FUs when the scalp is viewed from above.

With perpendicular grafting the FU is aligned such that the follicles tend to arise side by side from the scalp. Even if the follicles arise through a single point and/or in front of one another, the plane of the incision below the skin insures that the follicles will separate in a plane at right angles to the hair direction as they emerge from the skin.

In contrast FUs placed in a parallel slit will emerge one behind the other and any tendency for them to separate is such that they separate in a plane parallel to the hair direction. When viewed from above these follicles appear 'stringy' as the hairs pile up on one another (see Fig. 15.1C).

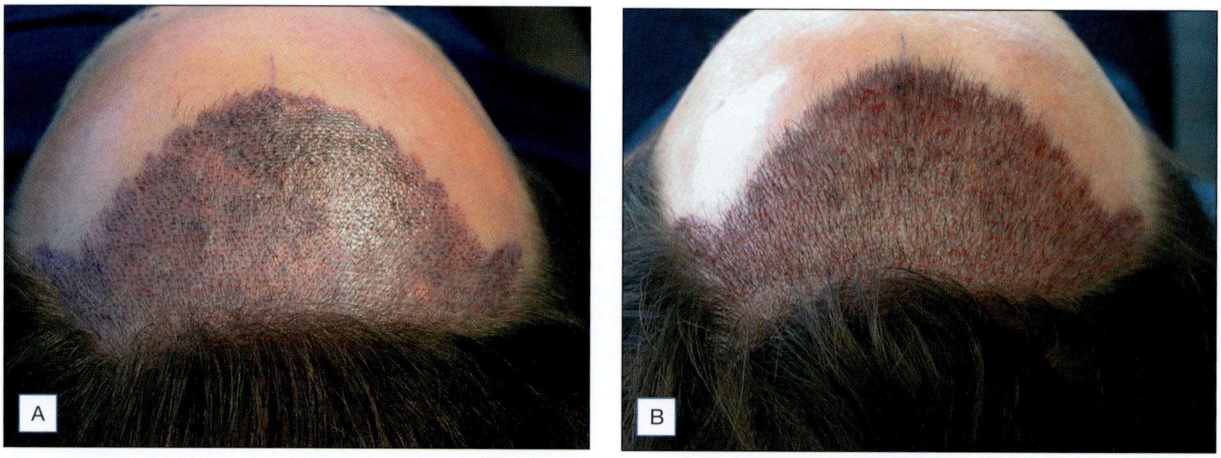


**Fig. 15.8** Perpendicular incisions. (**A**) Before and (**B**) after FU placement (approximately 3000 sites)

In this way with multi-haired FUs the coverage of the underlying scalp is multiplied as many times as there are follicles in the FU.

## Angle control

Since the angle of hair in the virgin scalp varies from area to area, the angulation of the unplanted FUs should be varied so as to match the angle of the existing or pre-existing hair.

The perpendicular incision allows for precise control of graft angulation by 'sandwiching' the FU between the anterior and posterior walls of the incision (Fig. 15.9A–C).

With parallel incisions the implanted FUs could 'rock' forwards and backwards within the incision as the graft is sandwiched between the lateral walls of the incision.

In addition with parallel incisions the effect of one hair arising behind the other causes a lifting effect of the hair from the scalp. Here the hair is seen to stand away from the scalp, which is particularly obvious closer to the hairline (Fig. 15.10).

There is no other type of incision that can maintain the hair lying flat against the skin in the temporal/parietal scalp.

The exact control of graft angulation allows for a smooth flow of hair in the superior scalp and a natural transition as the scalp angle becomes more acute in the lateral and posterior scalp.

## Increased density

The FUs may be safely transplanted closer together with greater resultant density with perpendicular incisions. The reasons for this are:

1. **Reduced injury to the subdermal vasculature.** For a given angle of insertion, the deepest level of penetration of the perpendicular-orientated blade for a given graft is shallower than the deeper penetrating parallel-orientated blade.
2. **Smaller incisions.** The surface incision is the same regardless of the blade angulation. With parallel blades the wound length increases with more acute angulation.

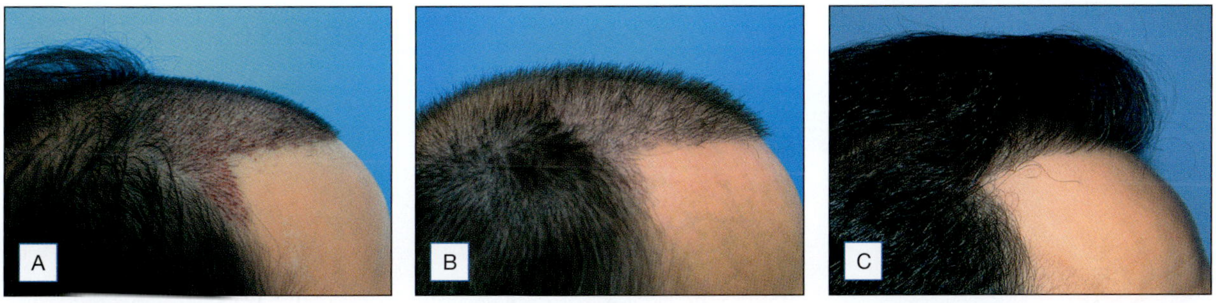


**Fig. 15.9** Control of graft angulation. **(A)** Immediately post surgery. **(B)** 10 days postoperatively. **(C)** 8 months postoperatively

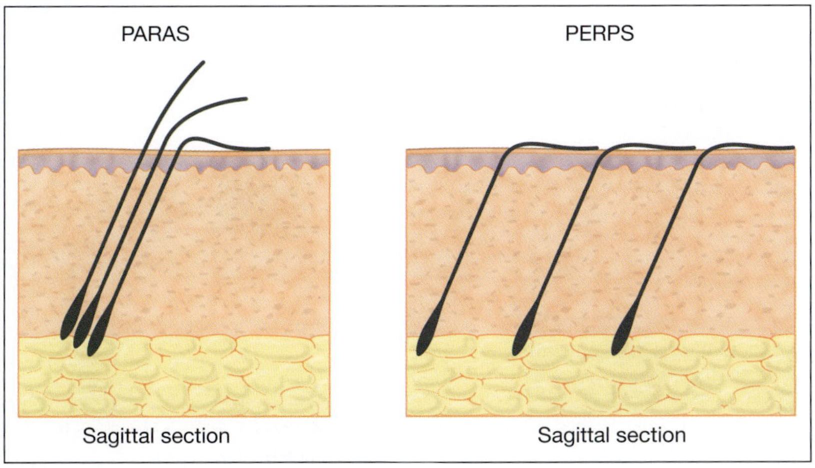


**Fig. 15.10** Effect of site orientation on lifting effect

3. **Reduced popping**. With parallel incisions the outward pressure created when a graft is placed is in a lateral direction. This lateral pressure is added to the pressure caused by the surrounding grafts, and when the grafts are tightly packed this combined lateral pressure will cause grafts to pop.

   With perpendicular incisions the pressure is largely in an upward and downward direction. There is free expansion in the upward direction so that there is no buildup of pressure as more grafts are inserted (Fig. 15.11).
4. **Reduced bleeding**. The shallower incisions reduce bleeding, which is a common cause of popping.

The interstitial hematomas that result from bleeding occupy space with resultant increased pressure. As the hematoma breaks down tissue, osmotic forces increase and more fluid is drawn

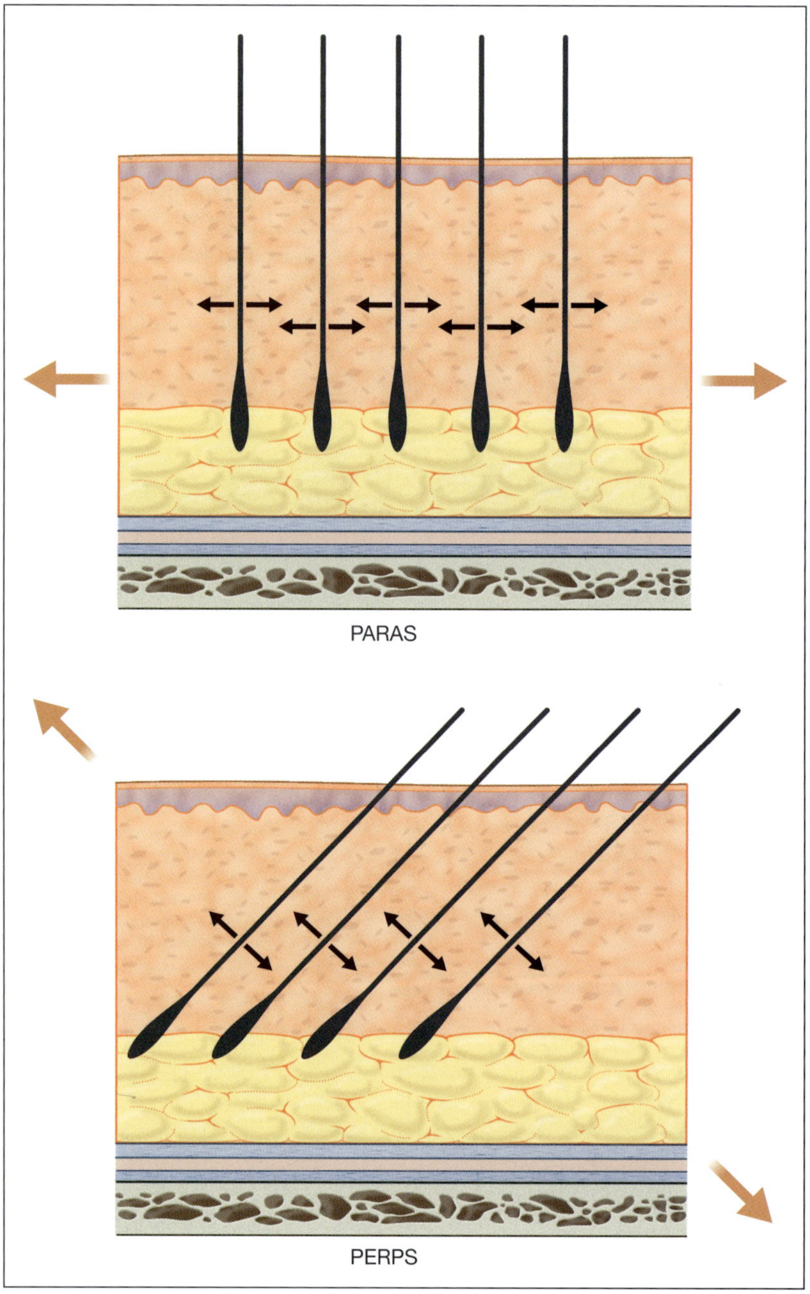


**Fig. 15.11** Pressure transmission in scalp after FU placement

from the vessels into the interstitial tissue, which further exacerbates the pressure problem.

5. **Improved naturalness**. In the author's opinion, hairs arising side by side from the scalp appear less pluggy and 'stringy' than those that exit one on top of the other. This is important when viewing the scalp from above. The appearance is further improved by single-haired FUs placed at the hairline.

## Conclusion

By recreating the natural orientation of the FU in nature, an attempt has been made to address many of the problems caused by parallel grafting with the goal of producing an esthetic result, which more closely resembles the original hair growth.

## Further Reading

Bernstein RM 1998 Measurements in hair restoration. Hair Transplant Forum International 8:27

Bernstein RM, Rassman WR 1997 The aesthetics of follicular unit transplantation. Dermatologic Surgery 23:785–799

Bernstein RM, Rassman WR 1997 Follicular transplantation: Patient evaluation and surgical planning. Dermatologic Surgery 23:771–784

Limmer BL 1994 Elliptical donor stereoscopically assisted micrografting as an approach to further refinement in hair transplantation. Dermatologic Surgery 20:789–793

# 16 Dense Packing Techniques

*David Seager*

## Introduction

Planting follicular units closer together than 30–35 follicular units (FUs) per $cm^2$ is usually regarded as dense packing. Many doctors do not dense pack and plant instead to a usual density of 15–25 FUs/$cm^2$. Even technicians with moderate experience can usually place grafts at this lower density quickly and easily. Planting FUs to densities above 35 FUs per $cm^2$ units is much more technically demanding, and risks poor growth unless a stringent protocol is followed.

## Dense Packing

Dense packing between 40 and 50 FUs/$cm^2$ is optimal for an average Caucasian man. This presumes that this average man has a hair shaft diameter between 67–77 μ and his FUs have an average of 2.3 hairs. Planting 45 FUs/$cm^2$ would therefore produce about 105 hairs/$cm^2$ (Fig. 16.1). This represents just less than 50% of average normal hair density in the frontal area. The human eye tends to perceive this density as that of early thinning. Most patients do not have adequate donor hair to justify planting greater densities.

Without even considering the success of extreme dense packing, there are three main concerns. First, the total donor supply could be depleted rapidly. For example, the area behind an extremely densely packed area would also have to be planted at high density to look balanced. As the balding area expands, more and more donor hair would be required. Second, the results could look unnatural and unbalanced, especially after aging and progression of hair loss. A narrow, extremely dense frontal forelock in front of a large, often dome-shaped bald head may look quite unnatural. Third, because it is visual perception that is dealt with, the law of diminishing returns applies. It takes much more transplanted hair to change the look from early thinning hair to thick hair than it does to change from bald to early thinning. Doubling the amount of hair in an area does not double the apparent cosmetic benefit.

## Dense-packing Methods

There are two main methods of dense packing. Either allows close placement of grafts.

The first and most commonly used method involves edematizing part of the recipient area with saline, then creating the required number of incisions per expanded $cm^2$ with a small blade or needle. When the edema dissipates and the skin shrinks, the number of incisions per $cm^2$ correspondingly increases. This is repeated until all of the recipient sites have been made. With experience, the surgeon learns how many incisions to make into the edematized recipient area to produce the desired degree of dense packing.

The second method is called 'stick and place.' The operator inserts a needle or blade into the recipient skin. As the needle is withdrawn, the graft is simultaneously inserted into the newly made tract (Fig. 16.6A–D). Commonly, 18–22 gauge hypodermic or solid needles, or sharply pointed or narrow chisel blades are used.

When dense packing, recipient sites must be kept small to preserve vascularity. It is widely believed that more superficial incisions are more sparing of the recipient blood supply than deeper incisions. Various proprietary instruments are made with depth-limiting capabilities (Fig. 16.2).

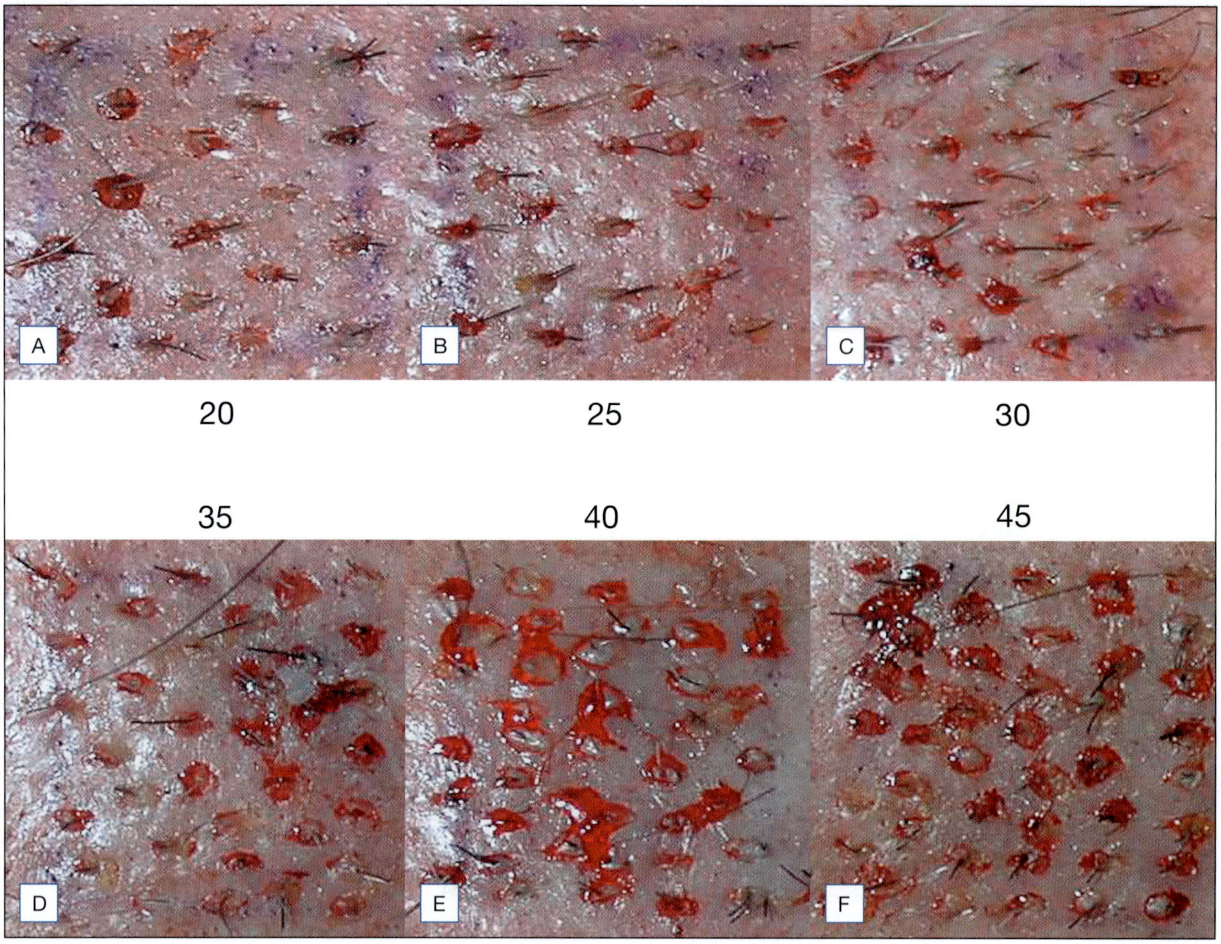


**Fig. 16.1** Photograph showing different densities of graft placement using the stick-and-place method. (**A**) 20 grafts/cm$^2$. (**B**) 25 grafts/cm$^2$. (**C**) 30 grafts/cm$^2$. (**D**) 35 grafts/cm$^2$. (**E**) 40 grafts/cm$^2$. (**F**) 45 grafts/cm$^2$

## Complications and Side Effects

Dense packing has the same general risks as any other type of transplantation. In addition, there is potential vascular risk if the dense packing overwhelms the blood supply.

General risks can be increased by dense packing. For example, it could be expected that there will be more and longer-lasting edema after transplanting 3000 grafts into a frontal forelock area than after transplanting 800 grafts, less densely, in the same area.

Similarly, when a large area is densely packed, the procedure can take more time. Dense packing takes longer per graft than regularly spaced planting. Care taken to avoid damaging adjacent grafts can slow down graft placement. In addition, the skin pressure during placement of a new graft can cause 'popping' up of the previously transplanted adjacent graft. More total time is required because more grafts must be transplanted to cover the same area more densely. A longer surgical time can increase medication use and associated complications, and the grafts are more likely to be 'out of the body' for longer.

Dense packing incorrectly can interrupt the recipient area's blood supply. This would then cause certain predictable complications, the first of which is poor growth of transplanted and/or pre-existing hair. With yet more severe embarrassment of the blood supply comes necrosis of skin. This is characterized by a black scab, which stays tightly adherent for up to 2–4 weeks. The necrotic area heals by granulation and eventually leaves white, shiny skin devoid of natural pores and hair, i.e. scar tissue. With lesser degrees of vascular embarrassment, frank necrosis may not take place, but poor or no growth of hair results.

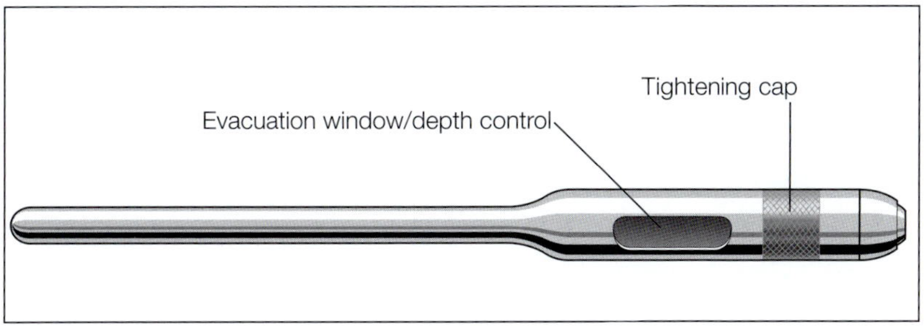


**Fig. 16.2** Photograph of the Versi Handle and depth-limiting capabilities

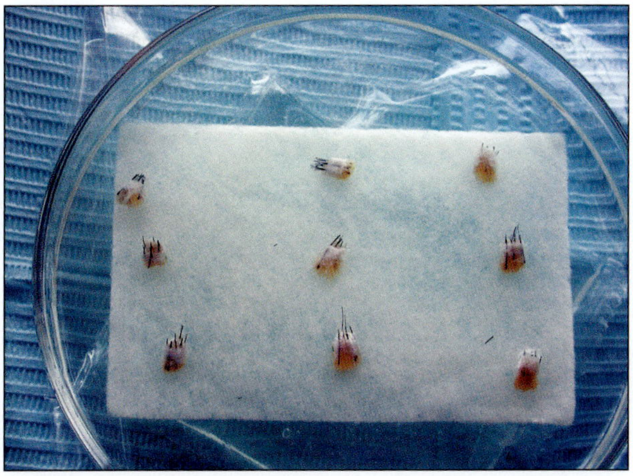

**Fig. 16.3** Photograph showing traditional graft storage of 4 mm grafts on moist gauze

Vascular impairment of the recipient area resulting in poor growth, no growth, or worse still necrosis, is more likely in patients with pre-existing vascular impairment such as diabetics, those with previous skin surgery in the area, smokers, and the elderly. Previous hair transplants in the area are a relative contraindication to dense packing. Before transplanting a recipient area that already has been transplanted, or has had its vascularity impaired in the other ways, it is important to assess the extent of vascular impairment. Factors to take note of when deciding how densely such an area can be dense packed will be:

- The color of the skin
- The presence or absence of hair in the area (either pre-existing or transplanted)
- The length of time this skin stays blanched after it is pressed
- The ease and rapidity with which the skin bleeds when incised.

Experience is the best teacher but, given the difficulty of treating vascularly impaired skin, it is better to err on the side of caution.

## Are There Any Disadvantages With Dense Packing? Why Are All Hair Transplants Not Dense Packed?

The answer is 2-fold.

First, dense packing requires meticulous attention to technique to be successful. If the operator is not highly skilled and does not adhere to a strict protocol, incomplete growth is extremely likely. Merely transferring skills, learned with regular density transplantation, to dense packing has led many experts to achieve only 70% growth. They erroneously blamed FU transplantation in general instead of their individual technique. For example traditional graft storage, as shown in Figure 16.3, is excellent for 4 mm grafts and multi-follicular unit grafts but breaks the most important rule for FUT, which is to 'keep the grafts moist.' Storing the grafts as in Figure 16.4 will lead to dry grafts and suboptimal growth whereas immersion in saline, as in Figure 16.5, will keep grafts moist and yield much better survival. With proper technique a few practitioners are able to consistently obtain greater than 100% growth (including the telogen hairs that are pushed into anagen). This has been independently verified on several occasions.

Second, dense packing is labor intensive and usually requires long hours, and a large number of highly trained staff.

## Conclusions

Dense packing of grafts, greater than 30–35 FUs/cm$^2$, is not for every patient or every practitioner. Dense packing FUs can achieve greater than 100% regrowth. The main complications of suboptimal

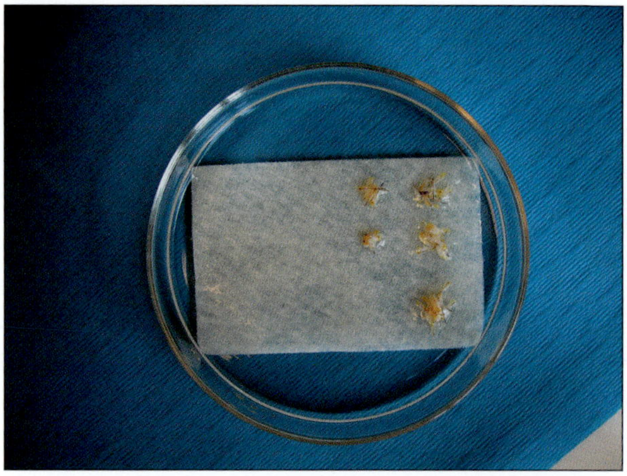

**Fig. 16.4** Photograph showing FUGs with traditional storage

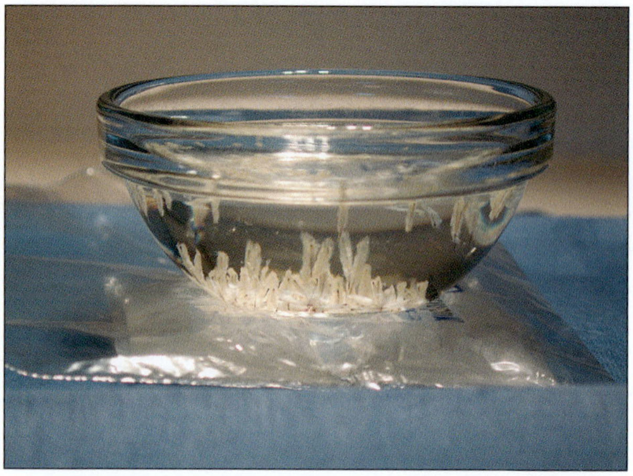

**Fig. 16.5** Photograph showing FUGs immersed in saline

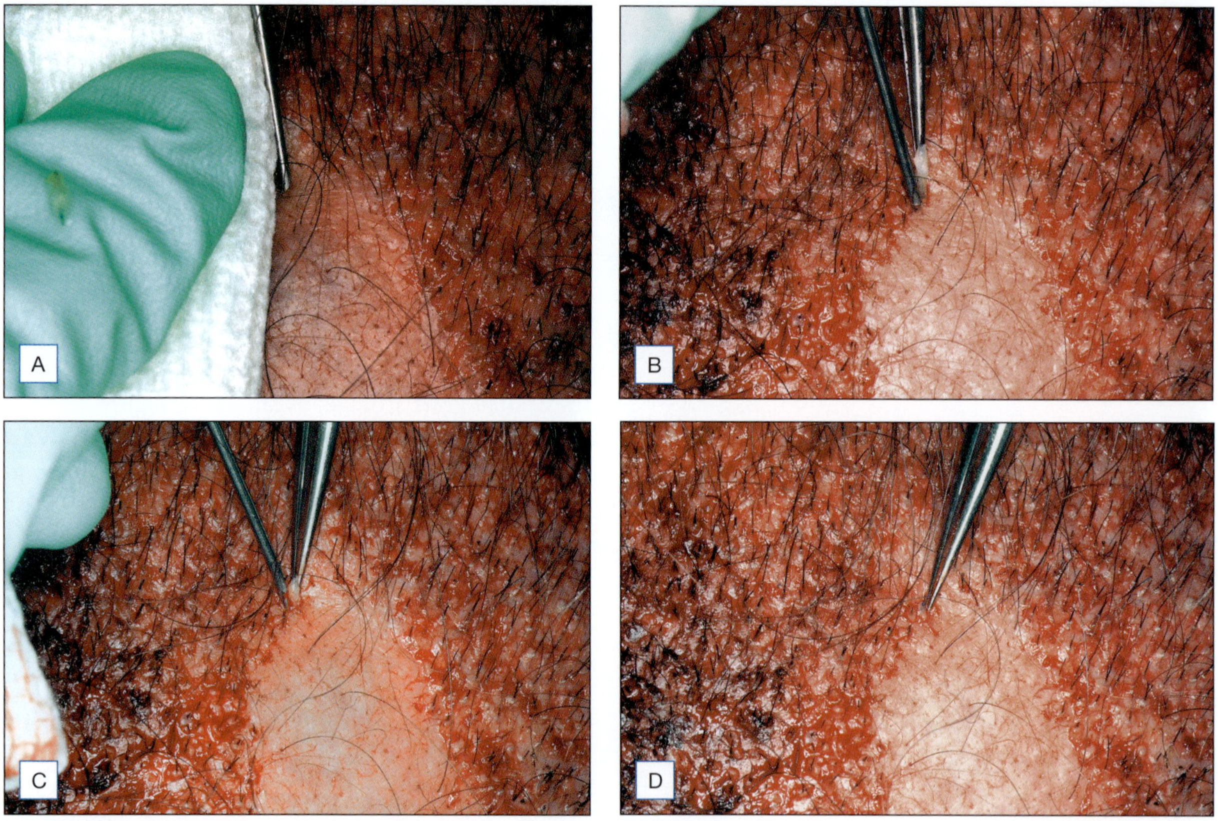

**Fig. 16.6** (**A**) Photographs showing insertion of needle into the recipient skin. (**B**) Photograph showing simultaneous withdrawal of needle and insertion of FUG into newly made tract. (**C**) Photograph showing insertion of FUG into recipient site. (**D**) Photograph showing the fine adjustment of the FUG in the recipient site

growth and vascular compromise can be avoided, if the necessary protocol is followed and the technique is performed by experienced and meticulous practitioners. Finally, it should be stressed once more that for the vast majority of situations, 40–50 FUs/cm$^2$ is dense enough. With current knowledge, extreme dense packing increases vascular risk, risk of poor growth, donor depletion, and the potential for unnatural results after further aging and progression of hair loss. In life and dense packing, moderation is best.

## Further Reading

Bernstein RM, Rassman WR 1999 The logic of follicular unit transplantation. Dermatological Clinics 17(2)
Limmer BL 1997 The density issue in hair transplantation. Dermatologic Surgery 23(9)
Seager DJ 1997 Micrograft size and subsequent survival. Dermatologic Surgery 23(9):757–761
Seager DJ 2002 The 'One Pass Hair Transplant' – A six year perspective. Hair Transplant Forum International 12(5)
Stough DJ, Whitworth JM 1999 Methodology of follicular unit hair transplantation. Dermatological Clinics 17(2)

17

# Follicular Unit Extraction

*William R. Rassman, James A. Harris, Robert M. Bernstein*

## Introduction

The follicular unit (FU) was first defined by Headington and the conceptual framework for using FUs in hair transplantation was laid out by Bernstein and Rassman. It became clear to most hair transplantation practitioners that the single-strip harvesting and stereomicroscopic dissection techniques developed by Limmer in 1988 were the best ways to both harvest and isolate FUs.

Although single-strip harvesting is an extremely efficient means of obtaining tissue for subsequent dissection into FUs, it results in a linear scar. Careful technique with thin donor strips will produce very fine scars, but if the strips are taken too wide, the scar can widen to an unacceptable degree. Covering the donor area with longer hair was the only solution to widened scars, as surgical repairs of these wounds generally proved to be ineffective. As a result, a number of patients became hesitant to undergo a procedure that had a potentially difficult-to-treat widened linear scar.

In the mid-1990s, Rassman set out to find a way around this problem by directly extracting FUs from the donor area using a small punch. Early attempts were frustrated by high transection rates in a significant number of patients until Richard Shiell brought the work of Masumi Inaba to his attention.

Inaba's technique varied slightly, using a similar punch but only partially cutting down on the hair follicle and then removing the remainder with forceps. Inaba's insight led to Rassman and Bernstein describing follicular unit extraction or the FOX procedure (FOllicular unit eXtraction), outlining an entire hair transplant procedure without strip harvesting.

After performing the FOX procedure on patients of various nationalities it became obvious that extraction proved to be quite variable. Histologic analysis was used in an attempt to elucidate the cause of patient variability and the FOX Test was introduced, an important surgical recommendation tool to determine patient candidacy.

Overall results showed that the FOX Test classified approximately 60% of all patients as candidates for the FUE procedure. However, even the good candidates had a strong possibility of follicle transection.

## Two-Step Technique

This process is comprised of two main steps. In the first step, a sharp 1 mm punch is placed over the follicular unit and aligned to approximate the angle of the hair shafts below the skin surface. A rotational motion of the punch is then used to cut through the skin and isolate FUs in the epidermis and upper dermis.

For a successful procedure, the incident angle of the punch cannot vary much from the hair shaft direction or some, or all, of the hairs in the FU will be transected. Since the hair bulbs in each FU splay outward in the deep dermis and fat, it is also important to limit the depth of the punch to the upper dermis, which proves difficult.

In step two, the extraction, fine rat-toothed forceps are used to apply gentle traction to the top of the FU until the unit is pulled loose from its deep dermal and subcutaneous connections. There is person-to-person variation with this procedure. To help limit variation effects, the technique was refined further, adding dissection when simple extraction proved difficult. If a graft cannot be removed with gentle traction, then the deeper part of the graft is separated from the surrounding tissue through dissection using a fine needle (with a U-shaped tip) while traction is applied with delicate forceps.

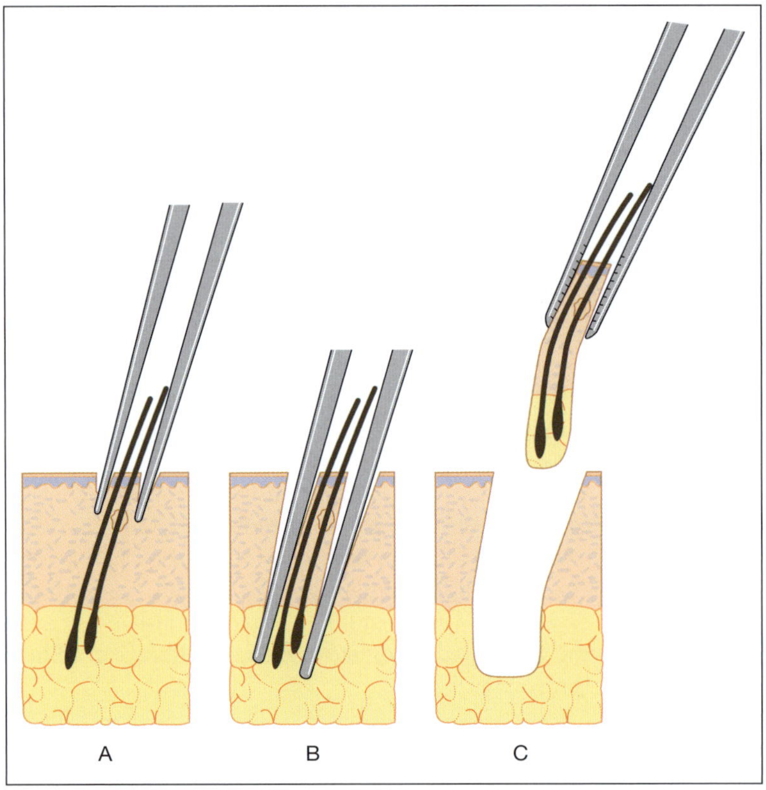


**Fig. 17.1** Three-step technique of FUE. (**A**) The epidermis and upper dermis is 'scored' to a depth of 0.3–0.5 mm with a sharp dermal punch. (**B**) A 'dissecting' punch is inserted to separate the follicular unit from the investing dermal tissue. (**C**) The follicular unit is removed with forceps

With this additional dissection step, percentages of positive FOX patients increased. Despite a significant yield improvement, a large number of patients still could not be shifted into 'FUE candidacy.' In many cases transection rates were still unacceptably high and dissection times for significant cases unacceptably long; the additional step slowed the entire process.

## Three-Step Technique

James Harris presented a paper and a new solution at an ISHRS scientific meeting, in which he added an additional third step requiring new instrumentation. In this new three-step procedure, a sharp punch is used to score the epidermis (rather than cut through the full thickness to the dermis) and then a dull punch is used (through a back-and-forth twisting motion) to bluntly dissect the FU graft from the surrounding epidermis and dermis (Fig. 17.1).

This variation has several advantages over the original two-step process. Using a dull punch avoids follicle transection and allows intact FUs to be extracted more easily. As the blunt-tipped punch is advanced into the dermis, splayed follicles are 'gathered together,' avoiding transection. In effect, the dull-punch technique allows a full realization of the 'extraction concept' with an easy-to-learn methodology. One untoward result of the three-step technique is a possible higher incidence of buried grafts, as discussed later. In addition, some of the FUs remain tethered to the subcutaneous tissue and require additional dissection.

One great advantage of this addition was that it opens the technique to the inherent FOX-negative population: those with very fine hair and those with African kinky hair types. Because the procedure is performed blindly, visualization is no longer an issue, potentially increasing yield for those with hard-to-see gray hair. In addition, it appears that this FUE modification has applicability for corrective procedures, removing FUs inside old plugs.

Indications for FUE have evolved considerably. Initially, FUE was limited to FOX-positive patients (that showed minimal transection) and in those in which the size of the balding area matched the surgical team's ability to perform the procedure in an acceptable time frame – essentially small procedures in select patients. With improved techniques, Rassman reported his largest case yet in 2004: 1903 FUs performed exclusively with the original two-step technique. Harris' modification should allow these large sessions in a greater number of patients.

## Nuances of three-step technique

Although the three-step technique is easier to master than the two-step technique, there are certain factors that will increase its efficiency and success.

Because the subcutaneous course of follicles cannot be ascertained with great accuracy, 'scoring' incisions should be limited to a depth of between 0.3 mm and 0.5 mm (approximately the level of the end of the bevel on a standard 1 mm Miltex punch) to decrease the risk of inadvertent transection. However, in patients whose follicles are slightly longer, scoring incision depths may be increased by 0.1–0.2 mm. This increase should facilitate insertion of the 'dissecting' punch and may decrease the incidence of 'buried' grafts.

Even though the use of a blunt punch provides protection for follicles and makes the angle of insertion less critical, follicles may be damaged if the angle is radically different from the follicle's direction. To prevent damage, scoring incisions can be created, and their angles reassessed to obtain a more accurate estimate of the follicle's direction and more accurately 'aim' the dissecting punch.

Follicle separation from the epidermis and upper dermis at the sebaceous gland may occur during extraction. This phenomenon, which has been called 'capping,' can be handled in three ways. If the subcutaneous attachment is significant, a second pass with a dissecting punch can be attempted. A second option is to grasp the unit at the sebaceous gland region and pull, applying a slow, steady force. The final option, if standard dissection fails, is to leave the graft in situ and allow the skin to heal by secondary intention.

Since a third step is required in this new method, the need for efficiency has increased. Rather than performing each of the three steps for each FU in sequence, a preferred method is to identify an area to be extracted, score 25–50 FUs, dissect each one, and then extract. Assistants may help with dissection and extraction but care must be taken to identify any buried grafts for subsequent retrieval efforts.

The need for tumescence varies from patient to patient, but for the most part, it has been found that tumescence may cause the dermis to become somewhat 'mushy' and impede the extraction process. The surgeon must make constant assessments of extraction success each step of the way with every patient. Ease of extraction also seems to vary with scalp location. The occipital area tends to be easier while temporal areas may require manual dissection due to a higher degree of tethering.

## Management of buried grafts

As previously mentioned, this technique has an inherent possibility of producing buried grafts. Incidence can vary from patient to patient depending on unidentified skin characteristics. It has been observed that in some patients and in some areas (the temples for example), slightly increasing scoring depths decreases the incidence of buried grafts.

When a buried graft is identified, immediately apply pressure around it in an attempt to 'force' the graft to the surface. If this maneuver fails, the surgeon should examine the circular incision to identify the follicle base, a key step in facilitating removal. If the follicle is not visible, use small, curved forceps with the tip directed towards the 'superior' aspect of the incision in an attempt to grasp the FU. Owing to punch insertion angles, the incision depth is shallower at the superior aspect of the incision. Grafts often invert at this location by tethering to a nonscored attachment.

If the graft still cannot be located, make a small incision towards the superior aspect to create a larger exploratory opening. If after these steps visualization still eludes the surgeon, the graft should be left buried. Exact incidences of graft burial and graft recovery are not available; however, in a 40-patient and approximately 10,000-graft study, only two instances of buried grafts resulted in hair-bearing inflamed cysts requiring removal (Fig. 17.2).

## Indications for FUE

FUE is indicated in the following situations:

1. When even a very thin linear scar is unacceptable (i.e. in those who shave their head or wear their hair very short)

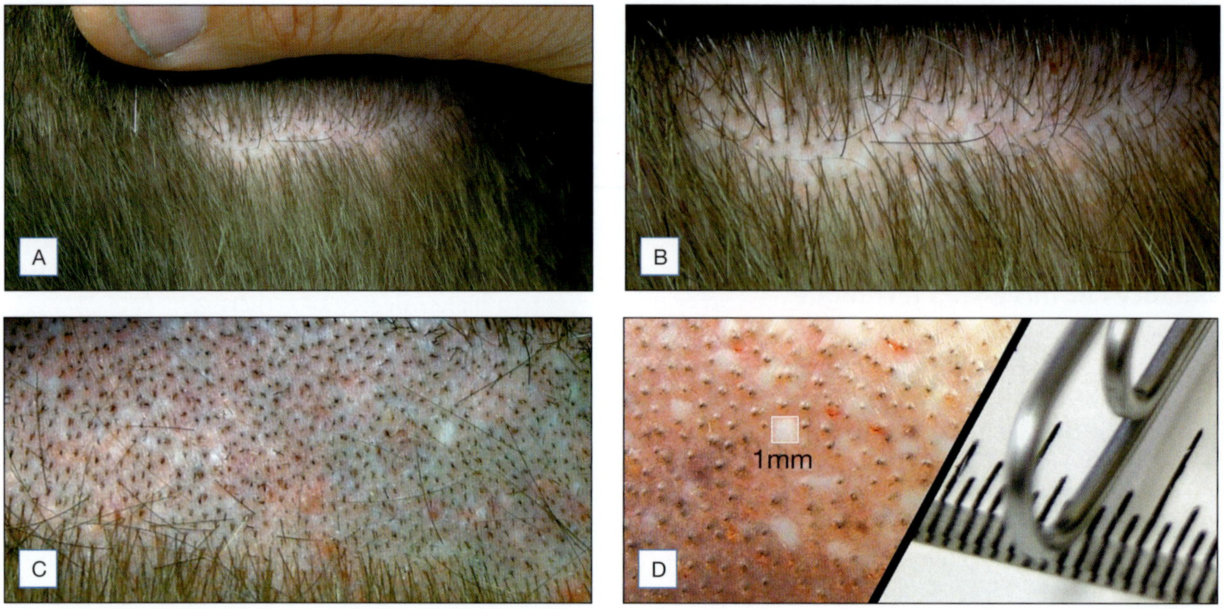


**Fig. 17.2** FOX procedure donor scarring: 1 year after ~1600 grafts in two sessions: (**A**) Normal view with natural short hair. (**B**) Up close with natural short hair. (**C**) Up close with clipped hair. (**D**) Extremely close with clipped hair

2. When a patient requests an FUE procedure and enough grafts can be harvested to meet his or her needs
3. In patients with limited hair loss or those who require small sessions. This group would include patients with male pattern hair loss in a Norwood Class 3 pattern or those with small vertex balding areas
4. For limited cosmetic areas, such as widow's peaks, eyebrows, eyelashes, mustaches
5. For limited areas of alopecia secondary to dermatologic conditions
6. In the treatment of widened scars resulting from traditional strip excisions
7. In patients without adequate laxity for a strip excision
8. For scarring from dermatologic conditions, trauma, or neurosurgical procedures
9. For individuals with heavily scarred donor areas making a linear incision problematic
10. In patients who tend to heal with wide or thickened linear scars
11. In athletes who must resume full activity soon after the procedure
12. For patients with an inordinate fear of pain or scars
13. When the body or beard serves as a donor area.

## Contraindications for FUE

Contraindications for FUE include:

1. Inexperience in performing FUE techniques
2. Unavailability of proper instrumentation
3. Inadequate and uninformed patient consent
4. Unrealistic patient expectations
5. Inadequate donor supply
6. Scarring that makes both the two- and three-step procedures problematic.

## Conclusion

FUE is an exciting advancement that propels the field of hair transplant surgery one step closer to the elite minimally invasive status. The promise of an almost scarless surgery is enticing to both patient and surgeon. For the surgeon who has to perform this tedious technique, there remain many vague issues ranging from ethical representations of patient results to practical realities of surgical indication. Training periods are extensive, risks of less than desirable results are high, and many technical problems have yet to be worked out.

FUE clearly has a valuable place in a growing number of hair transplant candidates. Although the techniques have improved, issues of patient

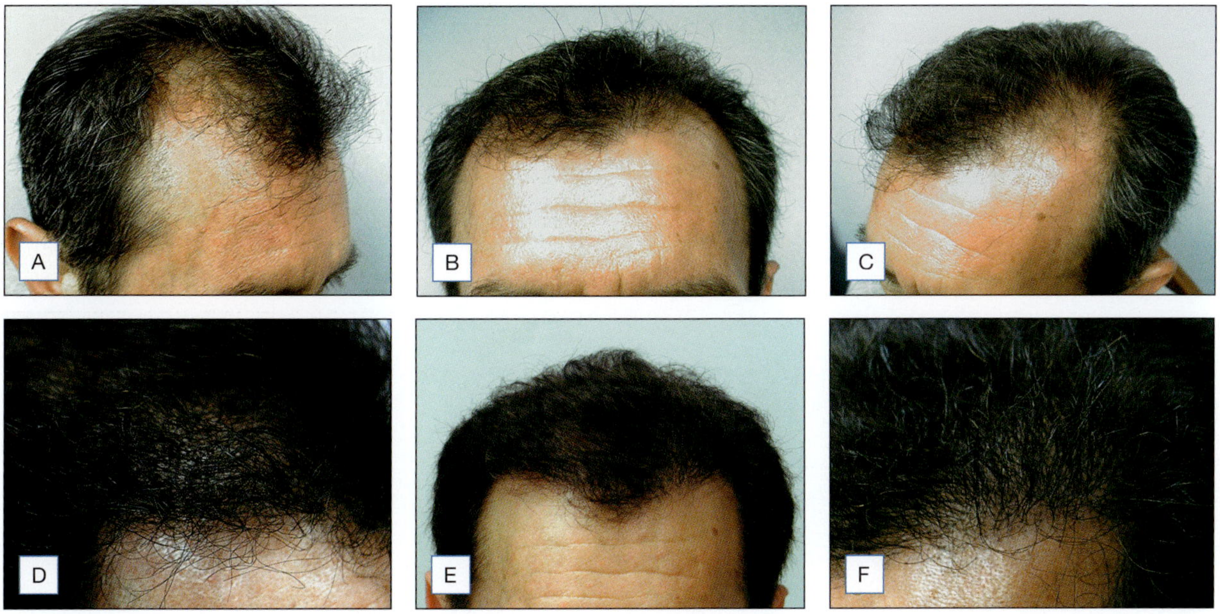


**Fig. 17.3** Results of FUE. (**A–C**) Pre surgery. (**D–F**) 19 months post surgery

selection, donor area healing by secondary intention after large sessions, and imbedded grafts still remain. The reasons for selecting FUE rather than a strip harvest may be the avoidance of a linear scar, the desire for a virtually pain-free recovery period, or simply the idea of having a minimally invasive procedure (Fig. 17.3).

## Further Reading

Bernstein RM, Rassman WR, Seager D, et al 1998 Standardizing the classification and description of follicular unit transplantation and mini-micrografting techniques. Dermatologic Surgery 24:957–963

Bernstein RM, Rassman WR, Szaniawski W, Halperin A 1995 Follicular transplantation. International Journal of Aesthetic Restorative Surgery 3:119–132

Bernstein RM, Rassman WR 1997 Follicular transplantation: patient evaluation and surgical planning. Dermatologic Surgery 23:771–784

Bernstein RM, Rassman WR 1997 The aesthetics of follicular transplantation. Dermatologic Surgery 23:785–799

Bernstein RM 1998 A neighbor's view of the 'follicular family unit.' Hair Transplant Forum International 8:23–25

Harris JA 2004 Follicular unit extraction: The SAFE System. Hair Transplant Forum International 14:157,163,164

Inaba M 1996 Androgenetic alopecia: modern concepts of pathogenesis and treatment. Springer-Verlag, Tokyo pp 238–245

Kim JC, Choi YC 1995 Regrowth of grafted human scalp hair after removal of the bulb. Dermatologic Surgery 21:312–313

Limmer BL 1994 Elliptical donor stereoscopically assisted micrografting as an approach to further refinement in hair transplantation. Dermatologic Surgery 20:789–793

Okuda S 1939 Clinical and experimental studies of transplantation of living hairs. Jpn Journal of Dermatologic Urology 46:135–138 [in Japanese]

Orentreich N 1959 Autografts in alopecias and other selected dermatological conditions. Annals of the New York Academy of Sciences 83:463–479

Rassman WR, Bernstein RM 2002 Follicular unit extraction. Minimally invasive surgery for hair transplantation. Dermatologic Surgery 28:720–728

Rassman WR, Carson S 1995 Micrografting in extensive quantities: the ideal hair restoration procedure. Dermatologic Surgery 21:306–311

Rassman WR, Bernstein RM 2002 Follicular unit extraction: Minimally invasive surgery for hair transplantation. Dermatologic Surgery 28:720–728

Sasagawa M 1930 Hair transplantation. Japanese Journal of Dermatology 30:493 [in Japanese]

# 18 Hair Transplantation in Women

*Marc R. Avram*

## Introduction

Tens of millions of women, representing 20–30% of all women in the United States suffer from female pattern hair loss (FPHL). Unlike men, hair loss in women has no social acceptance. All men would rather have their hair and millions seek medical and surgical options to correct hair loss, but bald men appear in movies, print ads and on the cover of magazines as the 'sexiest men alive.' Women with thin 'see through' hairlines often suffer in silence (Fig. 18.1). If a women expresses her distress to her primary doctor or husband their response is often dismissive. Too often physicians are unaware of the medical and surgical options available to treat FPHL. The majority of women with FPHL can be helped with a combination of medication and hair transplantation.

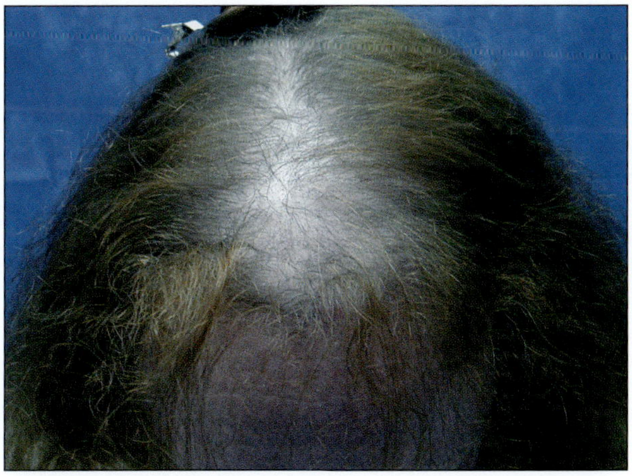

**Fig. 18.1** Telogen effluvium – diffuse thinning throughout scalp (not a surgical candidate)

## Medical Therapy and Hair Care

Minoxidil is the only FDA-approved medication to treat FPHL. The mechanism of action is unknown. The key to success with minoxidil is compliance and realistic expectation. It is important to emphasize maintenance over regrowth and to give the medication 6–8 months before judging its efficacy. If successful, it needs to be used long term except during pregnancy and breastfeeding. Many dermatologists report that topical minoxidil seems to show a more favorable response in women than men. Finasteride is contraindicated in women of childbearing years and has been shown to be ineffective in postmenopausal women. Many women with FPHL have accelerated loss from poor hair care. There should be minimal tension on hair follicles whether from tight braids, tightly pulled back hair or excessive chemical use in hair salons. A balanced diet is important for the entire body, including the hair on the scalp. If a patient reports poor diet habits, a multivitamin may be of benefit. Mega doses of vitamins are not helpful and may accelerate further hair loss.

## Surgical Therapy

From the 1960s into the late 1990s few women underwent hair transplantation. The diffuse nature of hair loss in women did not allow the creation of 2–4 mm recipient sites without a massive loss of existing hair follicles. Ironically, this limitation spared many women from the poor results many men received from 2–4 mm punch grafts.

The evolution away from 2–4 mm grafts to one to four hair follicular groupings has allowed women to benefit from hair transplantation.

Recipient sites measure in fractions of millimeters between existing hair follicles. Today the standard for men and women is consistently natural-appearing transplanted hair.

## Consultation

The success of any transplant begins with the consultation. The chief complaint of women with FPHL is the 'see through' appearance of the frontal hairline, which unlike in men is not socially accepted. A complete history and examination of the scalp are vital to confirm the diagnosis of FPHL before contemplating a hair transplant. If there are any questions on review of systems, a referral to endocrinology and/or gynecology is appropriate. The differential diagnosis of FPHL includes telogen effluvium, underlying hormonal imbalances, medications, poor diet, and diffuse alopecia areata. A scalp biopsy may be helpful in confirming a diagnosis for some patients.

The natural progression of FPHL needs to be reviewed during the consult. The net density from a transplant is the amount of hair follicles transplanted minus the number of hair follicles lost over the next 6–12 months. Minoxidil is the only FDA approved medication to maintain existing hair with FPHR and should be encouraged for all women undergoing a hair transplant. The majority of women undergoing transplantation use minoxidil. This allows the maximum density from the procedure.

A telogen effluvium from a hair transplant occurs in a minority of women. Women need to be aware before the procedure that they may have *less* hair 1–3 months after a procedure but after 6–12 months the lost hair will return with the transplanted hair resulting with a net *increase* in density. Women should also be aware that the transplanted hair will grow for as long as it was genetically programmed to grow. Over years or decades the donor density naturally thins in a majority of women and therefore the transplanted hair will slowly thin over years or decades.

## Procedure

To summarize, women: (1) have a more unpredictable donor region; (2) have an increased risk of postoperative effluvium; (3) often experience diffuse thinning with no bald regions; and (4) have relatively stable frontal hairlines. With stable hairlines and an increased risk of effluvium, placing the majority of one to four hair grafts in the frontal third of the scalp will address the 'see through' appearance of the frontal hairline while reducing the risk of effluvium. For those females with stable hairlines, the transplanted hair in the frontal third of the scalp should remain cosmetically appropriate indefinitely (Fig. 18.2).

## Procedural Differences

The preoperative care, instrumentation, anesthesia, donor harvesting, graft creation, recipient site creation and postoperative care are the same for men and women. Magnification to separate follicular groupings from a donor strip has been advocated for years, but there has been little or no emphasis on magnification when creating recipient sites. Women usually have existing hair that will never be lost in the recipient region. Magnification allows easier creation of recipient sites between existing hair follicles without damage to them (Fig. 18.3).

## Transplanting Scar Tissue

After FPHL the next most common reason for hair transplantation in women is to correct lost temporoparietal hairlines from face lifts. The chief complaint is the patient's inability to pull their hair back. A large number of one to four hair grafts at the natural angle of hair in the temporoparietal scalp will make a substantial difference for women (Fig. 18.4). Hair can also be transplanted to correct traction alopecia and inactive inflammatory scalp disorders with high patient satisfaction.

## Conclusion

Millions of women with thinning hair can be helped with medication and hair transplantation. A large number of one to four hair follicular groupings transplanted between existing hair follicles will create a natural increase in density for women.

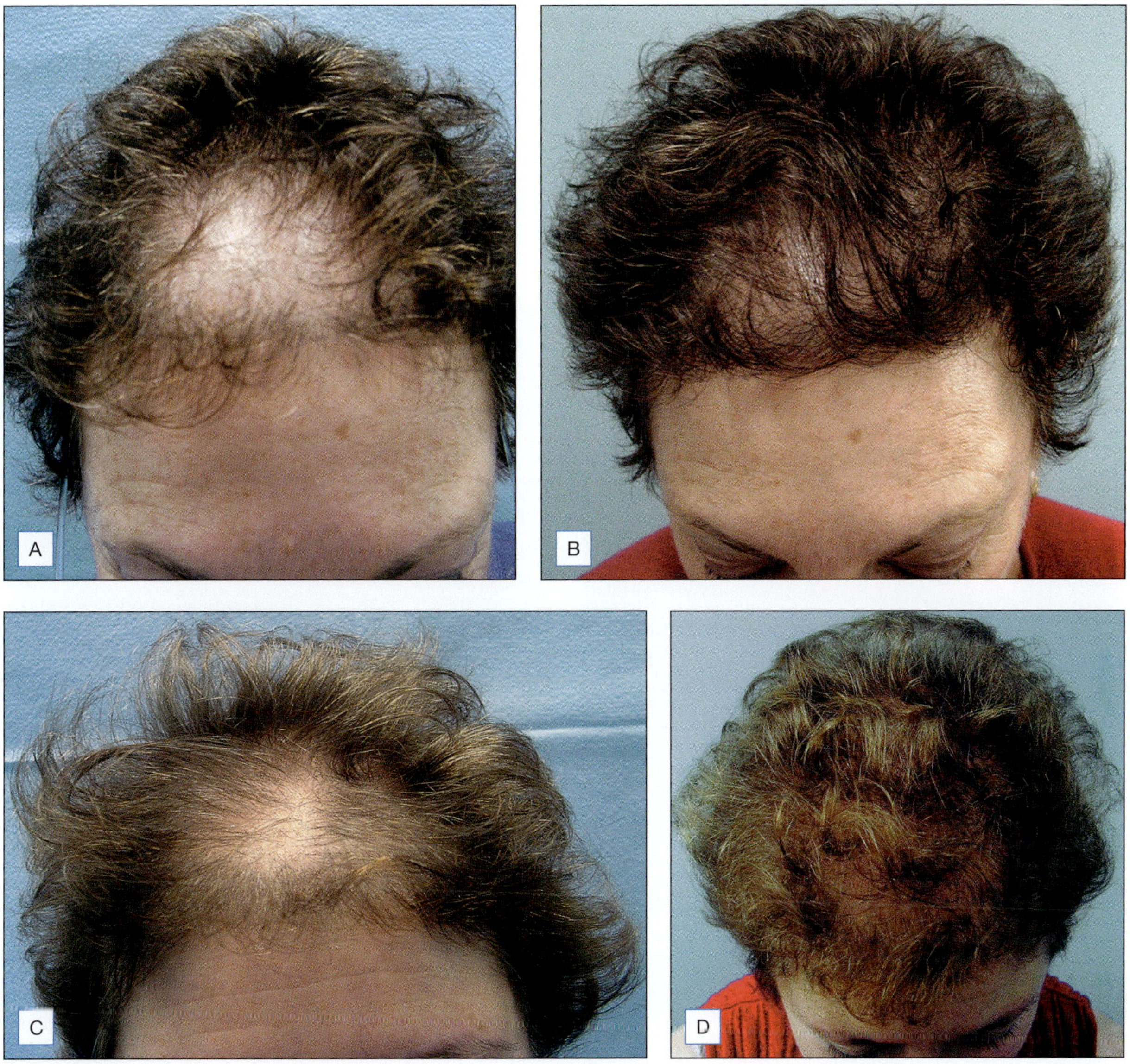


**Fig. 18.2** (**A**) Ludwig II before surgery. (**B**) After 850 grafts. (**C**) Ludwing II before surgery. (**D**) After 600 one to three hair grafts

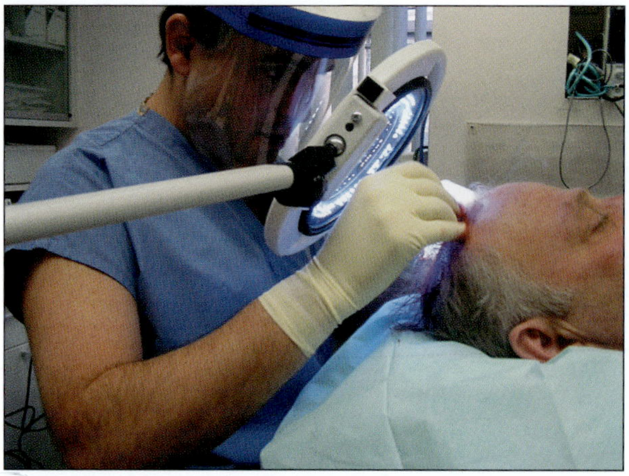

Fig. 18.3 Site creation using LED polarized magnification

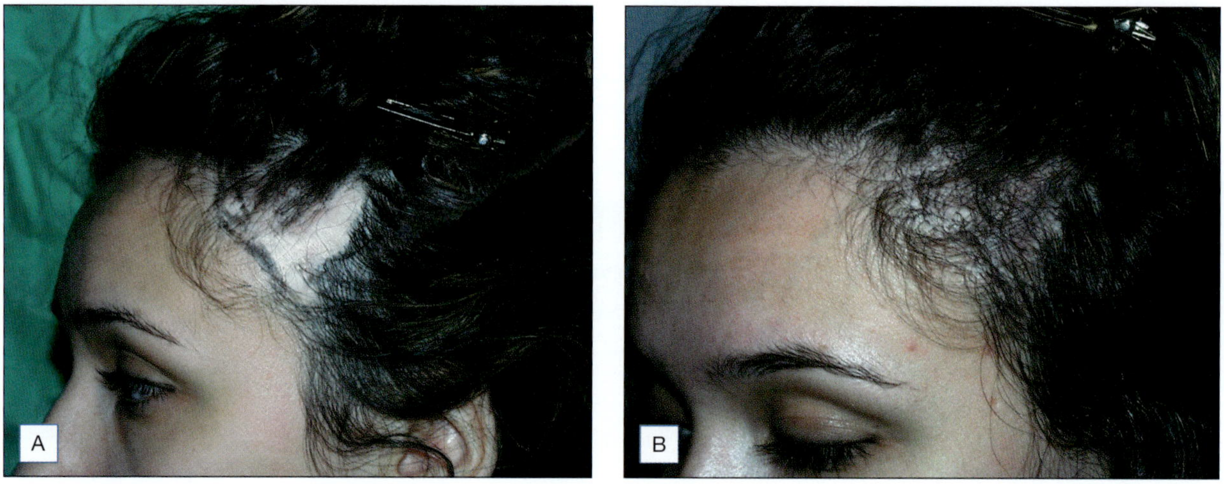

Fig. 18.4 (A) Scar after removal of tumor. (B) After 650 one two three hair grafts

## Further Reading


Avram MR 1999 Hair transplantation in women. Seminars in Cutaneous Medical Surgery 18:172–176

Avram MR, Cole JP, Gandelman M, et al 2002 The potential role of minoxidil in the hair transplantation setting. Dermatologic Surgery 28:894–900

Cash TF, Price VH, Savin RC 1993 Psychological affects of androgenetic alopecia on women. Journal of the American Academy of Dermatology 29:568–575

Epstein JS 2003 Follicular unit hair grafting – state of the art technique. Archives of Facial Plastic Surgery 5:121–126

Leavitt M 2004 Women and hair loss: A physician's perspective. Beautiful Media, Atlanta

Limmer B 1999 Elliptical donor stereoscopically assisted micrografts as an approach to further refinement in hair transplantation. Dermatologic Surgical Oncology 20:789–793

Lucky AW, Piacquadio DJ, Ditre CM et al 2004 A randomized placebo controlled trial of 5% and 2% topical minoxidil solutions in the treatment of female pattern hair loss. Journal of the American Academy of Dermatology 50:541–553

Olsen EA, Messenger AG, Shapiro J, Bergfeld WF, et al 2005 Evaluation and treatment of male and female pattern hair loss. Journal of the American Academy of Dermatology 47:795; 52:301–311

Olsen EA, Hordinsky M, Roberts JL, Whiting DA 2002 Dermatologic Consortium for Women's Health. Female pattern hair loss. Journal of the American Academy of Dermatology 47:795

Price VH, Roberts JL, Hordinsky M et al 2000 Lack of efficacy of finasteride in post-menopausal women with androgenetic alopecia. Journal of the American Academy of Dermatology 25:637–642

# 19 Hair Transplantation in Blacks

*Jerry E. Cooley*

## Introduction

The approach to hair transplantation in Blacks involves special considerations. This approach is based on differences in hair characteristics, types of alopecias, and possible complications compared to Caucasians. These differences effect the pre-operative evaluation as well as the surgical techniques used in these patients. While it is becoming increasingly more common to see patients who have a mixed or multiracial background, this discussion refers to patients whose characteristics are more Black than Caucasian, recognizing that it is a spectrum.

## Pre-operative Considerations

Alopecia is a common problem among Blacks. Typical male and female pattern hair loss presents as a nonscarring alopecia in a patterned distribution. Further hair loss can be slowed or halted with oral finasteride, which is approved for use in men, and topical minoxidil. In addition to pattern hair loss, other types of alopecias frequently occur in Blacks.

Traction alopecia results from long-term hairstyles (e.g. braids) in which chronic traction on the hair follicle results in permanent hair loss. The effect of these hairstyles should be discussed with the patient and discouraged.

Central centrifugal cicatricial alopecia (CCCA) is a type of scarring alopecia that may occur in all races and either gender, but is seen mostly in Black women. Clinically, it appears as hair loss in the central vertex that spreads outwards in all directions if it is not treated. In the past, it was sometimes referred to as 'hot comb alopecia' or 'follicular degeneration syndrome' before the current name was widely accepted. During the active stage, treatment for CCCA consists of intralesional or topical steroids. Hair transplantation is an appropriate option for CCCA when it is no longer active.

Styling and grooming practices are an important consideration in this group of patients. Seborrheic dermatitis may be more common in Blacks, possibly because of less frequent shampooing compared to Caucasians. Antidandruff shampoos that do not dry the hair (e.g. zinc pyrithione) are preferred over other types (e.g. tar, salicylic acid). Topical steroids are effective but the vehicle should be cosmetically acceptable to the patient. An ultrapotent steroid (e.g. clobetasol) can be used for several days to clear seborrheic dermatitis. A foam vehicle is generally preferred by patients over that of a gel, cream, or ointment. Patients are cautioned that these products should be used only for a limited time due to the adverse effects of chronic daily steroid use. Many dermatologists recommend that these products not be used for more than 7–10 days per month. Alternatively, a lower potency steroid (e.g. fluocinolone oil) may be used more regularly and has less risk, but takes longer to work.

In addition to properly diagnosing the type of alopecia and evaluating grooming and styling practices, another key pre-operative consideration is healing characteristics. Black patients may have a tendency to hyper- or hypopigment following trauma to the skin, which may be a problem if a hair transplant is performed.

Keloid formation appears to be an uncommon but important risk in Black patients (Fig. 19.1). Experienced surgeons have noted the rarity of this complication in the era of mini-/micrografting and follicular unit transplantation (FUT). If a patient does have a history of keloids elsewhere on the body, the surgeon is advised to perform a few test grafts in the scalp to see if they are likely to occur after a full hair transplant. The risk of keloid

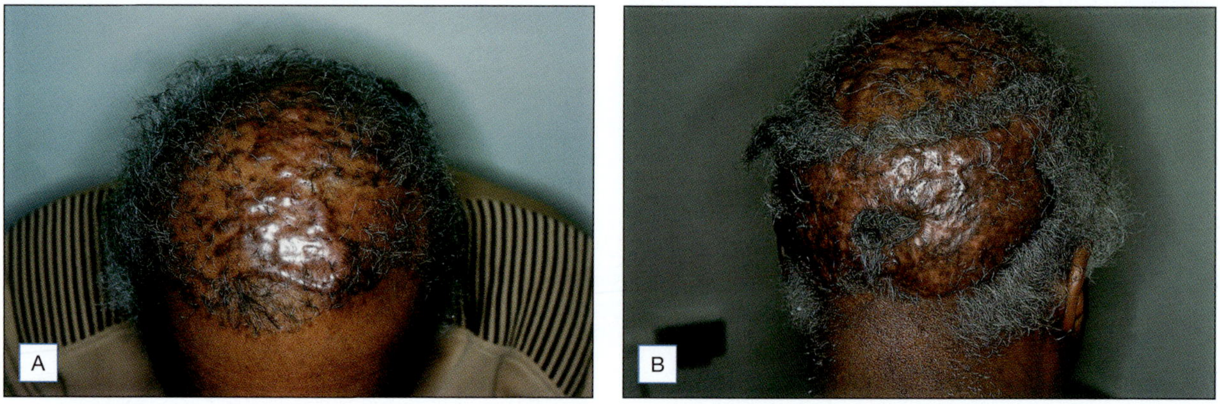

Fig. 19.1 (A) Severe keloid formation in the donor area after hair transplantation. (B) Keloid formation in the recipient area after hair transplantation. (Reproduced from Stough D, Haber RS 1996 Hair replacement: Surgical and medical. Mosby Year Book Publishing Company, St Louis. Fig 10.45, p 324, with permission. Courtesy of Dr Marc D. Brown)

formation in these patients should be fully discussed as part of the consent process.

Differences in hair characteristics are an important factor when considering hair transplantation in Blacks. The density of hair in the donor area is lower, generally about 170 hairs/cm$^2$ in Blacks, compared to about 230/cm$^2$ in Caucasians, although there is wide variation within the races. In terms of follicular units (FUs), Blacks have about 60 FUs/cm$^2$, compared to an average of 100/cm$^2$ in Caucasians. For a typical FUT procedure in which a 10 cm strip is removed, about 600 grafts can be created in the Black patient, compared to 1000 grafts for the Caucasian. The average number of hairs/mm$^2$ in Blacks is 1.6, compared to 2.0 in Caucasians. The average hair diameter in Blacks (60–65 μm) is also less than Caucasians (70–75 μm), but there is greater variation in this population, with some having diameters up to 85 μm. Unlike the hair shaft, which is oval, the Black Caucasian hair shaft has an elliptical shape (Table 19.1). The lower hair density in Blacks is offset by the curlier, elliptical hair shaft, which provides greater cosmetic coverage compared to that of Caucasians (Fig. 19.2).

Variations in hair characteristics among races

| Factor | Caucasian | Asian | Black |
|---|---|---|---|
| Hair shape | Wavy | Straight | Curly |
| Hair cross-section | Oval | Round | Elliptical |
| Hair diameter (average) | 70 μm | 80 μm | 60 μm |
| FU/mm$^2$ (average) | 1.0 | 1.0 | 0.6 |
| FU/cm$^2$ (average) | 100 | 100 | 60 |
| Hairs/mm$^2$ (average) | 2.0 | 1.7 | 1.6 |

Table 19.1 Variations in hair characteristics among races

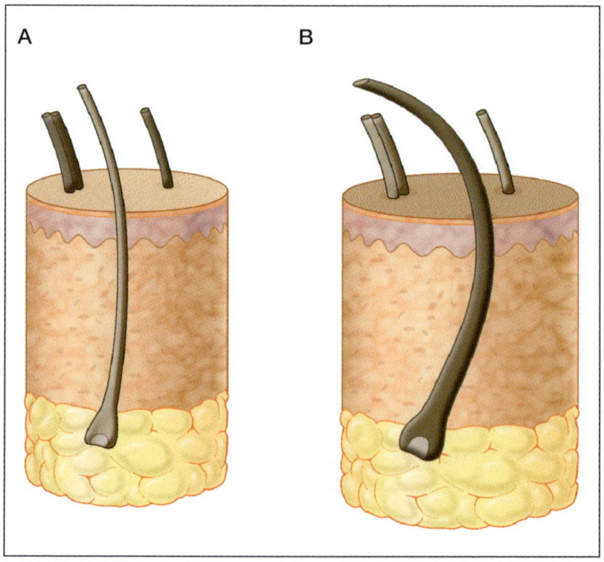


Fig. 19.2 (A and B) Schematic representation of Caucasian hair vs. Black hair characteristics. The Black hair is generally more elliptical and curlier than the Caucasian hair

## Operative considerations

The hairline in a Black male may be drawn in a flatter configuration compared to that drawn for a Caucasian male (Fig. 19.3), depending on the preference of the patient. Expert surgeons usually remove the donor tissue as a single strip excised with a single blade. The skin is first infiltrated with a generous amount of tumescent anesthetic solution

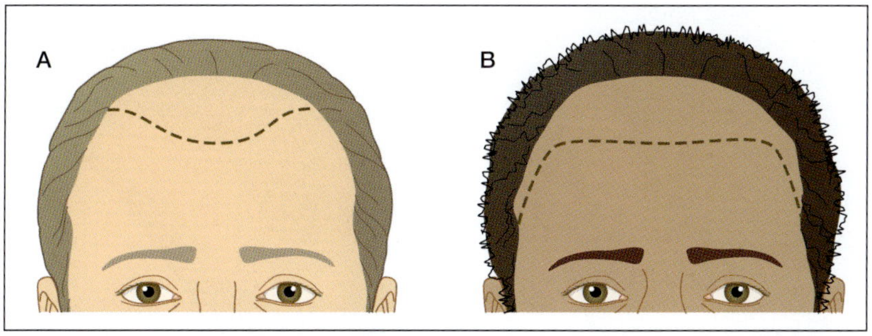


**Fig. 19.3** (**A** and **B**) Hairline design in Black patients. The hairline may be restored in a flatter shape compared to what is recommended for most Caucasian patients

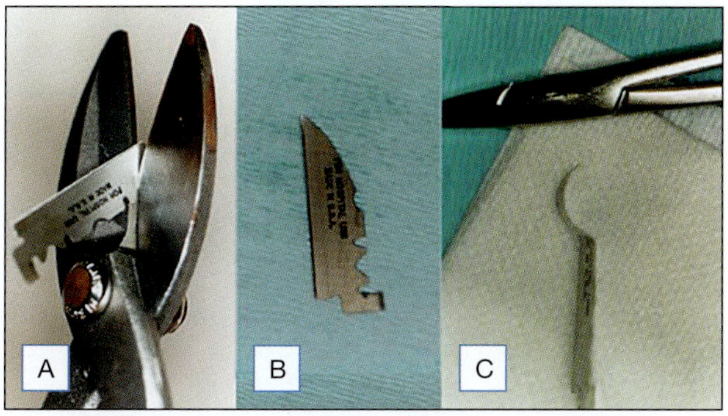


**Fig. 19.4** Making and use of a curved blade for donor harvesting. A surgical razor blade may be cut into a scalpel shape using wire snips (**A, B**). It is then bent using a needle holder to create a C-shaped blade (**C**). Alternatively, a flexible No. 15 blade may be bent using a needle holder.

**Operative considerations in Black patients**

- The hairline can be designed flatter than usual
- Excise the strip with a single blade technique
- Utilize a curved blade to match the curved hair follicle
- Use blunt dissection to minimize transection
- Close with minimal or no tension to avoid keloid formation
- Consider using more MFUs

**Box 19.1** Operative considerations in Black patients

to create firm turgor. Many surgeons including the author find it helpful to create a curved blade to match the curve of the hair follicle. This can be accomplished by bending a flexible No. 15 scalpel blade (Personna Plus, American Safety Razor Co., Staunton, VA) with a needle holder. Alternatively, a sterile razor blade can be custom made using wire snips and a needle holder (Fig. 19.4). Another approach is to use a standard scalpel, but limit the blade cuts to about 2 mm into the dermis, followed by blunt dissection using a needle holder or scissors (Box 19.1).

Regardless of the technique used, the blade is moved through the skin carefully, stopping frequently to visualize the edge of the strip and ensure that follicles are not being transected. The width of the strip should be such that the defect can be closed with minimal tension to avoid scarring and keloid formation (Fig. 19.5). A nondissolving suture is favored to ensure predictable healing.

Controversy exists over which method of grafting to use: multi follicular unit (MFU) grafts or pure follicular unit grafting. Some favor the former because of the difficulty in closely trimming FUs and because MFUs usually do not produce a tufty or 'pluggy' look because of the extreme curliness of the hair. Others, the author included, favor FU grafting (FUG) in which all grafts are created under the stereomicroscope (Fig. 19.6). Because of the decreased hair density, MFUs often contain more skin than hair in Black patients, requiring larger incisions. Well-trimmed two- and three-hair FUs can be placed at a density of about 20/cm$^2$ with excellent results in a single procedure. However, if the surgeon is not experienced at FUT or does not have the appropriate staff of trained assistants who can dissect grafts under the stereomicroscope, MFU grafting can be a viable approach. MFU grafting can be especially efficient at covering large areas and are less useful for creating a densely packed, 'single-pass' hairline.

Certain difficulties can arise more commonly when transplanting Black patients. Experienced surgeons note more bleeding and popping of grafts. Some find it useful to make a limited number of incisions, place the grafts into them, and then make another round of incisions. It is especially important when doing FUT in Blacks to test the fit between graft and incision site early in the procedure to make sure that the size and depth of incisions is appropriate. Some have tried to make curved incision

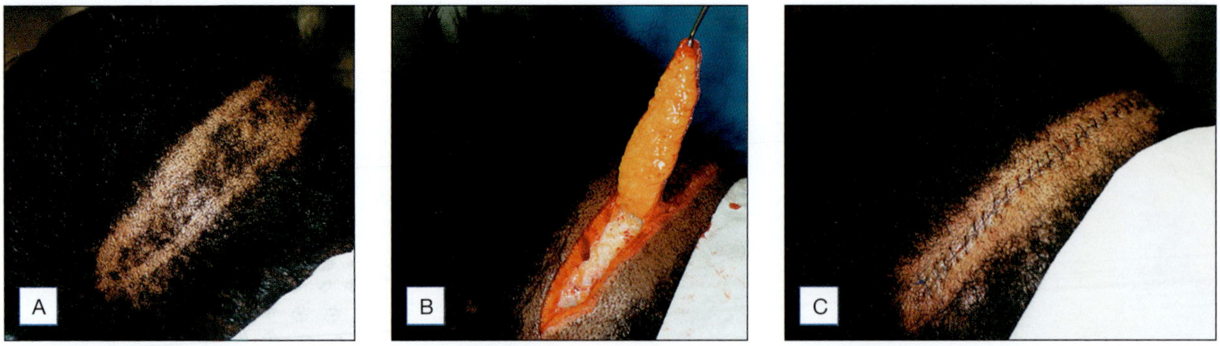


**Fig. 19.5** (**A–C**) Removal and closure of donor area. The width of the strip should be narrow enough to allow the wound to be easily closed and sutured without tension. Nondissolving sutures are recommended

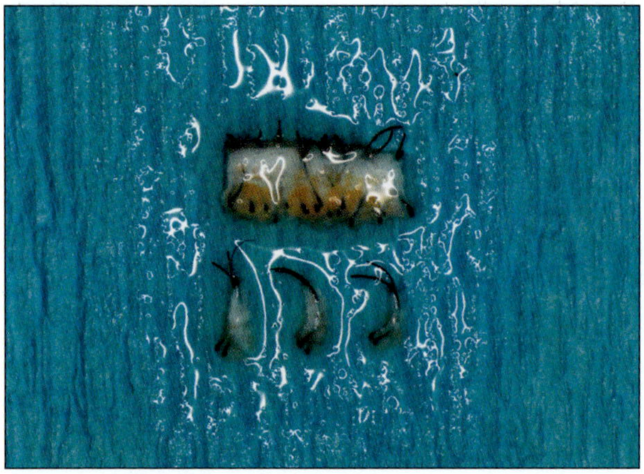

**Fig. 19.6** FUGs created with a stereomicroscope. The first step involves creating thin vertical 'slivers' from the donor strip. The individual FUs are then dissected to remove excess tissue

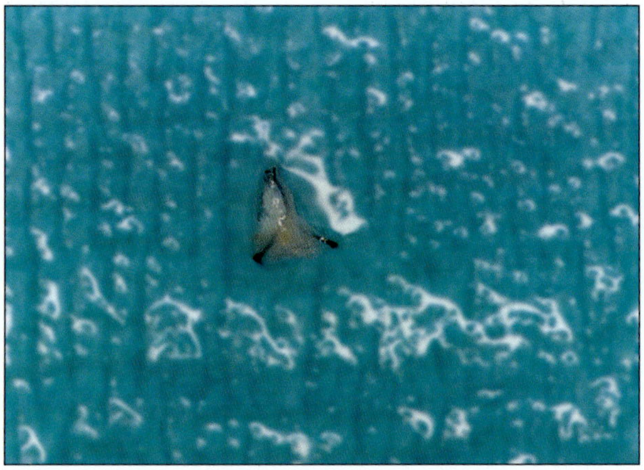

**Fig. 19.7** In some cases, splaying of the bulbs will occur with the grafts. This makes dissection and placement significantly more difficult

sites to match the curl of the hair, but this has not been widely adopted. In addition, some grafts when trimmed will splay out at the bottom, which makes placement extremely difficult (Fig. 19.7).

Excellent results can be obtained in most patients (Figs 19.8–19.10). If pattern hair loss is the underlying cause, patients must be counseled to continue their medical regimen (e.g. finasteride, minoxidil) to avoid further hair loss. Patients with CCCA must be aware of the possibility of recurrences and the need for medical treatment to avoid loss of the grafts to the inflammatory process. In the author's practice, these patients continue to use a once-weekly topical steroid to prevent future recurrences, even if the hair loss has stopped.

## Conclusion

Hair transplantation in the Black patient requires attention to the characteristic features of this population. Assuming that these issues have been taken into consideration and that proper technique is used, excellent results can be expected in the majority of cases.

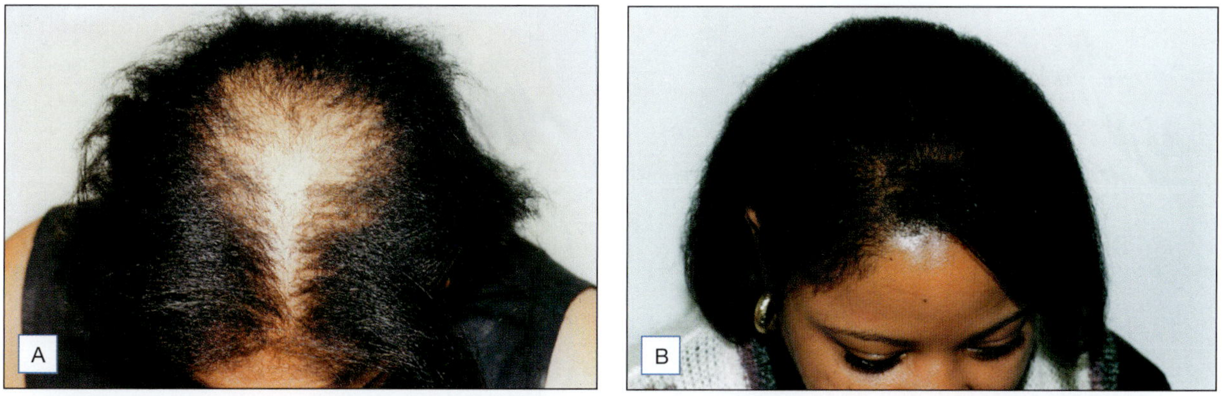


**Fig. 19.8** (**A** and **B**) Before and after MFU grafting hair transplantation procedures. This 34-year-old woman with inactive CCCA underwent two sessions of MFU grafts, with approximately 400 grafts per session

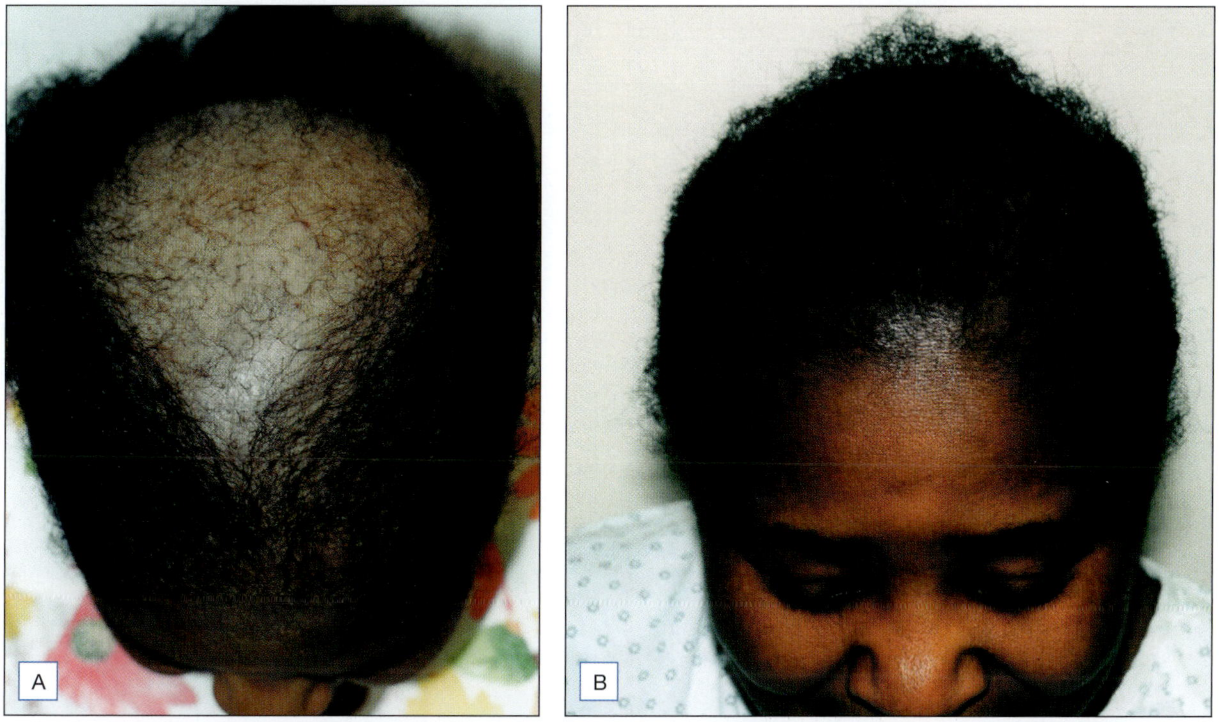


**Fig. 19.9** (**A** and **B**) Before and after FU hair transplantation. This 62-year-old woman had extensive scarring alopecia from burned-out CCCA. She underwent a single procedure of approximately 1000 one- to three-hair FUs. Although another procedure was recommended to improve density, the patient was very pleased with the improvement

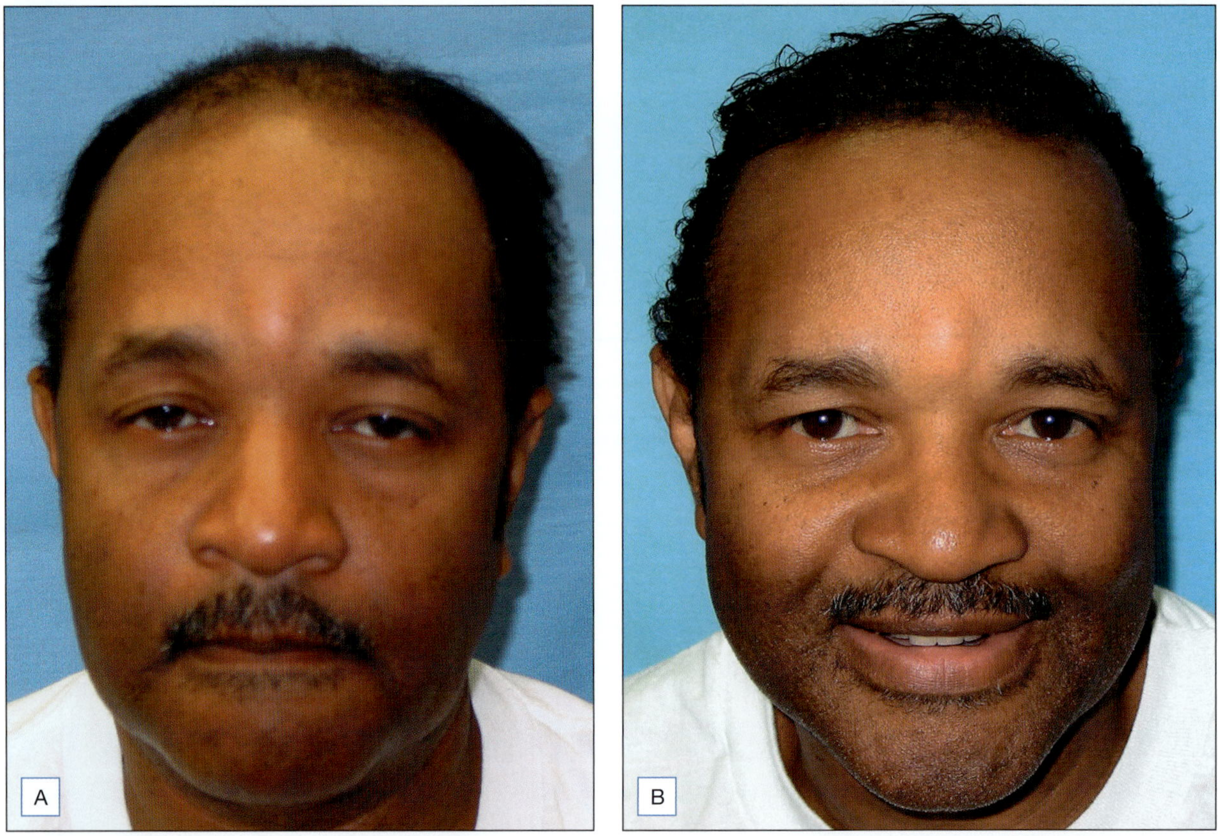


**Fig. 19.10** (**A** and **B**) Before and after FU hair transplantation. This 57-year-old man with androgenetic alopecia underwent a single procedure of 1500 FUGs to restore the frontal scalp. The flatter hairline, which appears natural in these patients, is demonstrated. (Photo courtesy of Dr William L. Parsley)

## Further Reading


Bernstein RM 1997 The aesthetics of follicular unit transplantation. Dermatologic Surgery 23:785–799

Callender VD, McMichael AJ, Cohen GF 2004 Medical and surgical therapies for alopecias in Black women. Dermatologic Therapy 17:164–178

Loussouarn G 2001 African hair growth parameters. British Journal of Dermatology 145:294–297

Holloway VL, Halder RM 2003 Ethnic hair and skin: What is the state of the science? Journal of the American Academy of Dermatology 48(6 Suppl)

Mayer ML 2004 Hair restoration in Black patients. In: Unger WP, Shapiro R (eds) Hair transplantation. 4th edn. Marcel Dekker, New York

Randall JK, Stough DB 1996 Hair restoration in Blacks. In: Stough DB, Haber RS (eds) Hair replacement: Surgical and medical. Mosby, St Louis

Sperling LC 1999 Hair density in African-Americans. Archives of Dermatology 135:656–658

# 20 Hair Transplantation in Asians

*Damkerng Pathomvanich*

## Introduction

Hair transplantation in the Asian population is increasing in popularity, but is associated with unique demands. Techniques include procedures and devices used elsewhere in the world, and include scalp flaps, the use of single and multifollicular unit grafts, Choi needle implanters, as well as various blades and needles. It is important to understand the Asian culture before performing hair transplantation surgery in this population.

In a study performed by the author, the incidence of male pattern hair loss in Asians was found to be similar to that of Caucasians (Fig. 20.1). This is in contrast to an earlier study by Takashima, which showed the incidence of male pattern hair loss (MPHL) in Asians to be one quarter that of Caucasians.

## Asian Features

### Anatomy

The Asian skull has less frontal and occipital projection than the more oblong Caucasian skull and therefore appears more round (Fig. 20.2). The Asian face also appears more round, posing a special challenge for hairline design.

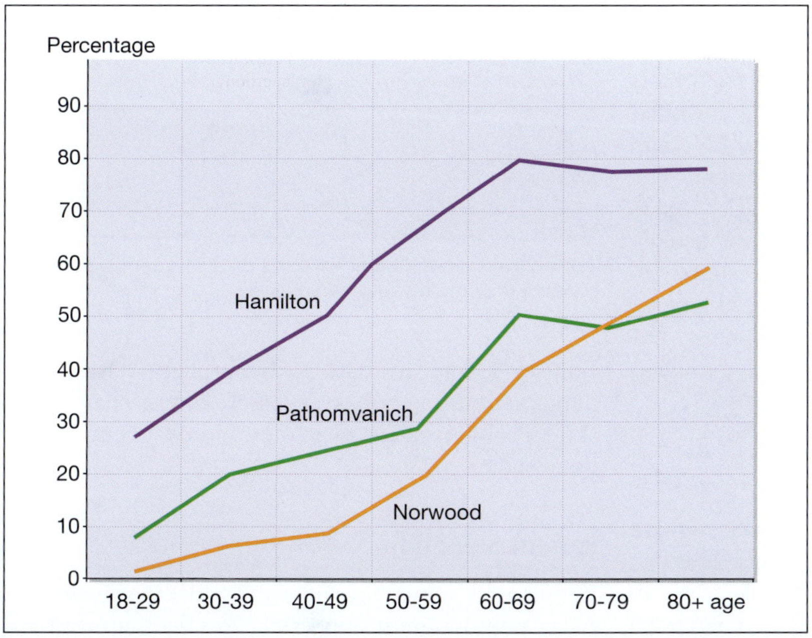


**Fig. 20.1** Comparison class IV–VII between Hamilton, Norwood and Pathomvanich

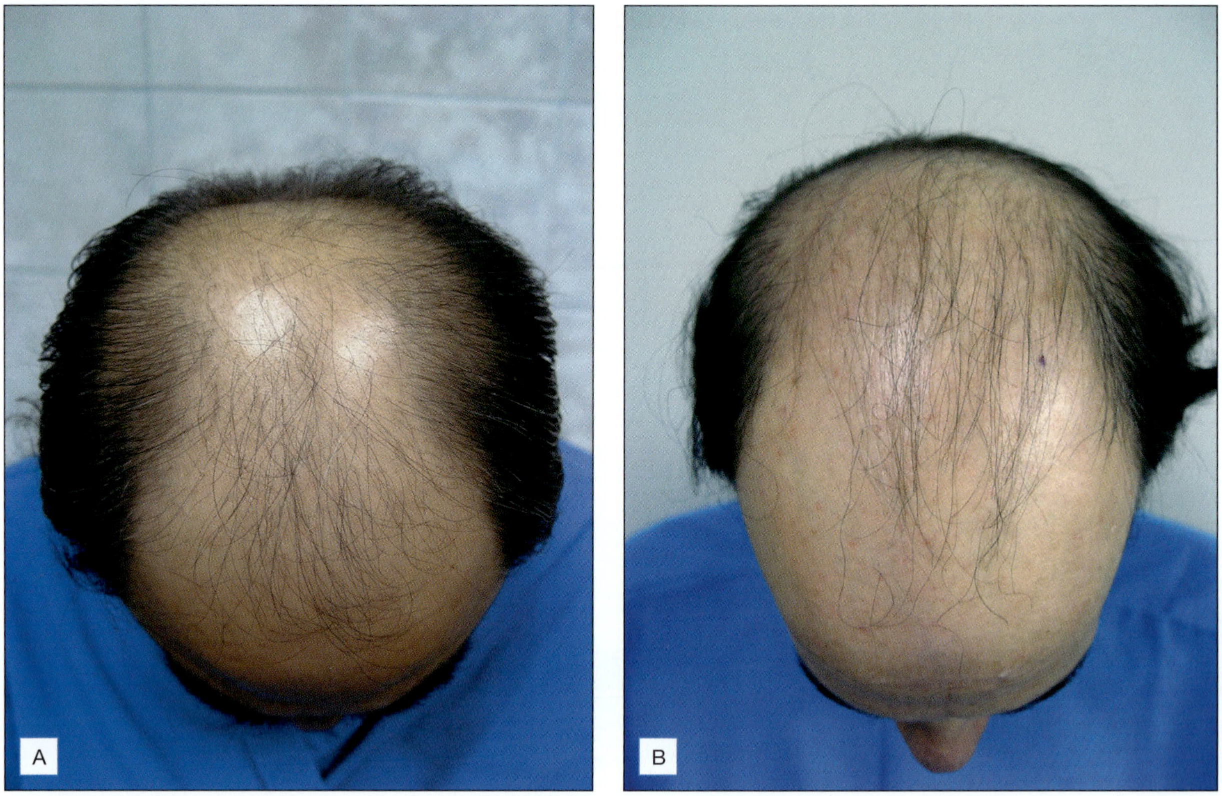

**Fig. 20.2** The Asian skull (**A**) has less frontal and occipital projection than the more oblong Caucasian skull (**B**) and the former therefore appears more round

## Hair

At the mid occiput, Asians have 90 FU/cm$^2$ or 170 hairs/cm$^2$, while in the parietal zone, they have 70 FU/cm$^2$ or 127 hairs/cm$^2$. This represents 1.8 hairs per follicular unit (FU). Caucasians have a similar density of FUs, but have 2.3 hairs per FU, and therefore a greater total number of hairs. The distribution of FU size is shown in Table 20.1. Asian hairs are coarse, of large caliber, and are usually straight. Studies of donor zone hair shafts in androgenetic alopecia revealed an average diameter of 71 µ, and a range of 63–79 µ. In Asians, the follicle length from epidermis to dermal papilla is 5.5 mm compared to 4.5 mm in Caucasians.

Distribution of follicular units in a series of 30 patients undergoing strip harvesting

| Number of hairs/FU | % |
|---|---|
| 1-hair FUs | 23.65 |
| 2-hair FUs | 63.83 |
| 3-hair FUs | 12.52 |
| 4-hair FUs | 0–1 |

**Table 20.1** Distribution of follicular units in a series of 30 patients undergoing strip harvesting

## Scarring

Asians often have black hair and white skin, which creates a contrast rarely seen in Caucasians. This can become a concern in individuals with wide scars. In addition, Asian skin is more prone than Caucasian skin to keloid formation, hyperpigmentation and depigmentation, but to a lesser extent than Black skin. Problem scars most commonly occur at the donor site.

## Patient Selection

Keeping in mind the inherent differences in the Asian population, it is possible to select appropriate surgical candidates. It is important to assess the likelihood of keloid formation by history and examination, but no test grafts are required. The high contrast between skin and hair is overcome with the exclusive use of FU grafts and by carefully selecting only the finest single hairs for transplanting the frontal hairline.

For patients with Norwood Class VII hair loss, a frontal forelock design with a connection to the temple zone will produce a cosmetically pleasing result in selected patients. True isolated frontal forelocks are not well accepted by the majority of Asians.

Asian hairlines are somewhat different from Caucasian hairlines in that the frontal projection of the hairline from a line joining both frontotemporal angles is shorter. Placing the hairline too high will leave no projection and produce a straight hairline. Most Asians desire a more rounded frontotemporal angle (Fig. 20.3).

Since the procedure can last 3–8 hours, some patients request more sedation during the procedure. As hair transplantation can now be completed in a few sessions with excellent results, scalp reductions and scalp flaps have fallen out of favor (Figs 20.4 and 20.5).

## Medical Management

Medical treatment is as important as surgical treatment, finasteride and minoxidil are routinely prescribed.

## The Consultation

In addition to a thorough discussion of the procedure, obtaining a family history of hair loss, medical illnesses, prior surgeries and complications, current medications, allergies, and a history of smoking, drinking, and abnormal bleeding are essential during the consultation. A routine check of blood pressures will identify several patients each year who require referral to an internist for evaluation.

## Donor Area

### Evaluation

To determine the amount of donor material required, the hair count is first measured under magnification, and expressed as follicular unit/$cm^2$ (Fig. 20.6A). The bald area is then directly measured using the Chang method (Fig. 20.6B; see also Chapters 13, p. 99). For a given desired recipient site density, the donor strip length is determined by the formula:

$$B \times \text{Proposed density}/cm^2 \div A$$

In high-risk patients, a heparin lock access is placed pre-operatively. This will prove useful if excessive bleeding or a vasovagal episode occurs and IV fluid replacement is needed.

## Donor Strip Dissection

The author has developed a method of donor strip removal that minimizes transection. While this method of removal is more time consuming, it is proven to be advantageous in minimizing transection along the superior and inferior borders. The donor strip is marked and anesthetized, then tumescent fluid is injected. A No. 10 blade is used to score the epidermis to a depth between 1 and 2 mm. Skin hooks are inserted inside the incision, roughly 1.5 cm apart. The tip of a No. 15 blade is then used to cut between the FUs from the epidermal portion to the dermal papilla while an assistant provides upward and outward traction (Fig. 20.7).

If high hair density is encountered or the follicles appear to interlock, the initial dissection should be carried only to the lower dermis for a short distance. During a second pass for further dissection with the skin hooks, the incision will be separated without transection (Dow Stough, personal communication). Tension must be maintained by the skin hooks to accomplish this separation. The operative area must be clear and dry to visualize the follicles, otherwise the risk of follicular transection is increased. The skin hooks are then advanced each 1–2 cm and dissection continues in the same fashion until 7 cm are fully dissected along both incisions. This portion of the strip is then removed. Strip dissection into slivers and FUs is then carried out under 10× magnification utilizing a video image on a monitor screen (Fig. 20.8).

The remaining portion of the strip is dissected, then the incision is closed with 4-0 running Vicryl Rapide sutures. A two-layer closure may be required for tight skin or subsequent sessions as described by Gerard Seery.

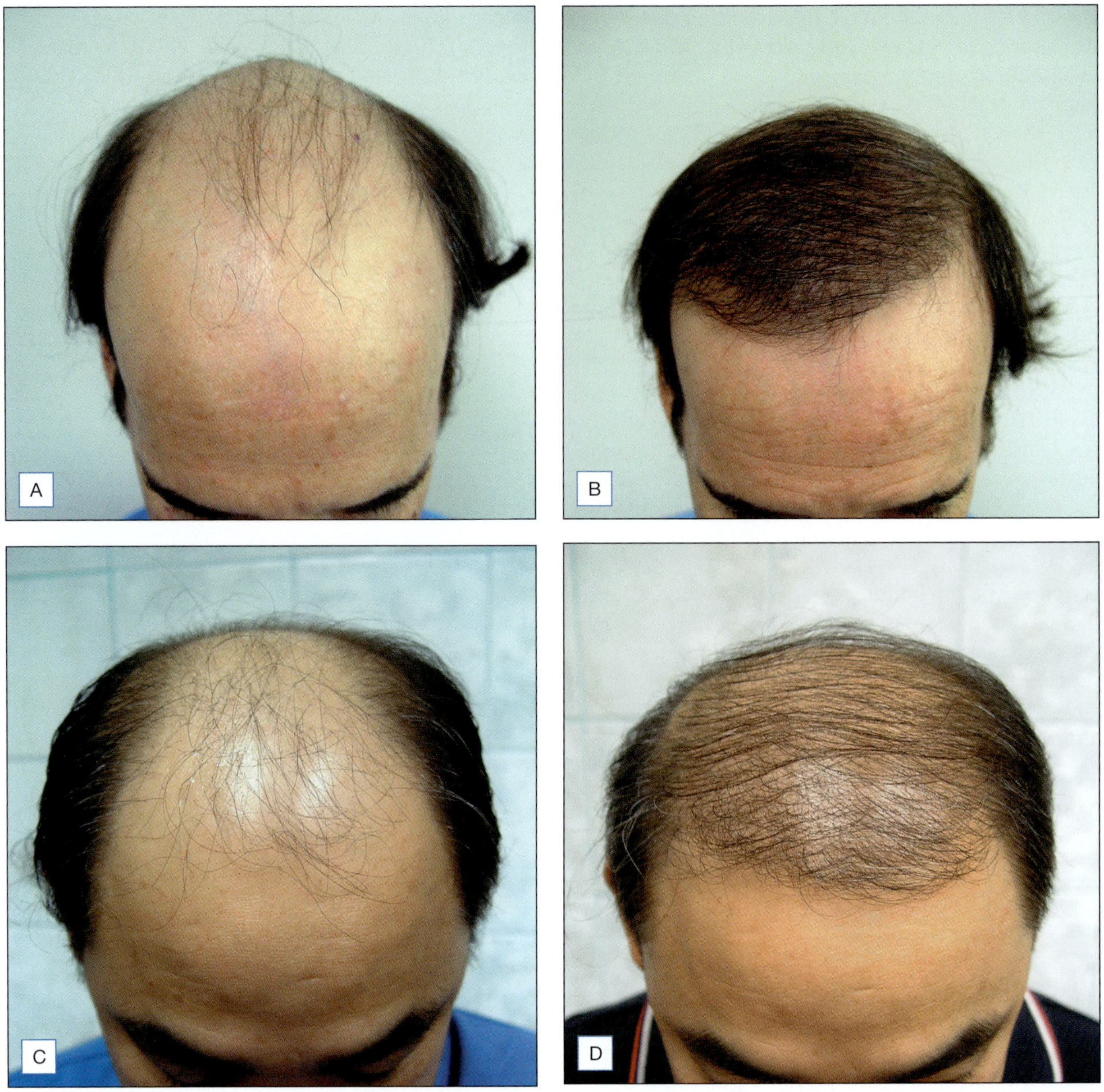


**Fig. 20.3** Comparison between Causasian (**A** and **B**) and Asian (**C** and **D**) hairlines. Note the more rounded frontotemporal angle in the Asian hairline

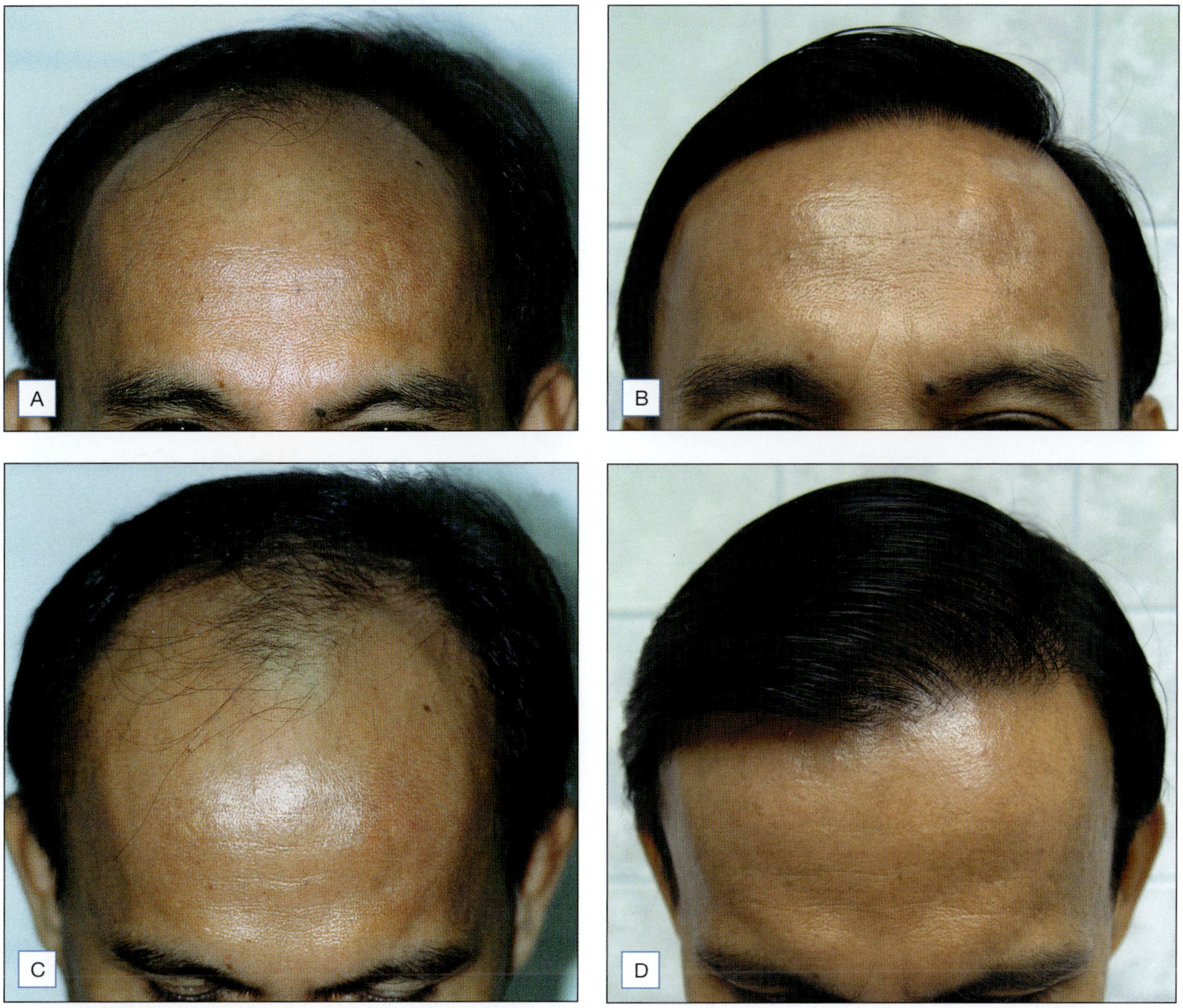


**Fig. 20.4** Before (**A** and **C**) and after (**B** and **D**) three sessions (5099 FUGs)

## Recipient Site

Supraorbital nerve blocks are useful, especially in megasessions. Ring blocks are also used. Most recipient site incisions are pre-made. At the end of the case, excess grafts are planted utilizing the 'stick and place' method. Single hair grafts are placed into 20 and 21 gauge needle sites in perpendicular orientation. Two-hair FUs are placed into 19 and 20 gauge needle sites, and three-hair FUs are placed into 19 or 18 gauge needle sites in a parallel orientation.

At the temple all perpendicular incisions are made with a flat angle. A headband is applied and maintained for a minimum of 2–4 days to prevent swelling. The patient returns to the clinic the following day for shampooing and wound care. The interval between sessions will be a minimum of 6 months.

## Complications

Other than an increased but rare risk of keloids and wide donor scars, complications are very rare and are the same as in Caucasian patients.

## Conclusion

Hair transplantation in Asians can produce results as good as those in Caucasians in spite of the high

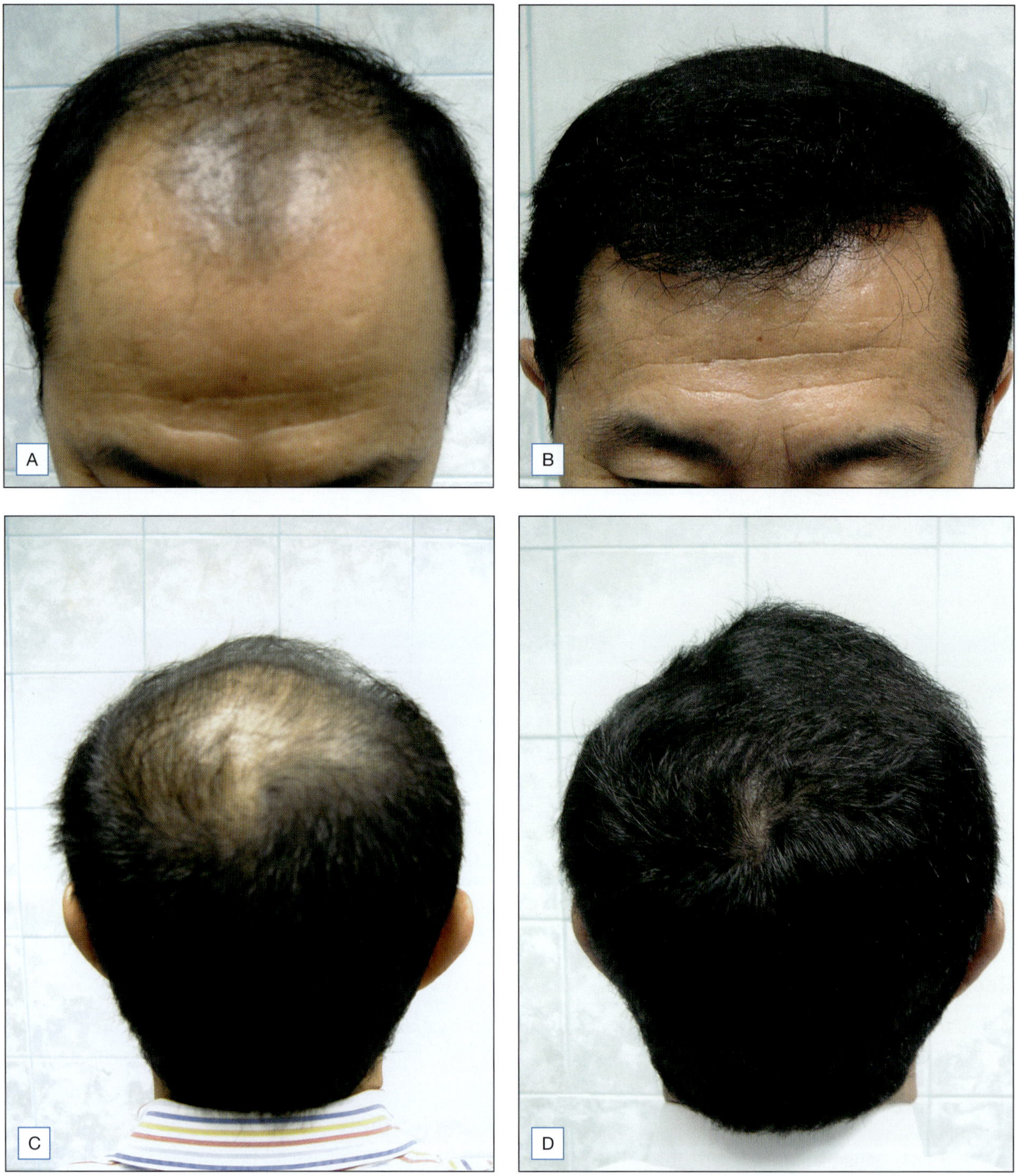


**Fig. 20.5** Before (**A** and **C**) and 10 months after (**B** and **D**) one session (2169 FUGs)

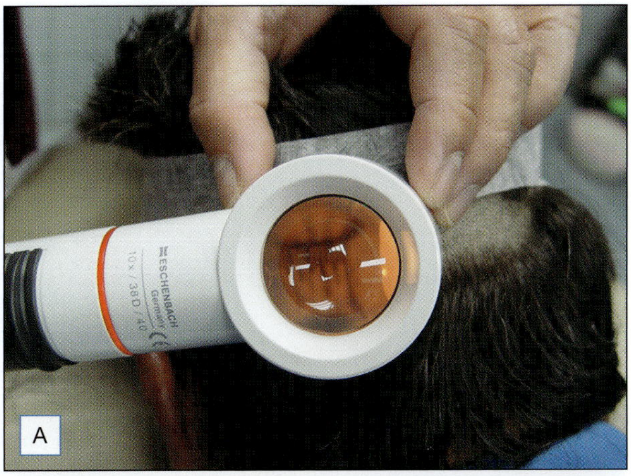


Fig. 20.6 (**A**) Measurement of hair count under magnification. (**B**) Measurement of the bald area using the Chang method

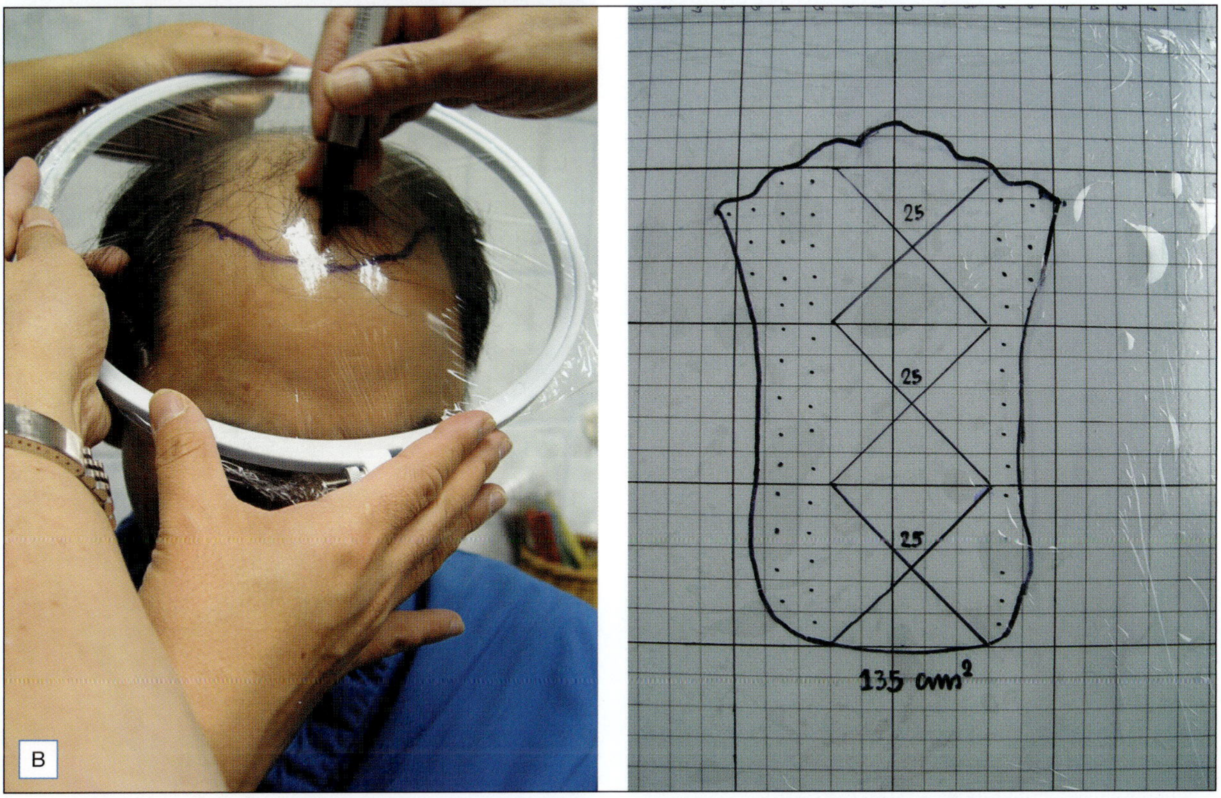

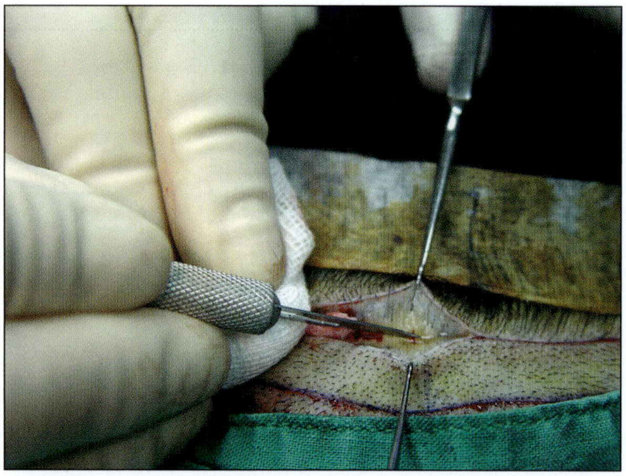

Fig. 20.7 Cutting between the FUs from the epidermal portion to the dermal papilla using the tip of a No. 15 blade. Assistant provides upward and outward traction with skin hooks

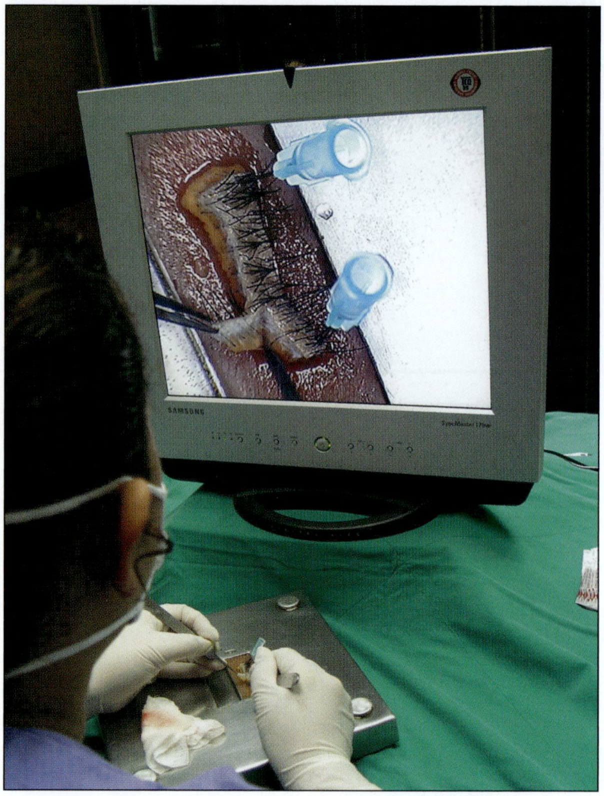

Fig. 20.8 Strip dissection into slivers and FUs is carried out under 10× magnification utilizing a video image on a monitor screen

hair/skin contrast. Low hair density is compensated for by larger caliber follicles and the use of more single-hair grafts for the frontal hairline. Special attention must be focused on the unique anatomical features of the Asian patient

## Further Reading


Bernstein RM, Rassman WR 1997 The aesthetics of follicular transplantation. Dermatologic Surgery 23:785–799

Chang S 2001 Estimate number of grafts and donor area. Hair Transplant Forum International 11(4), p. 97–102

Pathomvanich D 1998 Donor harvesting: A new approach to minimizing transection of the hair follicle. Hair Transplant Forum 8:1, 4–5

Pathomvanich D 2000 Donor harvesting: A new approach to minimize transection of hair follicles. Dermatologic Surgery 26:345–348

Pathomvanich D 2002 A random study of Asian male androgenetic alopecia in Bangkok, Thailand. Dermatologic Surgery 28:804–807

Seery G 2002 Transplantation: management of the donor area. Dermatologic Surgery 28:136–142

Takashima M, Iju, Sudo M 1981 Alopecia androgenetica – its incidence in Japanese and associate conditions. In: Orfanos CE, Montagna W, Stutgen G (eds) Hair Research Status and Future Aspects. Springer-Verlag, Berlin pp 287–293

Tang PH, Chia HP, Cheong LL, Koh D 2000 A community study of male androgenetic alopecia in Bishan, Singapore. Singapore Medical Journal 41:202–205

Yoo Jae-Hak 2004 Analysis of hair characteristics in Koreans using phototrichograms. Unger W, Shapiro R (eds) Hair Transplantation. 4th edn New York p 892–897

# 21 Renovation of Previous Transplants

*Russell Knudsen*

## Introduction

A significant portion of any hair transplantation surgeon's practice involves management of previously transplanted patients. These may be patients returning to the same surgeon, or frequently they are patients of other surgeons who performed their earlier surgery. A subset of this group is comprised of patients whose previous surgery was some years ago and utilized older, now outdated, techniques. The techniques described in this chapter apply both to **renovation**, or updating, of appropriately designed previous surgery or, equally, to surgical **repair** of poorly designed surgery. Renovation involves a variety of techniques ranging from infill with follicular unit transplantation (FUT) to soften and thicken the grafted areas, total excision of plug grafts, to partial de-bulking, or thinning, of plug grafts utilizing follicular unit extraction (FUE).

## The Problem

There are many potential problems with previously transplanted patients, even those with previous excellent surgical technique and design. Problems may involve plug grafts with gaps that require filling, plug grafts with too much density creating a frontal 'wall' (often the result of compression within the plug grafts), or harsh frontal hairlines lacking a scatter zone of single hair grafts. In addition, there may be incorrect angling of grafted hairs, inappropriately placed hairlines or widely scattered crown plugs in patients with extensive crown balding. Patients may also have developed further rim balding in the crown, **laterally** to previous grafts or there may be no useful amount of remaining donor hair to achieve all the patient's goals.

Every patient is potentially treatable to some degree as hair is quite resilient to being re-transplanted to other areas. The success of treatment depends upon factors such as the quality and quantity of potential donor hair (either remaining in the donor area or already grafted into balding areas), the potential for further significant balding, and patient expectations. As such, patient selection can be crucial to achieving a satisfactory outcome. The procedures to be discussed are included in Box 21.1. Alopecia reduction surgery will not be discussed in this chapter but is readily found in other textbooks.

## Patient Selection

The ideal patient is generally an older (40+ years of age) one who has had competent, appropriately designed surgery performed previously, has not lost much hair in recent years and has significant, good-quality donor hair remaining. The patients who should be excluded are those with no realistic chance of achieving their goals (unrealistic expectations) or those so devoid of adequate donor hair quantity or quality that no significant improvement may be expected. In some cases, the suggestion of a hairpiece is the best advice.

**Procedures of renovation of previous surgery**

1. Excision/dissection/relocation of standard plugs
2. Frontal elliptical reduction of standard plugs
3. De-bulking (thinning) of standard plugs (FUE)
4. FUT to soften and thicken between previous grafts

**Box 21.1** Procedures of renovation of previous surgery

Careful assessment is required during the consultation, with specific attention paid to the amount and quality (caliber, curl, color) of remaining donor hair, the potential impact of possible future progression of hair loss, and the patient's coverage priorities if balding is too extensive to satisfactorily cover all balding areas. In most of these cases, patients will choose to address their frontal balding and accept crown balding as the trade-off. It is also pertinent to note that the patient's budget may impact significantly on the surgical plan. Patient selection is summarized in Box 21.2.

## Expected Benefits

As long as adequate donor hair remains, significant visual benefits are routinely obtained from renovation. This improved cosmesis is based on better general coverage of the balding areas together with a more natural look from modern grafting techniques. If properly chosen, the donor hair from the lower scalp may confidently be expected to persist for many years (perhaps permanently). Nonetheless, careful attention to the possibility (indeed, probability) of future hair loss must be taken so that proper planning and proper patient expectations are achieved.

In patients with poorly planned or performed previous surgery, the improved cosmetic result is based in part on correction of these planning or surgical deficiencies. Once these deficiencies have been corrected, further benefits will again depend on the quantity and quality of the remaining donor hair. It is the author's experience that subtle improvements in cosmesis can generate great patient satisfaction in many cases.

Some patients present with both an exhausted donor supply and only moderate growth from previous grafts. Even subtle changes such as removal and relocation of previously grafted hair in the balding central crown may make a significant improvement in this area. The removal and relocation of crown grafts, together with softening the frontal hairline, may produce the greatest cosmetic benefit in the extensively bald patient.

Previously grafted hair is resilient to re-transplantation if carefully removed and relocated. The surgical impact on the patient is minimal and bandaging is usually not required. Infection remains uncommon and significant improvements in previous scarring in the balding areas can, in some cases, be achieved by simple excision of the scarring. The range of likely outcomes is described in Box 21.3.

## Overview of Treatment Strategy

The overall strategy is to achieve maximum impact within the budgetary constraints of the patient. This will generally be best achieved by improving coverage in the cosmetically significant areas, and improving the naturalness of these grafted areas. The patient's goals must be aligned with the amount and quality of any remaining donor area, together with prioritization of the surgical plan in the extensively bald patient. Adding hair via remaining donor area will usually make a more dramatic impact than re-distributing the existing grafted hairs. Approximation of the grafted density of standard plugs via new FUT in the gaps, perhaps with de-bulking of any compressed or super dense grafts, will together produce significant improvements in naturalness.

In patients with limited donor supply, discussion about preferred grooming often helps clarify the treatment plan. Generally, with limited donor hair, a side part will produce the best cosmetic result. The side of the frontal hairline containing the part has higher cosmetic importance and, in patients

**Patient selection for renovation surgery**

- Amount of remaining donor hair
- Quality of remaining donor hair
- Impact of future progression of hair loss
- Patient expectations
- Patient's coverage priority if balding too extensive
- Patient's budget

**Box 21.2** Patient selection for renovation surgery

**Likely outcomes of re-transplantation**

- Improved general coverage
- Increased naturalness of coverage
- Softening of frontal hairline
- Removal of central crown grafts
- Reduced area of coverage
- Correction of planning mistakes

**Box 21.3** Likely outcomes of re-transplantation

with limited donor supply, should receive higher priority for new grafts. The goal in these extensively bald patients is to achieve a result that mimics natural balding. For example, a Norwood classification of VI might be converted to a Norwood classification III vertex. As ever, grafting involves an area vs. density trade-off and this must be emphasized to the patient. A convincing result depends upon creating the illusion that greater coverage exists than actually is the case. Smaller areas of higher density help achieve this illusion.

Inappropriately placed grafts or an incorrectly placed hairline should be corrected prior to further thickening so that a coordinated surgical plan may be utilized. Every patient presents a unique picture and a combination of strategies and techniques will usually be required to achieve optimal improvement. Although the ultimate goal is to re-distribute all previously grafted hairs to improve the outcome, sometimes this is difficult to achieve with 100% success. Stray hairs from previous grafts are frequently left in spite of excision and, if inappropriately placed at the hairline, may continue to present a cosmetic problem. In certain cases, it may be advisable to consider laser hair removal to assist with these stray hairs.

Occasionally patients present with the stated desire of complete removal of previously placed grafts. Patients wanting complete reversals have, in the current author's experience, had small areas of temporal balding grafted at an early age and no longer wish to continue with any surgical option except reversal. Though this goes against the general inclination of the surgeon, if after careful explanation of the expected outcome, the patient is adamant in this desire, then removal and discarding of the grafted hair becomes the most appropriate option. It must be stressed to the patient that transplanted hairs are resilient and some can persist after removal attempts, possibly due to splaying of the grafts below the surface. As described later, care must be taken with punch removals and frontal elliptical reductions to include a margin sufficient to remove the entire FU.

## Major Determinants

All approaches involve relatively simple surgical techniques with, excepting a hair removal laser, minimal technical costs. As with all modern grafting techniques, the approaches are labor intensive and frequently time consuming. This is where the majority of the costs arise. Strategies usually revolve around the following factors:

1. Incorrect previous planning.
   a. If the hairline was created with multiple large grafts placed too low, a frontal elliptical reduction of the hairline (also known as strip excision of the hairline) and relocation of the hair may be preferred to individual excision and relocation of the grafts. This may in certain cases be combined with a brow lift.
   b. For widely spaced, large crown plug grafts or visible multifollicular unit grafts, individual excision and relocation would be preferred. Correction of incorrectly angled previous grafts is usually achieved by individual excision and relocation.
   c. Patients with frontal rotation flaps may require total excision of the flap (if possible) to correct inappropriately directed hairlines.
2. Correct previous planning.
   a. Filling of gaps, via FUT, if a significant donor supply remains.
   b. De-bulking (thinning), via FUE, of compressed or super dense grafts in highly visible areas.
3. Further expansion of balding since previous surgery. This limits the donor area and outcome.
4. Expected future expansion of balding. This limits the areas to be treated and reduces potential donor hair. Consider the role of medical stabilization therapy.
5. Available donor hair reserve. This determines priorities for donor hair placement.
6. Patient expectations and goals. This determines priorities for different treatment areas.
7. Patient budget. This determines priorities for any treatment offered.

## Patient Interviews

The most crucial aspects of the consultation prior to any surgery are to elicit the patient's feelings about their current surgical result and to clearly elucidate their goals. Some patients have clear expectations and goals; others are interested in generally exploring options that might give a superior outcome.

Some patients state a desire to start over again with newer techniques, others are happy to achieve a gradual improvement. Some patients have completely unrealistic expectations and must be carefully counseled as to expected outcomes. To blithely operate on an already unhappy patient, without a high probability of improving their outlook, is a surgical disaster.

Other patients are undecided about whether to proceed with further surgery or whether to completely reverse previous surgery. A careful exploration of the preferred outcome (more hair coverage or acceptance of balding) will help the patient decide what suits him or her best. Full reversal should be an option that is offered to the appropriate patient. In a few patients, no acceptable surgical outcome is possible and camouflage methods such as hairpieces should be explored. The following checklist of questions may be useful:

1. Are you happy with what has been done previously and simply wish for improved coverage?
2. Do you want a slight improvement or great improvement?
3. What budget do you have in mind?
4. What is the most important improvement you would like to achieve?
5. Have you considered the impact of any further hair loss?
6. Have you considered attempting baldness stabilization with finasteride or minoxidil?

## Treatment Techniques

### Excision/dissection/relocation of standard plugs

This technique involves the punching out of previous plugs using cylindrical punches of various sizes. The excised plugs are each dissected into follicular unit (FU) grafts, and then these grafts are re-implanted into the same area or another area that is more appropriate. The excised plug defect is sutured using interrupted sutures. One or two sutures may be required per excised punch graft.

### Patient Selection

The technique is suitable for improving the cosmetic appearance of appropriately placed plugs in highly visible areas or for relocation of inappropriately placed plugs.

### Equipment

- Carbonized steel or titanium punches
- Adequate magnification equipment plus dissecting blades
- Blades or needles for re-implantation
- Nondissolvable sutures (e.g. 4-0 nylon).

### Treatment algorithm

After ring-block local anesthesia (Lidocaine and epinephrine) of the required portion of the scalp, the plug graft hairs are trimmed to 2–3 mm to facilitate accurate removal. An appropriately sized very sharp cylindrical punch is chosen to just be of slightly greater diameter than the plug (i.e. 1 mm). The punch is angled parallel to the direction of the hair in the plug and rotated by hand or by a slowly rotating motorized handpiece. Once a proper full skin thickness cut has been performed, the plug is elevated by grasping the epithelium with a forceps and the subcutaneous fat is cut by a fine scissor.

The excised plug is handed to an assistant, who will dissect the plug under magnification into 4–8 single- or multi-follicular unit grafts, each containing 1–3 hairs. The excision 'hole' is sutured into a 'slit' by 1–2 interrupted nondissolving 4-0 sutures.

The resulting grafts are re-implanted into a new location using the surgeon's preferred technique with either fine blades or needles, creating the new incisions. Sutures will be removed 7–10 days postoperatively. This complete technique is shown in Figures 21.1–21.4.

### Troubleshooting

In areas of relatively closely spaced standard plugs, removal of numerous plugs in a small area creates tension problems in suturing the 'holes.' In this circumstance, it is wise to excise only some of the plugs (e.g. skipping some plugs near excision sites) so that a future staged excision can be performed for the remaining plugs.

Incorrect angling of the punch will result in transection of the peripheral hairs in the plugs and retained hairs in the excision hole wall. This will result in some re-growth in the excised area, which may be undesirable. A slightly larger sharp punch, careful angling of the punch, and increased tissue turgor by injection of normal saline into the graft prior to excision reduces the chance of this outcome.

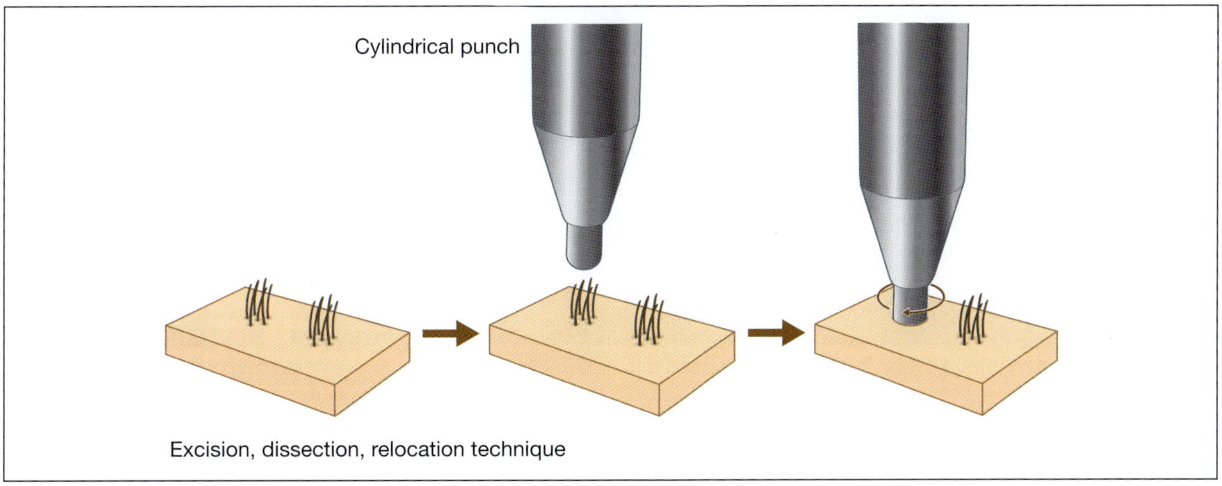


**Fig. 21.1** Punch excision of previous plugs

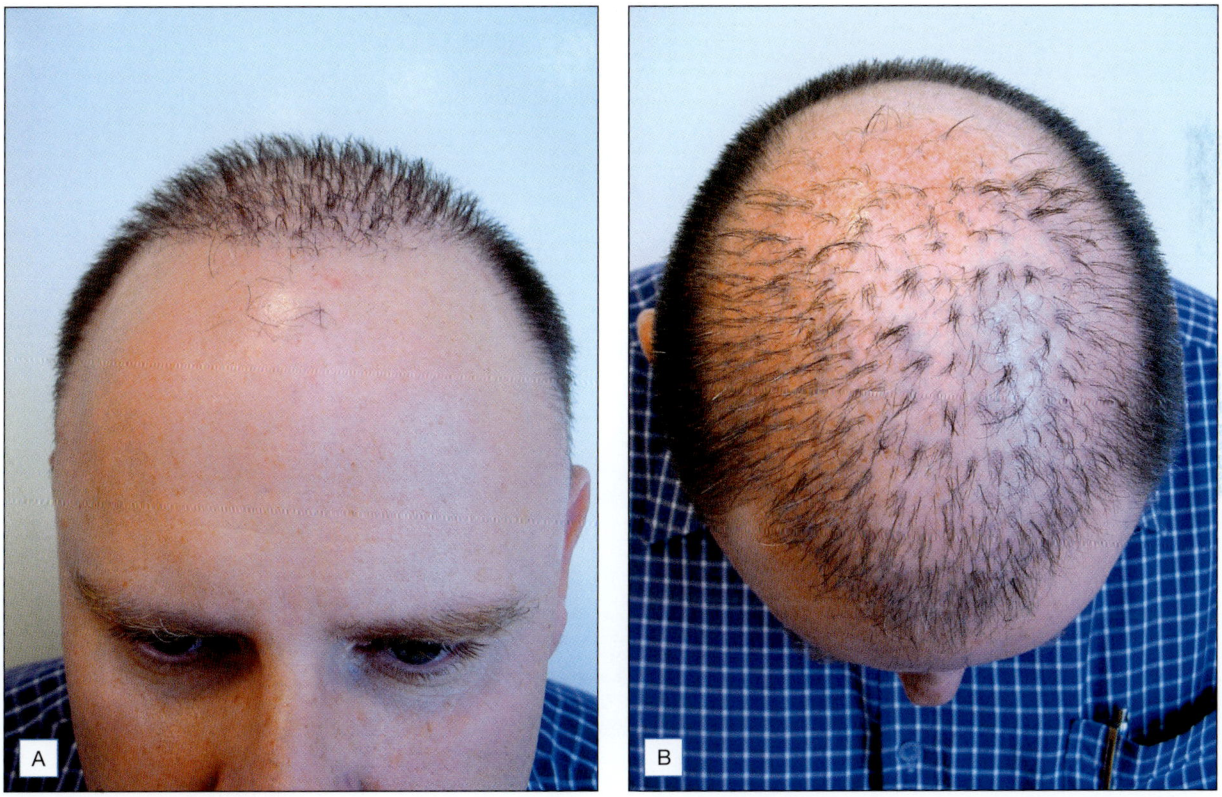


**Fig. 21.2** Face (**A**). Top (**B**)

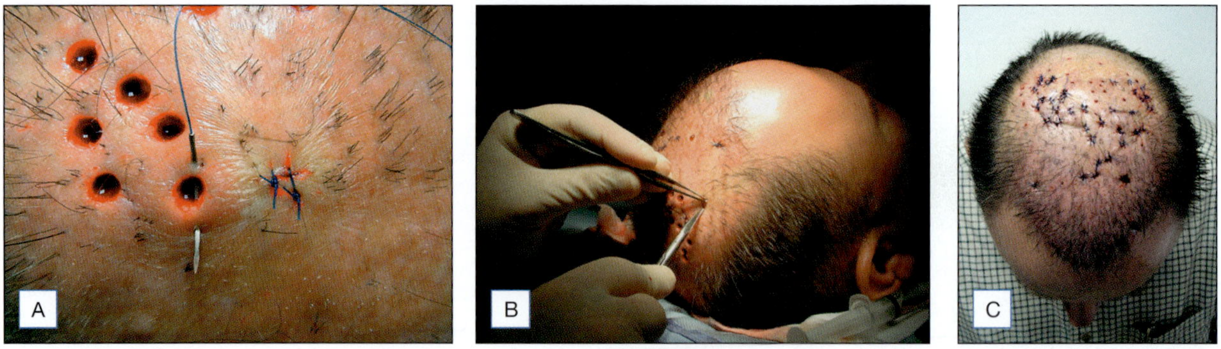


**Fig. 21.3** (**A**) Suturing punch holes. (**B**) Removal of punch micrograft. (**C**) Sutured plugs, unsutured minigraft excisions, frontal micrografts

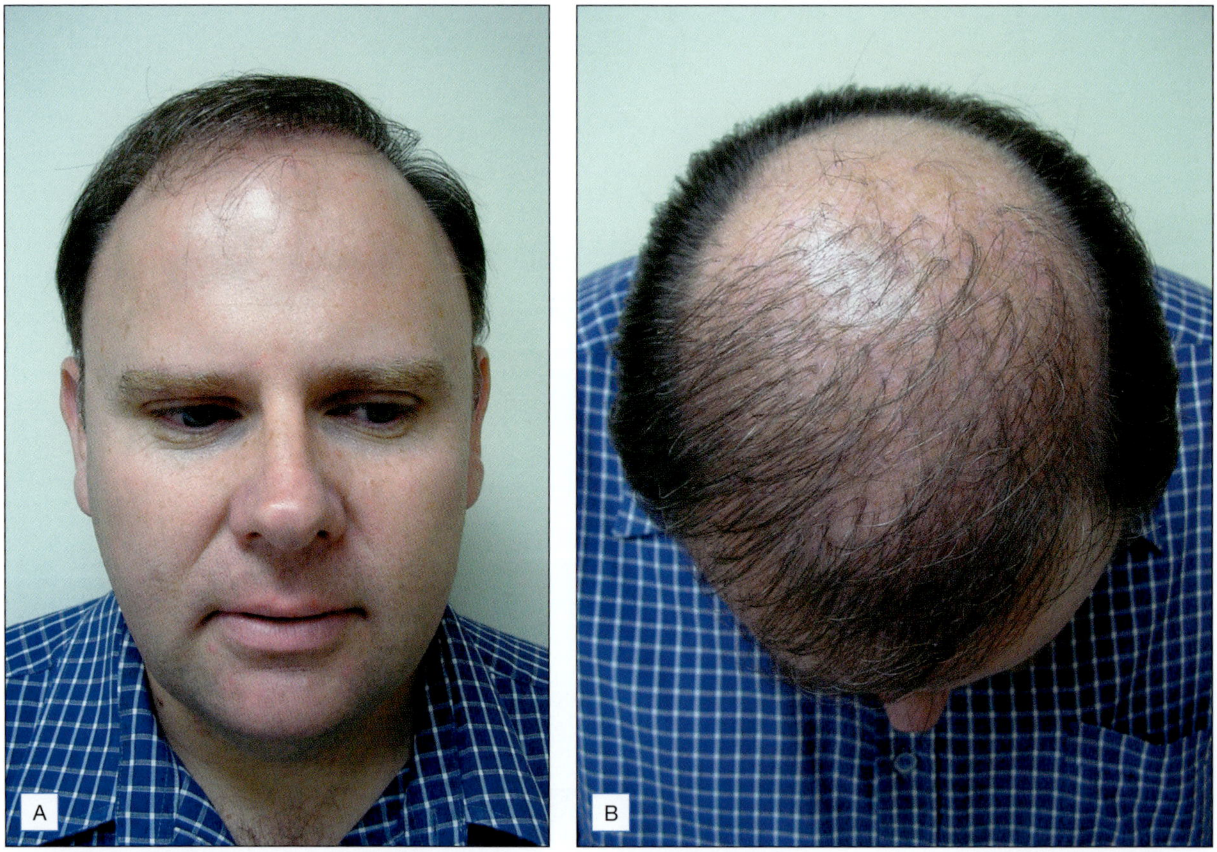


**Fig. 21.4** 5 months postoperatively. Face (**A**), top (**B**)

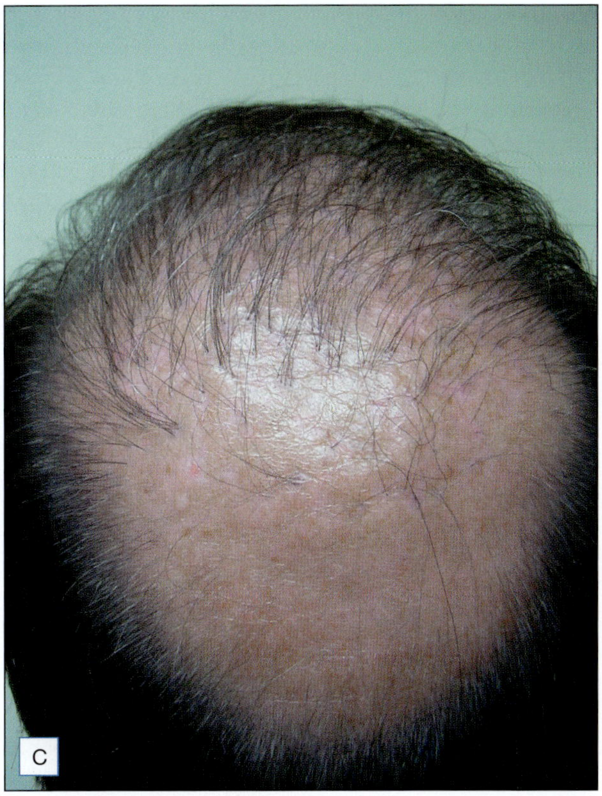

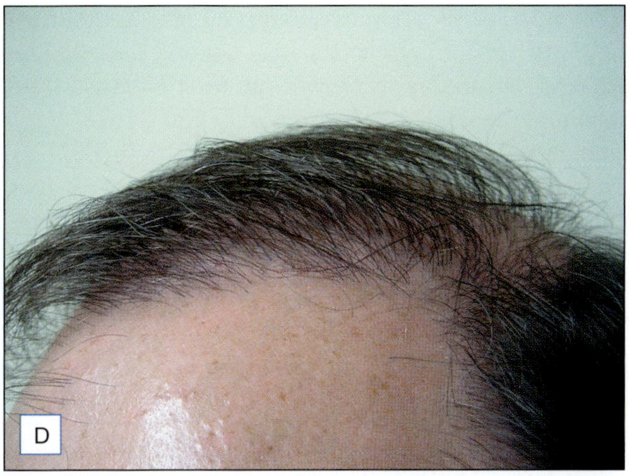

**Fig. 21.4** *Continued,* 5 months postoperatively. Crown (**C**), and hairline (**D**)

## Complications

Usually these relate to re-growth of incompletely excised hair, minor folliculitis or wound breakdown if sutures are applied under too-great tension with multiple closely spaced excisions.

## Frontal Elliptical Reduction of Standard Plugs, with Dissection and Relocation

### Patient selection

This technique is generally utilized to remove an inappropriately placed hairline or for an appropriately sited but significantly 'pluggy' hairline. The plugs are usually closely spaced (even touching each other) and form a row of grafts. The frontal elliptical reduction represents a relatively simple way to elevate the hairline and in some cases, single hair grafts can be scattered to cover the resulting linear scar.

### Equipment

- Scalpel blades (Nos 10, 11, or 15)
- Magnification for dissection
- Blades or needles for both dissection and relocation of micrografts
- Nondissolving suture (e.g. 4-0 nylon) for repair of the excision site.

### Treatment algorithm

A ring block with Lidocaine and epinephrine is performed. The scalp flexibility at the site of the proposed frontal elliptical reduction is assessed by manual palpation. Frontal elliptical reductions generally vary between 5–10 mm in width. A single ellipse is generally excised by scalpel with careful attention to make the incision parallel to the angulation of the frontal hairs so as to avoid transection of the hair. Excisions should be approximately 1 mm lateral to the marginal hairs in the plugs to avoid leaving retained hairs due to variations in angling, or splaying of the hairs subcutaneously.

The ellipse is handed to the assistant for dissection into appropriately sized single or multifollicular unit grafts. The excision wound is sutured in two layers, first with an interrupted absorbable galeal suture (e.g. 3-0 Vicryl). This provides fixation and minimizes the risk of scarline stretch. A surface nondissolving interrupted suture (e.g. 4-0 nylon) provides the second layer. The surface suture is removed at 7–10 days. The technique is shown in Figures 21.5 and 21.6.

It is possible to immediately graft single hair grafts to the area of excision to hide the scar **if** it is appropriate to have hair in this region of the frontal scalp. Slight variations of the shape of the excision can be made to restore frontotemporal angles if required.

### Troubleshooting

The most common mistake is to excise too wide an ellipse, making suture closure difficult. This then requires wide undermining, with tension applied only (if possible) at the galeal layer. This mistake can be avoided by conservative estimation of the appropriate ellipse and assessing flexibility after the inferior border of the ellipse is incised. The lower forehead edge is manually elevated to overlap the proposed ellipse excision. A tension-free closure is always the goal, and most mature scars seen after frontal elliptical reductions are almost imperceptible.

### Complications

Infection is uncommon but excessive wound edge tension may provoke wound breakdown. Otherwise, conservative excision is very safe.

## De-bulking of Plugs

### Patient selection

Some patients have hair characteristics (coarse caliber, dark brown or black color, straight) that may make standard plugs, or even MFUs, highly visible

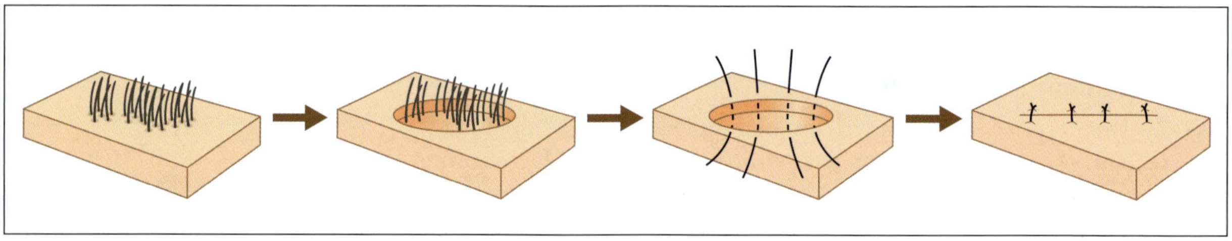

**Fig. 21.5** Frontal elliptical excision technique

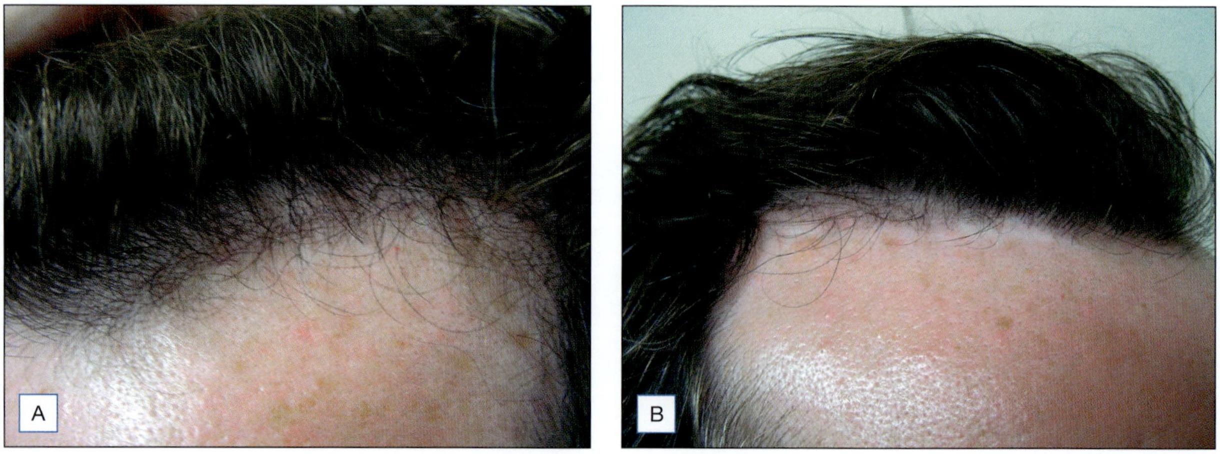



**Fig. 21.6** (**A** and **B**) Post-strip excision scar

in cosmetically important areas such as the hairline. In addition, some standard plugs and MFUs are prone to **compression** as a consequence of healing by contraction. This results in super-dense grafts that have higher density than the donor area. In essence, these grafts contain too many hairs to be cosmetically acceptable. In some patients, it is easier to de-bulk these plugs or MFUs than to completely excise, dissect, and relocate them. The decision to choose this option is generally a matter of degree; if a small de-bulking is likely to provide an acceptable result, and the position of the plug or MFU is acceptable, then this option is reasonable. Particularly if only a small number of plugs or MFUs are problematic. If, on the other hand, all the plugs or MFUs are cosmetically unacceptable due to compression, then total excision is more likely to provide an optimal outcome.

## Equipment

De-bulking is usually achieved by use of very small cylindrical punches (e.g. 0.8–1.5 mm).

## Treatment algorithm

Local anesthesia is achieved in the area and tissue turgor of the plug or MFU is achieved by injection of normal saline into the graft. A very sharp punch is used to incise the epidermis to 1 mm depth. A **blunt** cylindrical punch of the same diameter is then applied to the incision, carefully following the hair angulation, and a blunt cut performed by a circular rotating motion of the punch to full depth of the skin. The 2–4 hair graft is elevated by forceps and separated at the subcutaneous fat by scissors (Figs 21.7 and 21.8).

The position of the cut may be either central to the plug or at the periphery (Fig. 21.8). More than one excision per plug may be performed, if necessary. The excision sites are left to heal by secondary intention.

## Troubleshooting

It takes significant practice to accurately remove portions of larger grafts during de-bulking without significant transection of the hairs. A complete description of the technique of follicular unit

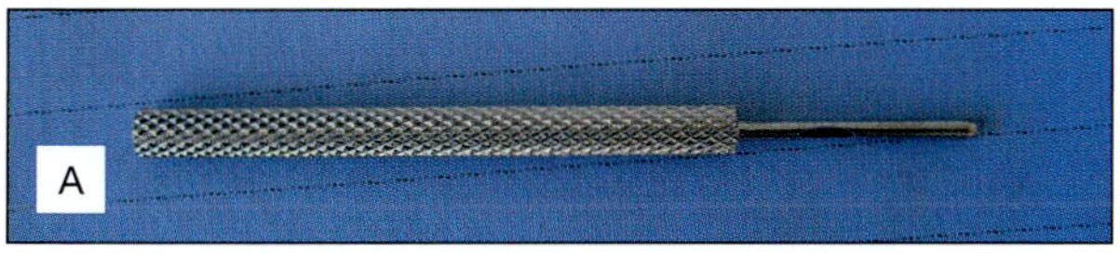


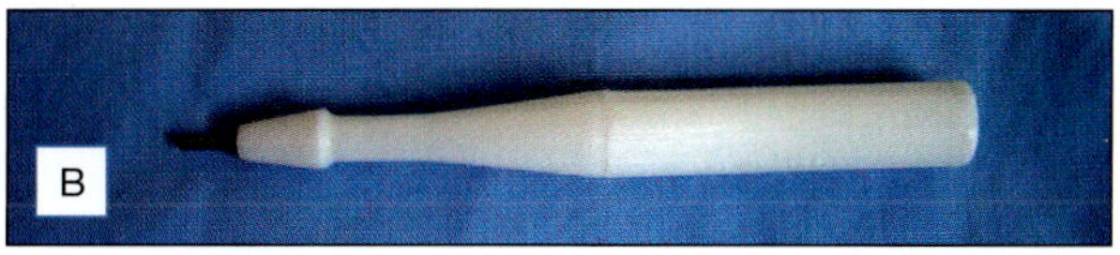


**Fig. 21.7** 1 mm punches: sharp (**A**) and blunt (**B**)

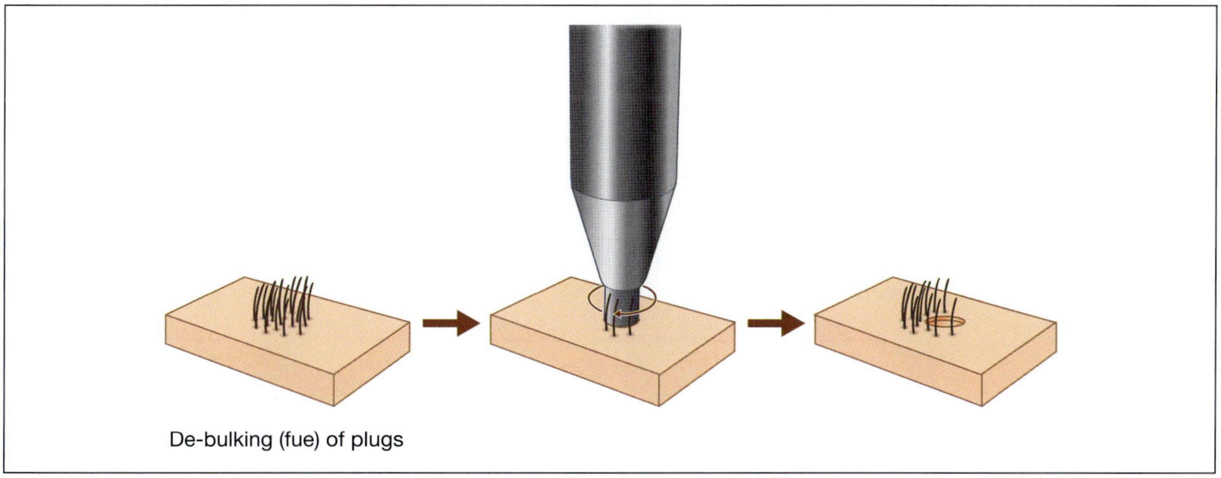


**Fig. 21.8** De-bulking (FUE) of plugs

extraction (FUE), of which this is a variation, is found in Chapter 17 of this text. Transection of hairs produces some loss of hairs, which might be crucial in patients with little donor hair remaining. Burying the excised graft subcutaneously is possible during the blunt incision phase and delicate downward pressure should only be applied at this stage.

### Complications

Generally, there are none if the areas excised are washed thoroughly with antiseptic shampoos on the first few days following surgery. Continued bleeding from the sites is rare.

## In-fill with FUT

### Patient selection

This technique is most preferable in patients who have significant remaining donor hair. The goal is to soften the cosmetically important areas by filling the spaces between the previous standard plugs or MFU. Generating a relatively even density through the area creates the best cosmetic outcome. This may require significant donor hairs. Nearly every patient who wishes renovation has some remaining donor, so this technique is generally part of the surgeon's armamentarium for nearly every renovation.

### Equipment

Identical to the normal requirements for this type of surgery and described elsewhere in this text.

### Treatment algorithm

FU grafts are planted with significant density between the standard plugs and MFUs. Single hair grafts are inserted **anterior** to the frontal row of the previous grafts. The number of grafts utilized often is only slightly reduced from the number required in a similarly sized, totally bald area! An example is demonstrated in Figures 21.9 and 21.10.

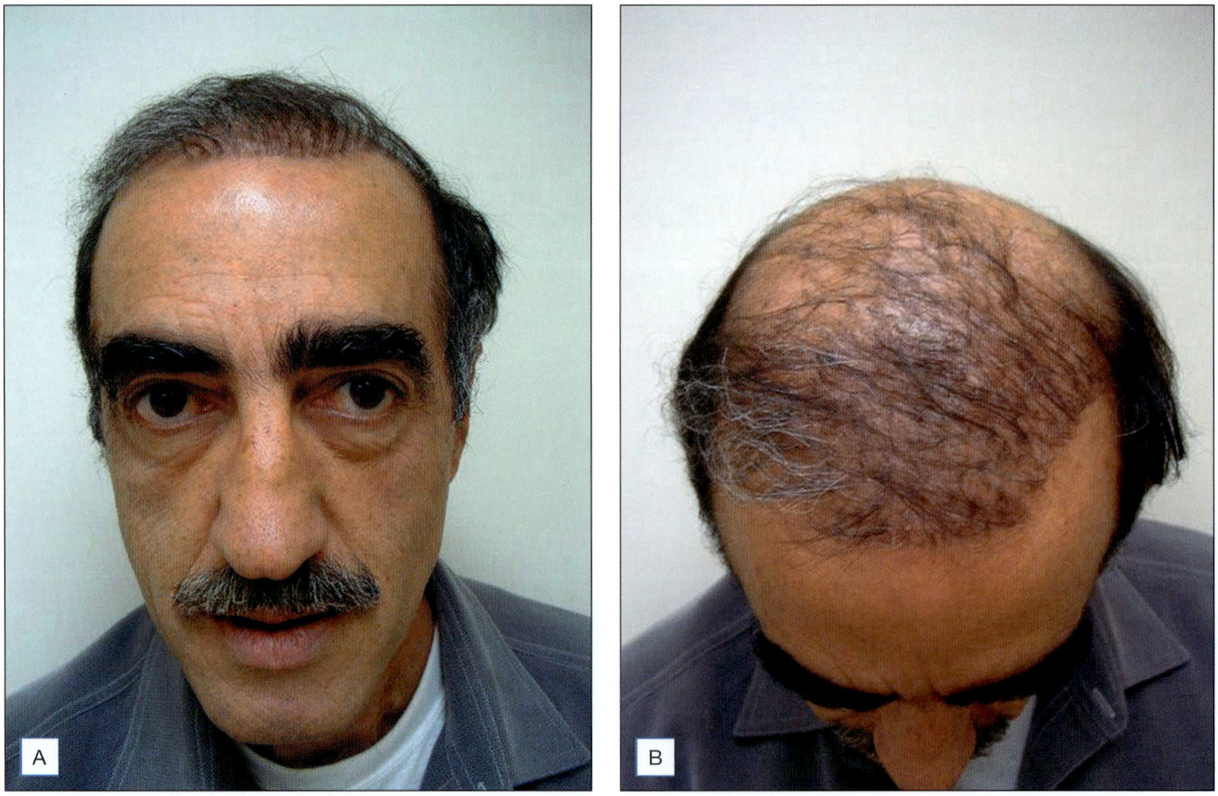


**Fig. 21.9** (**A** and **B**) Densely placed plugs prior to infill correction

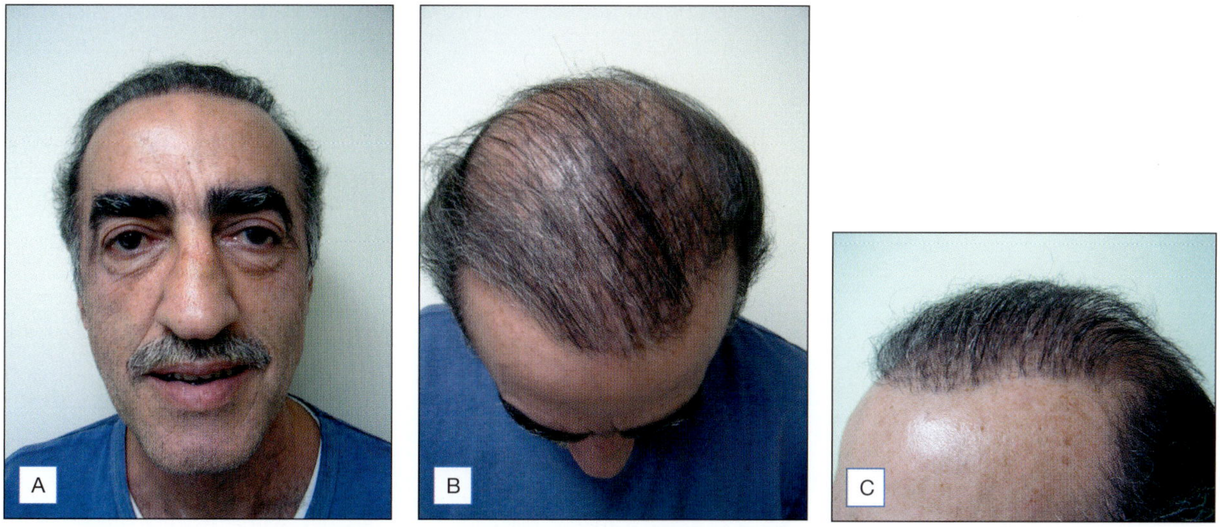

**Fig. 21.10** (**A–C**) After 1500 FU transplantation. Face (**A**). Top (**B**) and close-up after infill (**C**)

## Troubleshooting

The main mistake is to underestimate the number of grafts required to in-fill an area. It is therefore wise to prioritize areas of need and proceed in an orderly fashion if donor supply is restricted. Apply a density of grafts that will best approximate the density of the plugs or MFU in the area. Graft sorting is also useful (i.e. three-hair grafts in areas needing greatest density).

## Complications

There is no greater risk of complication with in-filling previously grafted areas than with a virgin bald scalp.

## Further Reading

Bernstein R, Rassman W, Rashid N, Ascione S, Shiell R 2002 The art of repair in surgical hair restoration. Dermatologic Surgery 28:873–893

Unger W 2004 Correction of cosmetic problems in hair transplanting. In: Unger W, Shapiro R (ed.) Hair transplantation. Marcel Dekker, New York, pp 663–687

Vogel JE 2004 Correcting problems in hair restoration surgery: an update. Facial Plastic Surgery Clinics of North America 12:263–278

# 22 Hair Transplantation in the Genetically Male Transsexual

*Richard Shiell*

## Definition

Transsexualism has been defined as the adoption of a social sex role opposite to that of the biological sex. It is characterized by a persistent and irreversible conviction that the affected individual does not belong to their biological sex but rather to the opposite sex. It is important to stress the difference between transsexuals and homosexuals, who are not distressed with their biological sex but prefer to express their sexuality differently than heterosexuals.

The adult man who rejects his gender and desires sexual reassignment is a rare, although increasingly common phenomenon. The present incidence is estimated to be from 1:5000 to 1:50,000, and although most who receive medical attention for this condition are men, Swedish studies suggest that the sex incidence is almost equal. Some of these persons have gained considerable publicity and notoriety, but from the author's experience the vast majority wish to remain anonymous and pass silently from being a man to being a woman without fanfare or fuss.

Unfortunately such a luxury is rarely permitted because transsexuals have parents, siblings, or even wives and children, all of whom must confront this issue. Their reaction is generally predictable and is one of shock, hurt, and outrage that their son/brother/husband/father could humiliate the family in such a manner. As a result, many of these individuals, in addition to the distress of feeling 'like a woman trapped inside a man's body,' have the problems of rejection by those whom they love most. On rare occasions family members may accept the man's desire for gender reassignment with sympathy and understanding, and they may even continue to live under the same roof.

Transsexuality encompasses quite a spectrum of behavior, from a man who enjoys putting on women's clothing in the privacy of his apartment to the man who likes to shop and socialize while dressed as a woman. Later the individual may gain the courage to commence living and working full time as a woman and take hormone therapy to soften the skin and increase breast development. The final phase, which is sought by only a small percentage of transsexuals, involves surgical removal of the male genitalia and construction of a functional vagina.

At any stage in this progression the individual may seek cosmetic surgery for a variety of feminizing procedures such as breast augmentation, removal of a prominent jawline, augmentation of the cheekbones, and removal of a prominent cricoid cartilage ('Adam's apple'). In addition, the older patient may seek surgical correction of wrinkles, baggy eyelids, and a 'turkey neck' to appear younger.

Male pattern baldness is particularly distressing since it emphasizes the very attribute that the individual is trying to deny, namely masculinity. For this reason the hair transplant specialist is frequently asked for assistance by the genetically male transsexual.

## Role of Physician

The transsexual patient requires empathy and understanding. It is not the physician's place to be critical or judgmental about the patient's choice of lifestyle. That decision was made years earlier, and the patient has often paid for it dearly with loss of old friends, family, and associates. The physician's role should be to provide sympathy, understanding, support, and an honest assessment of what is and is not possible with regard to hair replacement. If the surgeon is unable to feel comfortable with this situation, these cases should be referred to a more sympathetic colleague.

## Hairline Design

The male transsexual is generally seeking to acquire a frontal hair zone that is as near to that of a genetic female as possible. It must be pointed out to the patient that there are a variety of 'normal' female hairlines and that some compromise from his ideal may be necessary, depending on the extent of the baldness and the available donor hair (Fig. 22.1).

There are distinct differences between the hairline of the male transsexual and a genetic female with thinning hair. The latter generally retains the hairline and thins immediately behind this region. The transsexual male has male temple recession or more advanced balding of the typical Norwood patterns (Fig. 22.2).

## Type of Transplant Procedure

Follicular unit grafting as described throughout this textbook is ideally suited for conversion of a male to female hairline. While flaps have also been used successfully, they run a risk of long-term problems, specifically the hair behind the flap is lost, leaving the patient with an abnormal appearance.

There are many variables to consider when advising the patient about the best possible course of action. First, these patients are generally very good at hairstyling and thus can often get by with minimal surgical interference and clever styling. This fact is important because these patients are frequently in financial difficulty as a result of loss of regular employment or divorce and have much other cosmetic surgery to undergo in addition to hair transplantation. Second, the site of the donor scars is very important. Most patients want the option of being able to wear their hair up as well as down, so scarring at the lower hair margins is unacceptable.

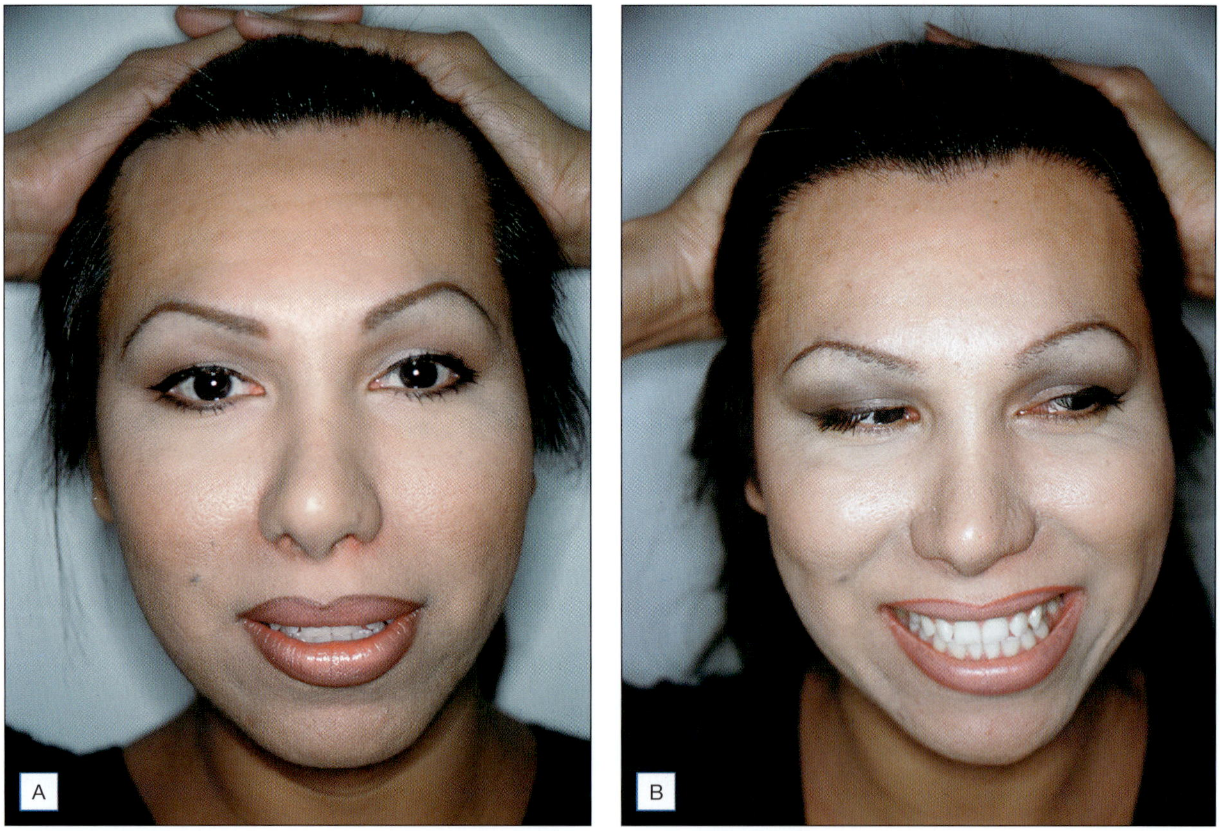


**Fig. 22.1** (**A**) Preoperative view of transsexual showing masculine hairline. (**B**) Postoperative view showing more rounded feminine hairline. (Photos courtesy of Dr Bobby Limmer)

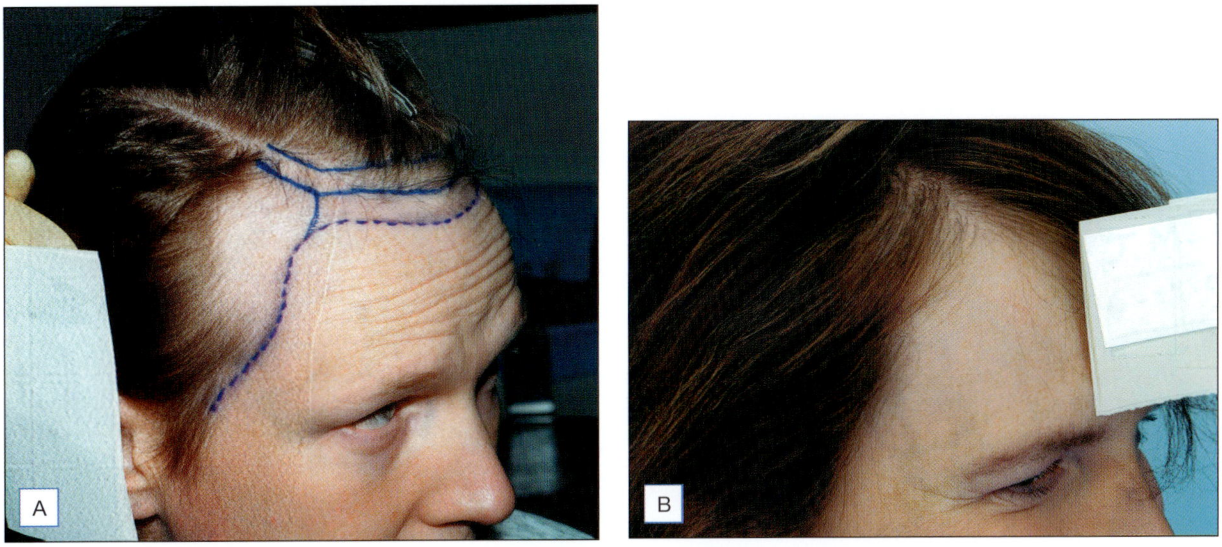


**Fig. 22.2** (**A**) Preoperative view of transsexual showing existing male pattern hair loss (MPHL) and planned surgical correction. (**B**) Postoperative view showing new hairline. (Photos courtesy of Dr Michael Beehner)

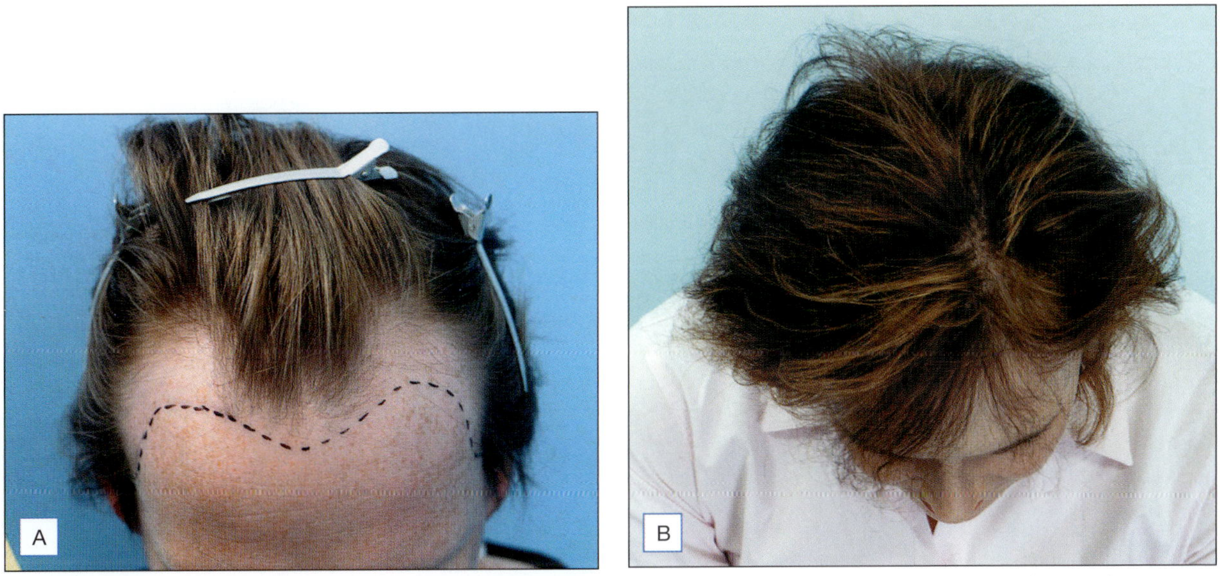


**Fig. 22.3** (**A**) Preoperative view of transsexual showing existing male pattern hair loss and planned surgical correction. (**B**) Postoperative view showing excellent density and feminine hair styling. (Photos courtesy of Dr Michael Beehner)

Generally these patients want a hairline that is low and rounded at the temples. This is feasible in most cases, but occasionally in middle-aged transsexuals the temple hair has receded too far to allow such a hairline. However, if the surgeon does their best, the patient is usually grateful for the extra hair and can usually work miracles with artful hairstyling (Fig. 22.3).

## Progression of Baldness

The male transsexual seeking hair transplantation is almost invariably undergoing estrogen therapy and is taking a 5-alpha-reductase inhibitor such as finasteride or dutasteride as well as antiandrogens. As a result of these medications, the progression of baldness is very slow unless the individual is required to cease therapy. In this case it is not uncommon for hair loss to begin rapidly and continue until estrogen therapy is resumed. Some older transsexuals have attained Norwood type V or VI baldness before seeking therapy, and these individuals provide the biggest challenge to the hair transplant surgeon because the available donor hair is so limited. It may be best to advise these patients to wear wigs because even after a lengthy series of operations the cosmetic results would still not pass as a convincing female hairstyle.

## Use of Surplus Face-lift Skin

It is common for the older male transsexual to undergo meloplasty for the removal of facial wrinkles and a sagging neck. Modern face-lift procedures attempt to conceal the posterior scars within the parietal hair-bearing zone instead of placement at the posterior hair margin as in older procedures. This scar placement allows the patient to 'wear her hair up' and thus increase the variety of hairstyles that are possible.

When the scar is placed in the parietal zone, much good hair-bearing skin is excised, whereas in the older procedure bald skin or hair of inferior quality on the nape of neck was removed. It is essential that the hair transplant surgeon work with the cosmetic surgeon to utilize these precious hair follicles, as well as those from the surplus temple skin. Occasionally the plastic surgeon is skilled at hair transplant procedures, but generally after a 4–5-hour meloplasty with upper and lower blepharoplasties will be in no mood to proceed with a further 1–2 hours of hair transplantation. The plastic surgeon would be well advised to seek the assistance of a skilled hair transplant team at this point.

## Coordination of Effort

In the current author's experience, co-operation between the two surgeons makes the transplant a simple add-on procedure to the face lift. The transplant surgeon can time their arrival to whenever the cosmetic surgeon estimates the first section of hair-bearing skin will have been removed. This donor section is then dissected into follicular units, and the grafts are kept moist in cool saline solution. The skin from the contralateral side will be available shortly thereafter and is similarly dissected and stored. As soon as the plastic surgeon has finished the meloplasty, the hair transplant surgeon gains access to the patient's scalp. Because the patient is usually under general anesthesia, analgesia is no problem, but it is advisable to infiltrate the recipient zone with the usual mixture of saline solution and epinephrine to gain optimum vasoconstriction before graft placement.


### Acknowledgment

This chapter is based on one that appeared in Stough D, Haber RS 1996 Hair Replacement: Surgical and Medical. Mosby Year Book Publishing Company, St Louis


### Further Reading


Harish D, Sharma BR 2003 Medical advances in transsexualism and the legal implications. Am J Forensic Med Pathol 24(1):100–105

Olsson SE, Moller AR 2003 On the incidence and sex of transsexualism in Sweden, 1972–2003, Arch Sex Behav 34(4):381–386

Swaab DF 2004 Sexual differentiation of the human brain: relevance for gender identity, transsexualism and sexual orientation. Gynecol Endocrinol 19(6):301–312

Walinder J 1971 Incidence and sex ratio of transsexualism in Sweden. British Journal of Psychology 119:195–196

# 23 Complications

*Mario Marzola, James E. Vogel*

## Introduction

Complications are part of any surgical procedure, but unfortunately, these are seldom discussed openly. Discussing complications is important if the science of hair transplantation surgery is to be advanced. Each complication must be dealt with individually. The philosophy and unique ideology behind the procedure must be critically evaluated, as well as the steps necessary for correction. It is only through the process of seeking the truth that avoidance of this same problem can eventually be found. Able clinicians should manage the adverse events professionally, minimize the damage, and help their patients to finally achieve the results that are expected by both parties. Fortunately follicular unit transplantation, if performed with care, is exceedingly safe and has a low complication rate.

## Planning and Concept

### Inadequate consultation

The majority of complications seen today occur during the consultative process. This statement may seem absurd, but underscores the fact that patient expectations are oftentimes unmet due to an inadequate consultation. The patient may expect more than the operation is able to deliver if the consultation has been brief, rushed or incomplete. Often more than one consultation is necessary to assimilate all the information, especially in anxious patients. It is strongly recommended that brochures be supplied and the patient be directed to informative websites.

### Poor patient selection

Patients who are in their early 20s or younger where the hair loss pattern is unclear and where their psychological maturity is unclear should be made to wait for surgery. Medical treatment should be given until the earlier mentioned aspects become more clear. At the other end of the spectrum where hair has been lost to Norwood VII or more, there may not be enough donor hair to make a difference. Another category of patients who should be avoided are those with body dysmorphic disorder, where a minor hair problem creates a maximum concern. It is oftentimes very difficult for surgeons to identify an individual with body dysmorphic disorder. Some individuals with this diagnosis will inadvertently be transplanted, and they will never be satisfied regardless of the surgical outcome.

### Ongoing hair loss

With the advent of finasteride it is tempting to promise a full head of hair to patients heading to a Norwood VI type of hair loss pattern. Unfortunately there may be side effects or the patients may simply change their minds and cease medical treatment. Always therefore plan the donor harvesting and the placement pattern with an eye to an advanced eventual hair loss pattern.

### Low unesthetic hairline

The center of the hairline should be 7, 8 or 9 cm above the glabella, not lower, and should not be rounded in the temples (Fig. 23.1). The hairline should remain horizontal as it is extended posteriorly. If the planned hairline does not connect to the lateral fringe, the fringe should be elevated by creating parietal humps. The hairline should not be lowered to meet the fringe, nor rounded to meet the temporal peaks.

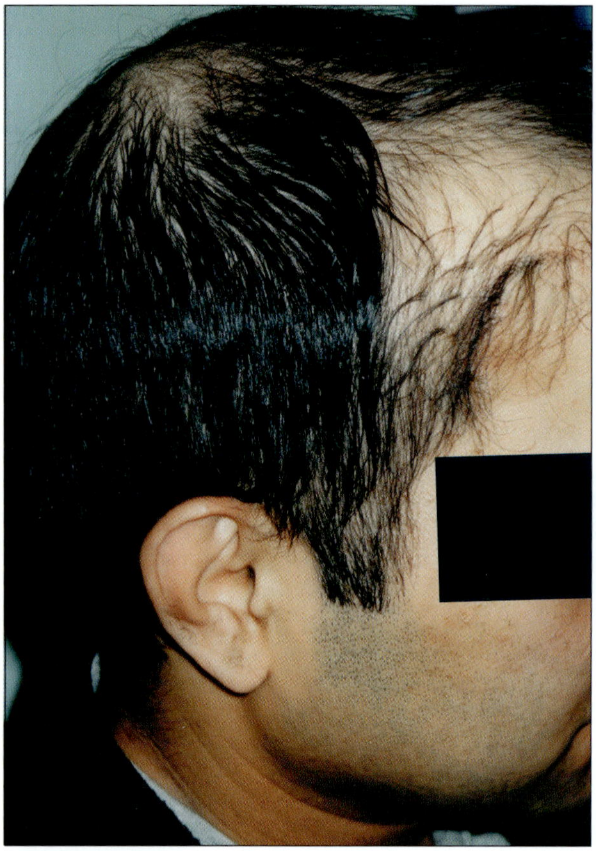

**Fig. 23.1** This hairline is too low and too rounded at the temples. These grafts are too large and hair is growing in the wrong direction

### Incorrect positioning of donor scar

The best donor material is usually sited in the middle of the back and sides of the permanent fringe. The scar should follow the shape of the fringe and not be too high or too low. Oftentimes, a novice surgeon will harvest the donor area in a slanted or nonhorizontal fashion. The resultant angled scar will present a problem in donor strip harvesting in future sessions.

### Bad hair direction

The sites should be made in a direction and exit angle that mimics the natural growth. The hairs on the grafts should be left a millimeter or two long so their angulation can be ascertained and all are planted going in the correct direction, not sideways or backwards (Fig. 23.2).

## Surgical Issues

### Pain

If the patient has been made to feel comfortable with the scheduling and the facility ambience is pleasant, he or she may be anxious but should not be agitated. Oral sedatives can be given if necessary. Local anesthetic with epinephrine may be injected slowly into the donor and recipient areas with ice or a vibrating instrument to minimize discomfort. Tumescence in both areas is essential to achieve

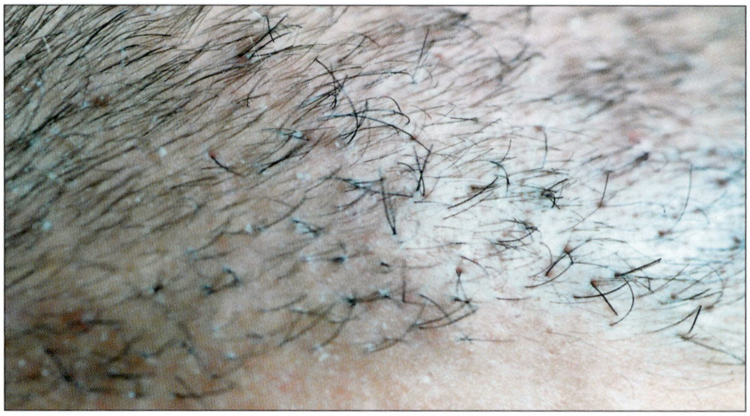

**Fig. 23.2** The great variety of hair direction is most likely due to inconsistent site creation. Another possibility is grafts moving around in sites that are too large for the grafts

longlasting analgesia and bleeding control. In this way pain will not be an issue during the operation.

## Bleeding and popping

Some patients bleed more, especially those who exercise aggressively. Grafts often pop up again, floating up in the bleeding site. Tumesce using saline with epinephine 1:500,000 and wait about 15 minutes. Tumescence takes time to exert its effect. The patient should be comfortable and completely anesthetized. A constant dialogue with the patient helps put them at ease. In cases of 'mushy dermis' the bleeding and popping can be minimized but not eliminated.

## Restlessness

This is usually a manifestation of the patient's anxiety state, but always monitor the vital signs. Sedatives are routinely given to patients. All patients respond differently depending on gender, size, and other factors, thus some individuals will need additional sedatives to achieve the same anxiolytic effect.

## Hiccups

Extremely rare, hiccups have been found to occur during or after the transplant procedure. They are thought to occur due to irritation of an aberrant branch of the vagus nerve. Hiccups have also been found to occur with the intravenous administration of midazolam.

## Quiet death of uncounted donor follicles

Each step from harvesting to placement places the hair follicle at risk. Transection, manipulation, dessication, oxygen starvation and reperfusion injury can all be fatal to the graft. Constant supervision and incremental improvement in handling techniques will minimize this loss.

## Donor area

### *Effluvium*

Hair in the anagen phase can suddenly be shed possibly due to a temporary lack of oxygen during the surgery. It varies from a small amount of loss along the suture line to a massive loss above the suture line when significant blood vessels are cut (Fig. 23.3). The hair loss will be noticed at 2–3 weeks postoperatively and regrowth will occur at the same time as the transplants grow, at around 3 months. Severe effluvium is rarely encountered now that the donor area can be raised above the blood vessels with large volume tumescence.

### *Infection*

This is exceedingly rare and will only occur when mitigating circumstances are present, such as a very tight closure or compromised immunity (Fig. 23.4). A gentle, clean surgical technique in a normal patient with a normal scalp will result in a cleanly healed wound without infection. Most transplant surgeons do not recommend the routine use of antibiotics preoperatively.

### *Dehiscence*

This is very rare and only due to poor surgical technique where the edges of the wound are rolled in on each other, resulting in epidermis-to-epidermis contact rather than dermis-to-dermis contact. Dehiscence can also occur with tight closures, infection and necrosis.

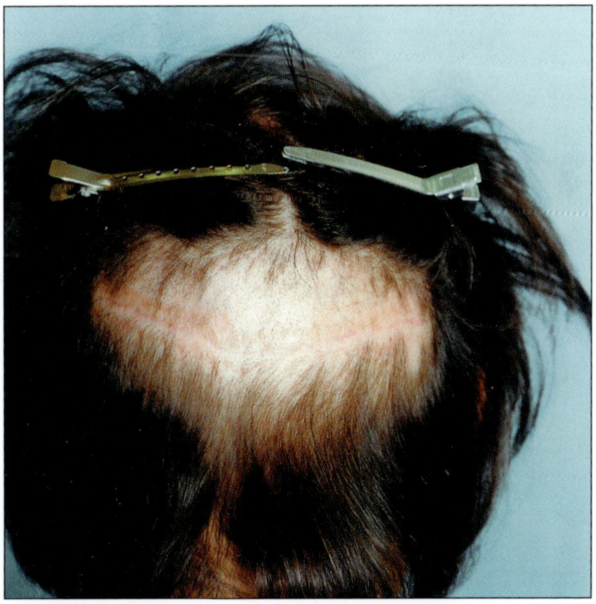

**Fig. 23.3** Massive hair fall-out resulting from both occipital arteries being cut at donor strip harvest. The hair regrew but the patient was unhappy for 3 months

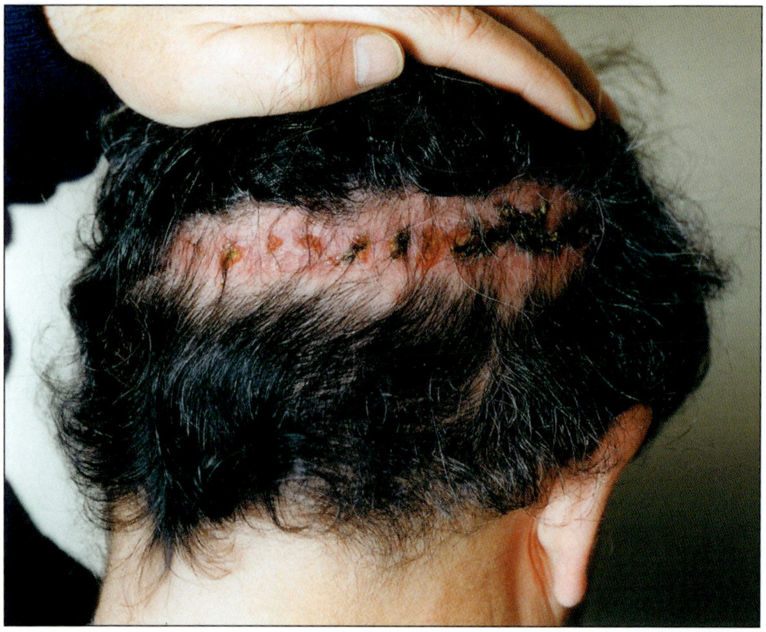

**Fig. 23.4** Red and crusty suture line with associated effluvium 3 weeks after surgery. Closure was under maximum tension. *Staphylococcus aureus* cleared with antibiotics

### *Necrosis*

Figure 23.5 illustrates the result of exceeding the limits of tissue mobility. When too wide a donor strip is harvested, this will result in an extremely tight closure. This will cause a massive compromise of the circulation and tissue death. Making the donor strips as long and as thin as possible will minimize tight closures, as will undermining of the edges. It is also preferable to leave the wound covered with a dressing but unsutured until the end of the operation, when the anesthetic and tumescent fluid will have dissipated. If the edges will still not come together comfortably, it is best to suture the wound as close as possible and leave the rest to heal by secondary intention. This will produce a much better scar than forcing a difficult, tight closure (Fig. 23.6).

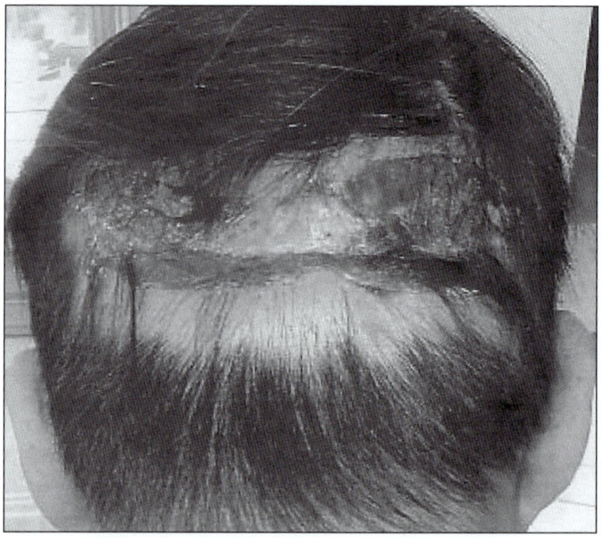

**Fig. 23.5** Massive necrosis and effluvium caused by the surgeon overpowering the scalp and closing the donor defect with too much tension

### *Hyper- and hypoesthesia*

Cutting the occipital nerves during strip harvesting should no longer occur, as tumescence will lift the follicles high above the neurovascular bundles. The scalpel should never cut deeper than the base of the follicles. When the donor strip is harvested at this level only minor and temporary numbness from cutting the very superficial nerve fibers will be experienced.

### *Undesirable scars*

Sound surgical principles of accurate approximation and closure with little or no tension will give us fine scars nearly all the time. Double-layered closures, trichophytic closure where the top edge is trimmed

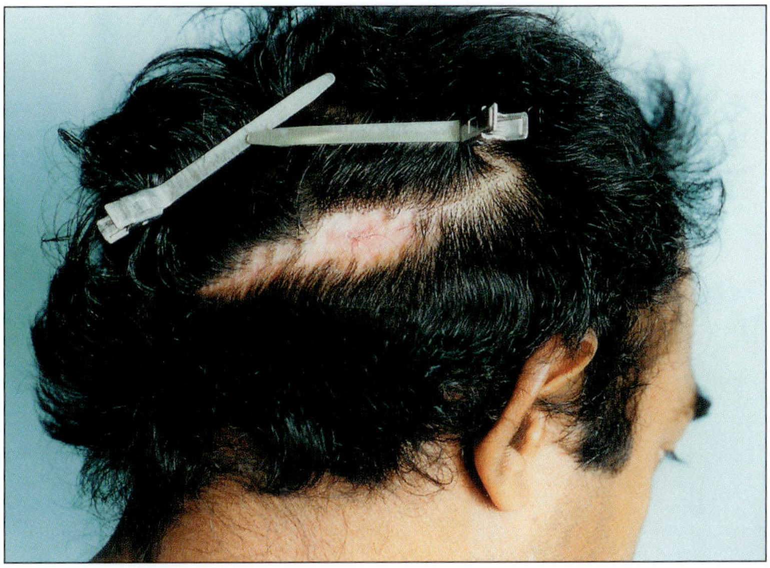

**Fig. 23.6** The tightest area on closure is always over the mastoid. Here a wide scar from tight closure is made wider by necrosis over the mastoid area

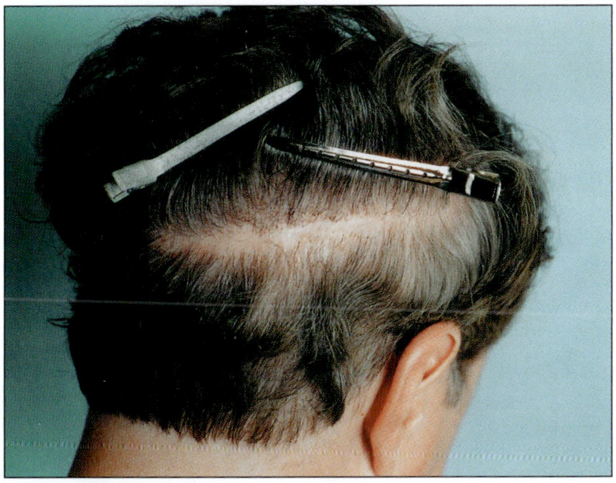

**Fig. 23.7** This 7–8 mm scar is the result of six harvests at the same site excising the previous scar. It began to widen at the fourth harvest

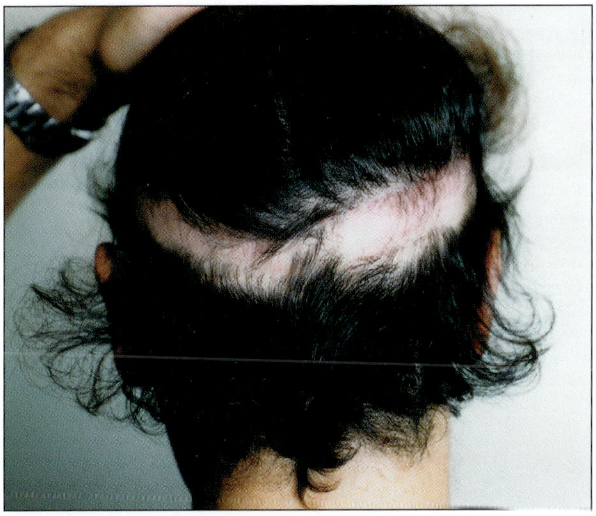

**Fig. 23.8** Three donor harvests at the same site after four alopecia reductions had already stretched the scalp. Bad donor scars are far more likely after reductions

off, and dissolvable sutures or not, can be used to extract even further improvement. All things being equal the first scar produced in the donor area will heal the best. Most practitioners today excise the previous scar during subsequent donor harvests and note that each closure is tighter and the scar gets a little wider each time despite best efforts (Fig. 23.7). When a scar becomes 3 mm wide, consider harvesting elsewhere or with follicular unit extraction (FUE). Tight donor closure can result in cosmetically unacceptable scars and should be avoided (Figs 23.8–23.11). Scar revision by serial excision has been singularly unsuccessful. W plasty with no excision will help to disperse the scar but in the end balloon expansion is the only way to successfully revise wide scars and maintain the improvement. FUE with planting into the scar is being increasingly used.

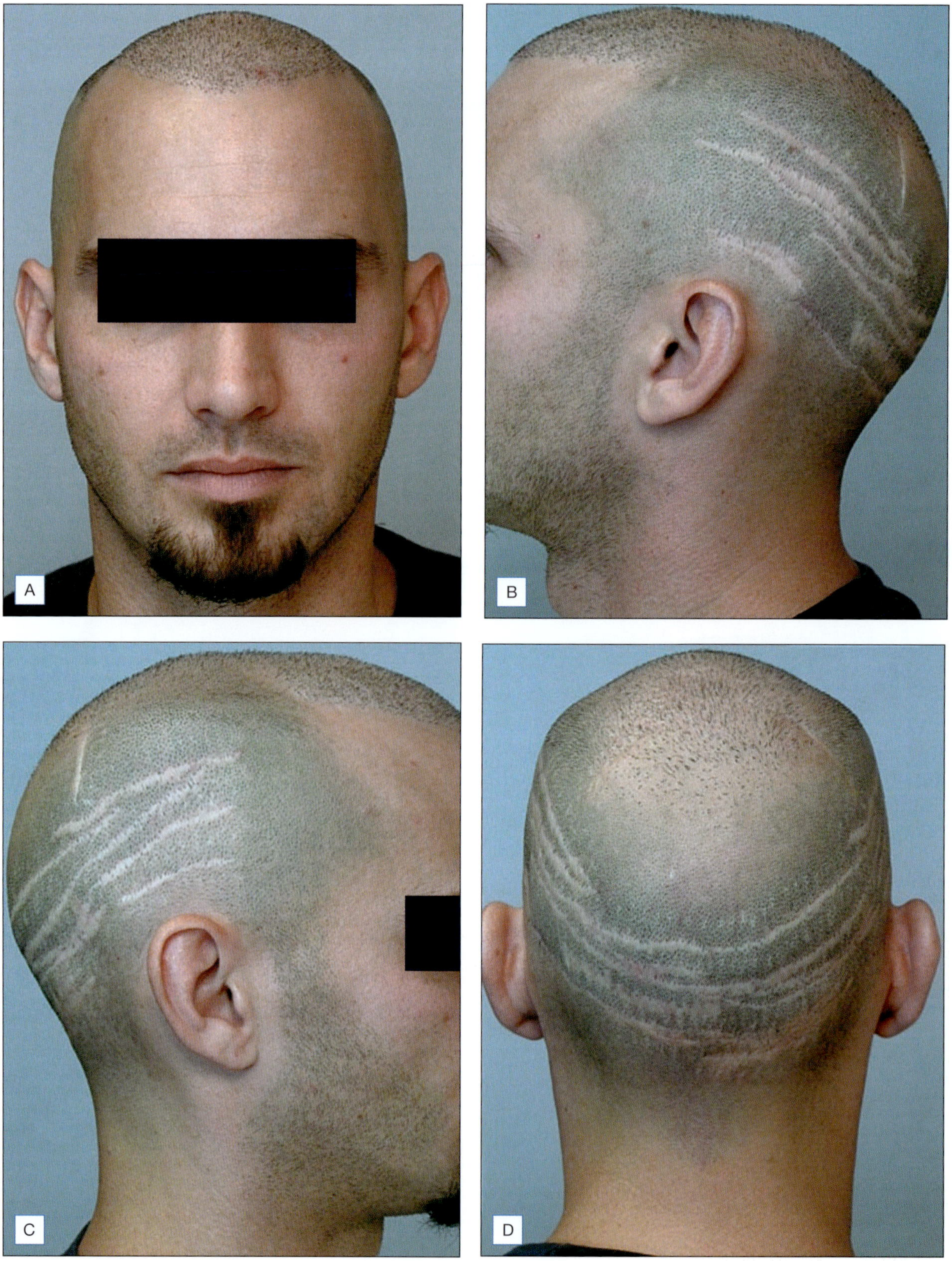


**Fig. 23.9** Example of an insoluble problem. This patient has had 12 hair transplant procedures. There has been complete disregard for the donor area and it is impossible to help this patient with the donor scars, which was his request

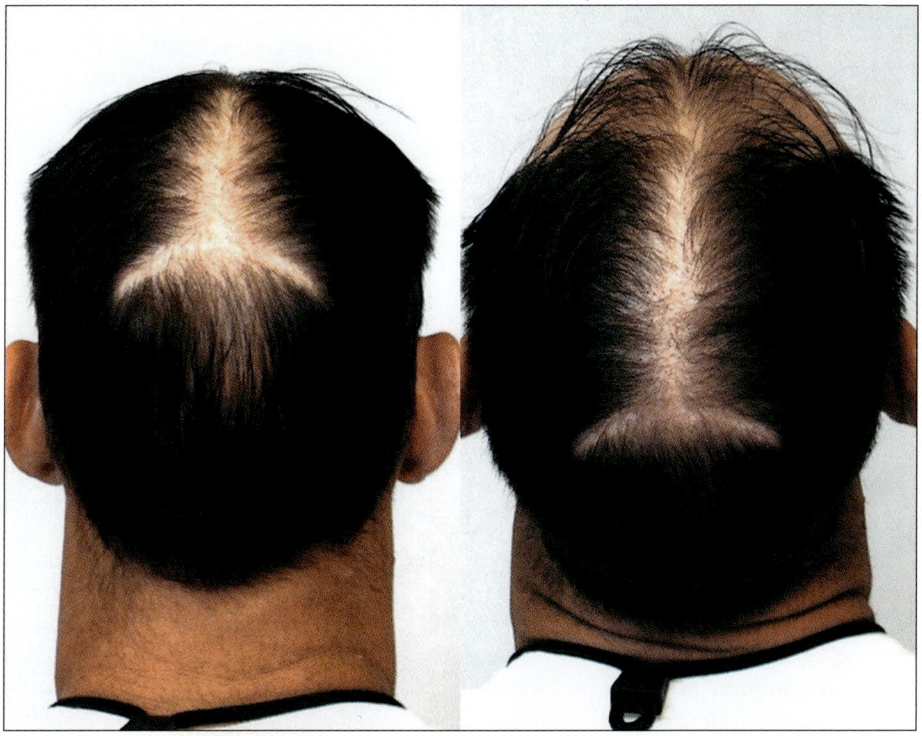

**Fig. 23.10** A scalp reduction has been performed using a Mercedes shaped excision pattern. Because of the different direction of hairs on either side of the scar, a slot deformity has occurred

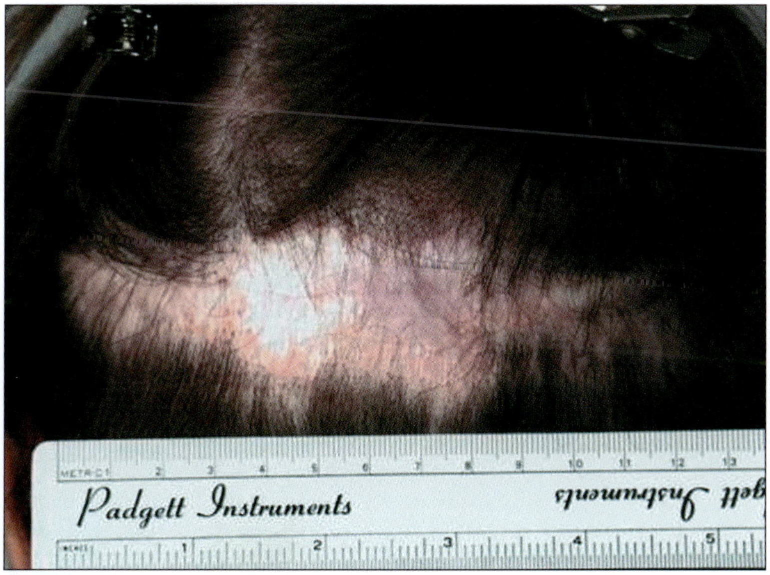


**Fig. 23.11** Result of a secondarily healed donor wound that necrosed following a third harvest attempt in the same location

Hypertrophic scarring is rare and keloids are seen occasionally in Blacks. Once flattened with steroid injections (e.g. triamcinolone) these scars are also best treated with planting after FUE as excision revision may lead to the same problem.

Patients with connective tissue disorders such as Ehlers–Danlos syndrome will always heal with wide, stretched scars so there's no point in revising these with excision either. Again, FUE offers hope in these difficult cases.

## Recipient Area

### Forehead swelling and ecchymosis

This most frequently happens when we work in the frontal area, especially the hairline. It begins on the second postoperative day and can last 3–4 days, gradually spreading downwards to the eyelids, bridge of the nose, and cheeks. It is worst in large cases, and in those patients who do not rest post-operatively. It can be reduced by including cortisone in the local anesthetic solution used at the hairline, applying a pressure bandage, and by the use of 50 mg prednisolone for 5 days postoperatively. Postoperative edema can also be reduced with the use of a turban-style wrap.

### *Surgical effluvium*

Shedding of the existing or 'native' hairs in the recipient area is most unwelcome, especially in female patients, where it is even more likely. It is the same process seen in the donor area where anagen hairs go into telogen en masse, falling out 2–3 weeks postoperatively and regrowing with the grafts at 3 months (Figs 23.12–23.14). However because these native hairs in the recipient area are miniaturizing due to the balding process, they are likely to grow back finer and paler than before so the end result may be little to no improvement in coverage when they and the grafts regrow. It seems to happen more in highly strung, highly motivated individuals and females. Minoxidil use 1 month before the procedure seems to help and certainly second and third procedures in these people should be at longer intervals, the grafts planted more sparsely and with less epinephrine used. Warning of the possibility of effluvium preoperatively can help avoid an angry patient.

### *Cysts, pustules, pimples, and folliculitis*

Many patients will experience one or two eruptions in a field of a thousand or more grafts, but eruptions of dozens or hundreds is quite distressing (Figs 23.15 and 23.16). The onset is about 1 month following surgery and can continue for up to 6 months. The patient can become quite annoyed by this. Fortunately these eruptions eventually clear and rarely reduce eventual growth, although it can be delayed. Obvious causes are piggy-backing one graft upon another or burying of grafts by making the recipient holes too deep. Burying epidermis during site creation, transecting hair during site creation, and planting hair spicules with the grafts is also believed to cause inflammation. Acne-type treatments have been of some benefit but time is the best healer.

### *Pitting and tenting*

Where the hair exits the scalp the epidermis is either inverted in the shape of a pit or elevated in the shape of a tent (Figs 23.17 and 23.18). A mild form of this is seen in natural hair growth but a large amount of it attracts attention, especially at the hairline. There may be variations in the healing characteristics of different patients but it is most likely due to placement errors. Grafts are placed too deeply in pitting and are placed too superficially in tenting. Appearance can be improved by further planting between the irregularities with obvious attention to the depth of planting. Tenting can also be improved by dermabrading the area while punch excision may be required for severe pitting.

### *Poor growth*

This can be apparent or real. Apparent poor growth happens in individuals with very fine hair. Though the growth of FUs may be excellent, the fine, 'see-through' hair gives the appearance of poor growth. FUs in fine hair cases should only be used at the hairline with larger grafts used behind the hairline to achieve more density. In real terms there may be more cases of poor growth than surgeons realize because it's so difficult to assess growth accurately.

With the expert graft handling techniques available today, greater than 90% growth should be managed in the first procedure but somewhere less than that with subsequent procedures. Occasionally there is a very disappointing growth rate (Figs 23.19 and 23.20). When this happens, it is important to carefully evaluate each step in the transplant procedure: the personnel involved, protocols followed, every aspect of postoperative care, and anything that may have affected the result. Good operative notes will help. The patient may be a little aggressive at this time. The practitioner should share with the patient their own disappointment and the fact that aggression is ineffective.

The patient's honest co-operation is needed to try to solve the mystery. Ask whether any of the grafts

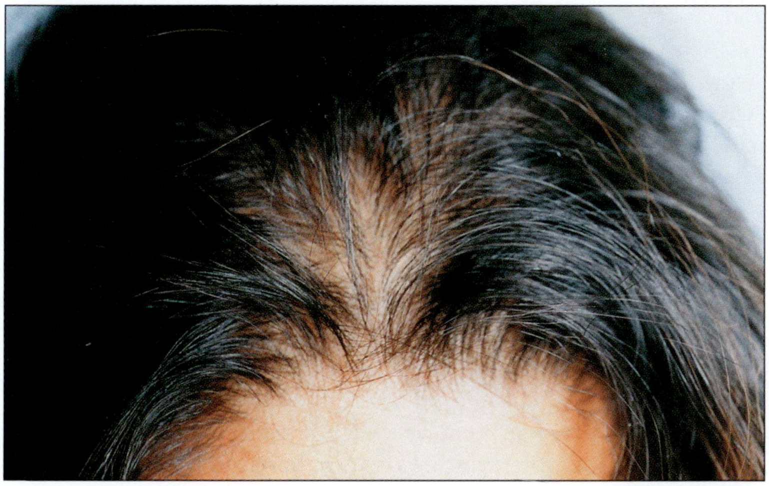

**Fig. 23.12** Typical female pattern hair loss in a 30-year-old highly successful but highly stressed businesswoman

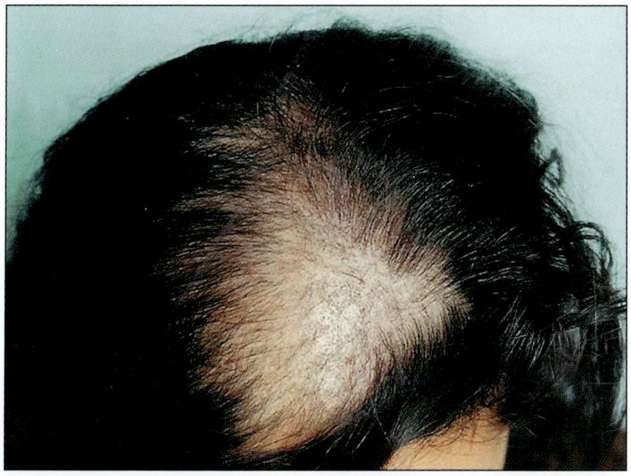

**Fig. 23.13** Three weeks after 1000 FU grafts to the frontal area she presents with massive fall-out of the native hairs and a massive increase in anxiety. Camouflage sprays and powders with judicious styling carried her through until regrowth

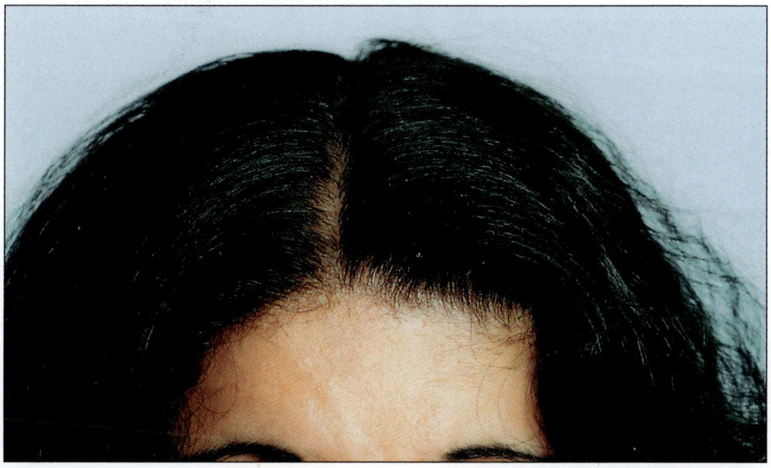

**Fig. 23.14** The expected result was achieved 6 months after the surgery. The effluvium was a real personal crisis for this patient, made bearable only by lots of practical and personal help along the way

fell out in the week after the operation, in the shower or through combing and brushing. Ask the patient if a hairpiece or a hard hat was worn. Find out if he is a closet smoker. Ascertain whether he had effluvium of his native hairs, which now produce less coverage. It is wise at this stage to wait at least 1 year before any final assessment can be made as late growth can make a huge difference.

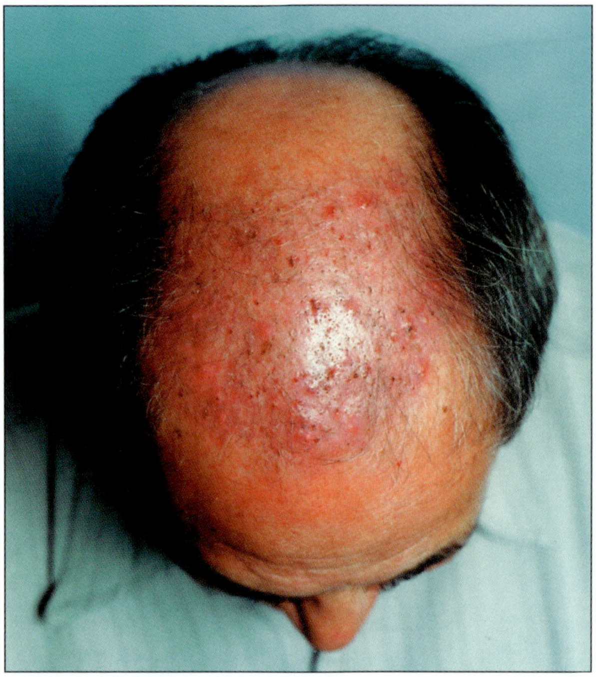

**Fig. 23.15** This patient had waited many years and needed many consultations before he had the courage to proceed to surgery. He was totally devastated by the postoperative inflammation

At 12 months measure the graft growth per cm$^2$. If the operative notes say '25 grafts per cm$^2$' were planted but only 15 can be counted on average, then 60% growth has been achieved. If there is no apparent cause, tell the patient. Share the fact that in rare cases this does happen. Offer free of charge, the numbers of grafts that may not have grown, with the assurance that every aspect will be closely monitored to try to discover the cause, but that if despite all this attention a similar growth rate of 60% is achieved again, then there may be a growth problem that is not understood. This has been described as 'X Factor' in previous articles and texts.

## *Ridging and hypertrophic scarring*

A raised band or ridge is seen at the hairline and for a centimeter or two within the hairline after transplantation. It's not seen with FU transplants but in cases where larger grafts, especially 4 mm punch grafts, were used. Excessive scar tissue is deposited in these cases, causing the raised appearance. It is unlikely to be a simple volumetric addition to the areas as punch grafts replace tissue which is removed, and dense, packed FUs into slits would add tissue volume to the hairline but do not produce ridging. If the ridging is unsightly it may have to be excised. Less dramatic treatments include steroid injections and planting of FUs to hide the ridge.

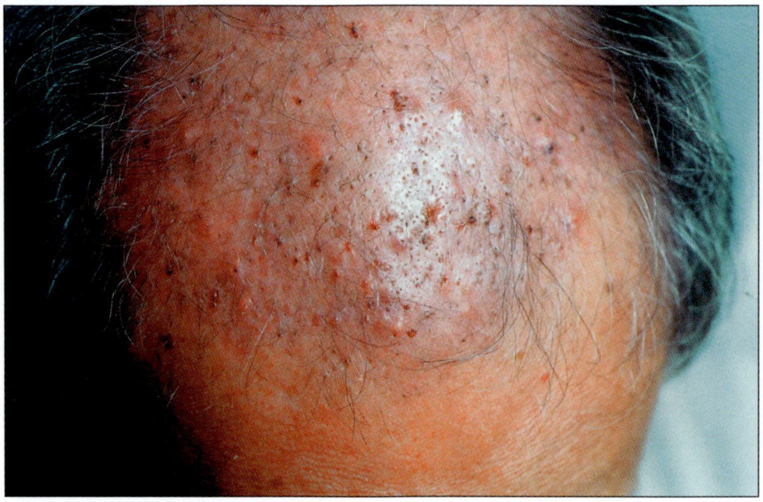

**Fig. 23.16** Close-up shows sebaceous plugs and pustules similar to acne, which were gradually settled with acne treatment. Growth began at 4 months but was not complete in the worst areas until 18 months postoperatively

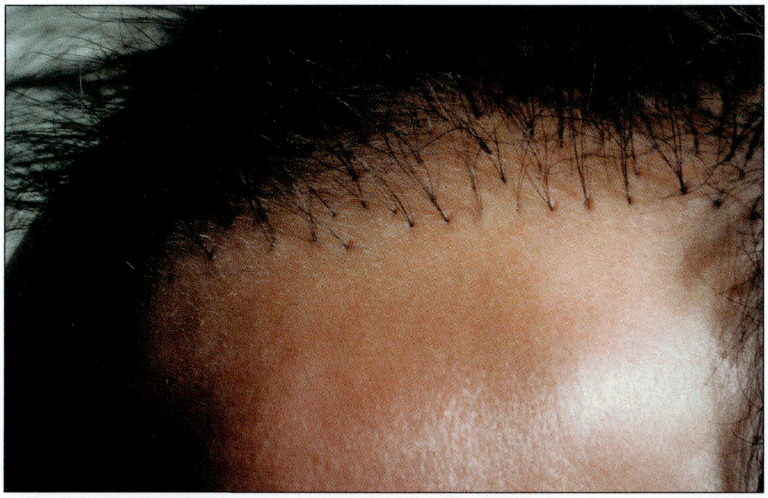

**Fig. 23.17** Minigrafts planted too deeply, resulting in pitting where the hair exits the scalp

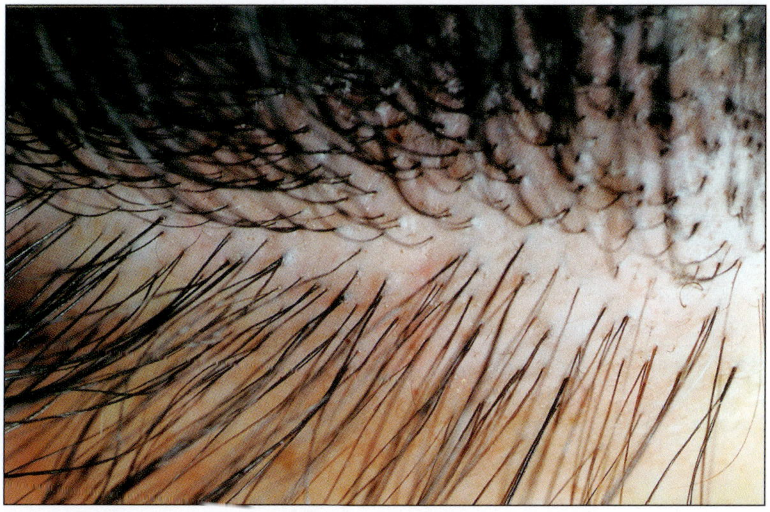

**Fig. 23.18** Most of these grafts display tenting at their site of exit. This patient's strong, coarse hair may have contributed but planting too superficially is the most likely cause

## Infection

Infection is almost unheard of. As in the donor area if it does happen, mitigating circumstances will be present such as compromised immunity, diabetes, excessive sweating under a hairpiece or very poor postoperative hygiene. Antibiotics should not be routinely prescribed. The use of antiseptic shampoo such as surgical scrub is appropriate for a few days postoperatively.

## Necrosis

This occurs when too many sites are made too close together, compromising the blood supply. It is most likely to happen in the center of the mid-scalp, where the blood vessels are at their most distal end, and when there has been previous surgery that left scars that interrupt the blood supply. It is fortunate that the scalp has a great supply of blood vessels and many anastamoses, but it is important to know its limits as necrosis is totally preventable. The authors deal with many unusual characters as patients, some of whom may injure themselves. Factital injury will occur if a patient has a fixation about a certain area and keeps picking at it. Surgeons need to be aware that factital injury can mimic necrosis.

## Pressure necrosis

Prolonged pressure applied to the scalp can result in permanent alopecia, thus the term 'pressure necrosis.' Pressure necrosis with resulting permanent alopecia can result from a myriad of etiologies. The most common cause of alopecia due to focal pressure in the hair-bearing region of the scalp is due to a hair piece attached with tapes, glues, and fastener devices. An unusual cause of pressure necrosis is due to anesthesia. Prolonged anesthesia, where the head is supported by a small surface area, can result in necrosis of the skin within 1 week after surgery (Fig. 23.21). The resulting alopecia is oftentimes permanent.

## *A-V fistula*

Rarely, an artery and vein injured side by side during site creation will lead to A-V fistula formation. This is a rare occurence. The fistula will be easily

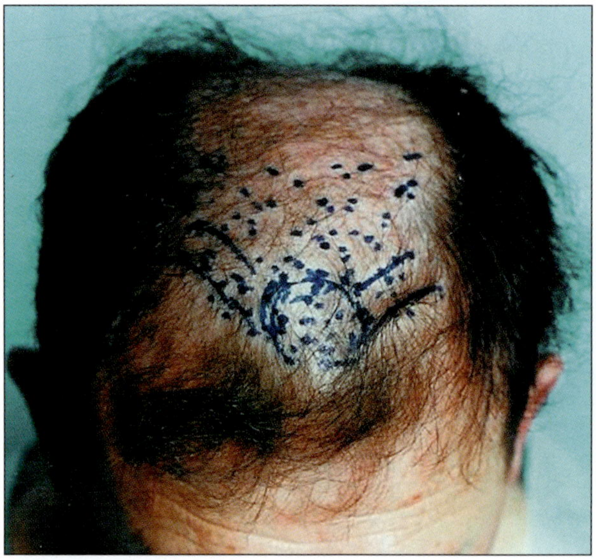

**Fig. 23.19** Patient with Norwood Va pattern with remaining forelock. The plan is to plant 1000 FU transplants to the frontal scalp behind his forelock

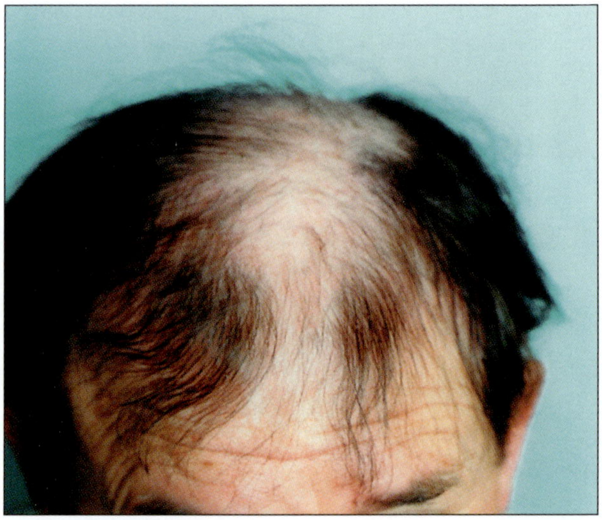

**Fig. 23.20** Nine months later the same patient as in Fig. 23.19 presented with less hair! Only about 50% of the grafts have grown and most of his forelock suffered effluvium and did not regrow. Planting of another 500 grafts free of charge also resulted in very poor growth. Could this be the X factor?

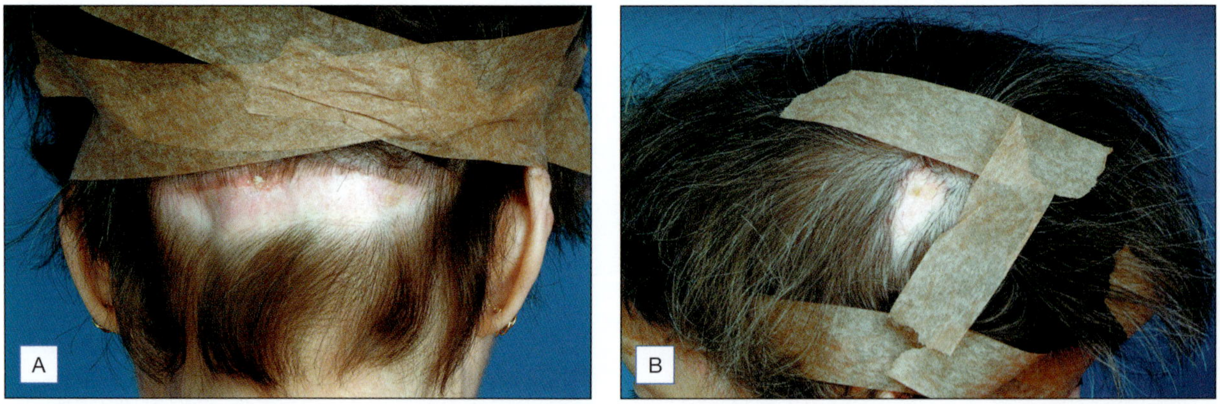


**Fig. 23.21** (**A**) Pressure-induced necrosis secondary to prolonged anesthesia. The patient, a 57-year-old female, underwent a prolonged operation in which general anesthesia was employed. (**B**) Approximately 3 or 4 days after surgery, the area became red and edematous. This was followed by sloughing of the skin and resultant alopecia as shown in the photographs

identified and should be left to heal spontaneously unless large and troublesome. Simple tying of the artery through a small incision will solve the problem. With no major vessels cut, A-V fistulas should not be seen in the donor area.

## Authors' Note

Some of these complications occurred to patients in the authors' hands while others came from elsewhere. We thank all our colleagues who contributed images and stories to help cover the broad range of complications.

## Further Reading

Bernstein RM, Rassman WR, Rashid N, Shiell RC 2002 The art of repair in surgical hair restoration Part I: Basic repair strategies. Dermatol Surg 738–794

Bernstein RM, Rassman WR, Rashid N, Shiell RC 2002 The art of repair in surgical hair restoration Part II: The tactics of repair Dermatol Surg 873–893

Cooley JE 2004 Complications of hair transplantation. In: Unger WP, Shipiro R, Eds. Hair Transplantation. 4th ed. Marcel Dekker 568–573

Vogel JE 2004 Correcting problems in hair restoration surgery: an update. Facial Plast Surg Clin N Am 263–278

Vogel JE 2001 Correcting frequently seen hair transplant problems. Hair Transplant Forum International 11(1)

# 24 Follicle Facts

*Matt L. Leavitt*

"Beware of her fair locks, for when she winds them around a young man's neck, she will not set him free again."

*Johann Wolfgang von Goethe, Poet (1749–1832)*

## Introduction

North Americans spend in excess of $7 billion each year attempting to fight hair loss with drugs, surgery, cosmetics and nonsurgical hair replacement. Hair transplantation accounts for nearly 1 billion dollars annually.

**Alopecia**, the medical word for hair loss, is Greek in origin and literally translated means 'fox.' It refers to the wild animal's mangy fur that often fell out in patches. Hair grows on virtually every part of our body except the lips, the palms of the hands and the bottoms of the feet.

## Historical Record of Hair Importance

- Stone Age: Discovery of a comb made of boxwood in a burial site dated 10,000 years ago. Many heads found at the site were adorned with bones and feathers.
- **Egyptians:** Statues, pyramid burials, and cave paintings dating 5000 years ago depicted the significance given to hair and stressed the importance of tresses.
- **Romans** battled hair loss at the beginning of the 1st millennium, including Caesar, who wore a laurel wreath to hide his lack of hair. He instituted the practice of cutting his enemy's hair as a sign of submission. Also in Rome, prostitutes were licensed, taxed, and forced by law to either dye their hair blonde or to wear a blonde wig.
- **The Dark Ages** continued to reveal hair's importance: Queen Clotild (d.554) of Gaul allowed her grandsons to be killed by the sword of enemies rather than have their hair shorn.
- **The Renaissance period** often depicted women covering their hair or using a net or fabric to collect the long hair at the back called a **balzo**, while English men and women began wearing wigs, a trend made popular by Queen Elizabeth I. In Shakespeare's tragedies, hair loss was portrayed as a weakness.
- **The 17th and 18th centuries** had Louis XIII of France top his bald dome with the 'big-wig' that became more outrageous and excessive with time as his subjects joined in the new fashion. The first ladies' salon appeared in France in 1635, some 1300 hundred years after the men's and was appropriately named 'Champagne.'
- **The American Colonies:** In 1655 the president of Harvard delivered his commencement sermon reiterating that long hair was forbidden and that it would not 'be lawful for anyone to wear long hair, locks or foretops' or 'to use curling, parting or powdering.'
- **Early 20th century:** Short hairstyles for women became popular, with more than 2000 women per day cutting their hair into the 'bob.' The University of Arkansas disclosed that it had proven through experimentation that longer hair was a sign of female intellect. Madam C.J. Walker, the first African–American millionaire, introduced haircare products for Blacks.
- **Late 20th century:** In 1989 the FDA reviewed 300,000 over-the-counter products claiming to grow, replace, restore or save hair. All of these products were determined to be ineffectual and 'not especially safe and/or effective.' There are

only two FDA-approved medical treatments to treat hair loss: **minoxidil** (topical), approved since 1988 (introduced to the public as Rogaine), and **finasteride** (oral), branded as Propecia, approved since 1998.

## History of Surgical Hair Transplantation

- **1897:** Scalp tissue is surgically transposed from one area of the head to the other to cover a denuded area (wound). This is considered to be the initial premise for hair transplantation.
- **1926:** The first scalp reduction is performed.
- **1931:** For the first time French surgeon Passot moved hair from a viable hair-bearing section of the scalp to a bald area, creating what is believed to be the first hair transplantation.
- **1939:** Japanese dermatologist Shojui Okuda published his results from hair transplantation. His technique of inserting grafts into small needle-stick recipient sites is similar to modern techniques.
- **1940s:** Dr James B. Hamilton began research into male pattern baldness. His work supported the androgenetic theory of common baldness, and he further developed the Hamilton Hair Loss Chart system for classification and identification still in use today.
- **1960:** credit is given for the founding and popularizing of hair transplantation to Dr Norman Orentreich, for his work in the early 1950s and later, his published material in 1959. He developed the theory of 'donor dominance,' whereby hair grafts were transplanted from the hair-bearing occipital area to the frontal balding area. Grafts maintained their integrity and behaved as they did at their original site.
- **1970s and 1980s:** introduced punch grafts or 'plugs,' which were responsible for the 'corn row' and 'doll-hair' appearance of frontal hairlines. This technique left the donor area with many small, round scars. Scalp reductions were routinely performed in order to save precious grafts for frontal transplantation.
- **1990s**: Dr Bobby Limmer is credited for developing the modern technique for hair transplantation. This technique allows for transplantation of 1000–3000 grafts at one time. The donor strip is examined with high-power magnification and cut into naturally occurring groups of follicular units (FUs), each usually containing one to four hairs.
- **1998** Board Certification for Hair Transplantation is awarded for the first time
- **2000s** Research scientists press forward with stem cell research, hair multiplication, and cloning.
- **2005** Most individuals receiving hair transplants have exceptional, natural results not visibly detectable as hair transplants.

## Follicular Facts

- **Hair** shafts grown in a lifetime would extend over 700 miles if placed end to end.
- **Hairs** on our body surpass 5 million; most never grow more than $^1/_2$ inch or exceed 0.0035 in diameter.
- **Hair** grows approximately $^1/_2$ in per month, or 6 in per year.
- **Hair** grows at the rate of: 0.00000001 miles per hour.
- **Hair** grown everyday on the body: 40 yards.
- **Hair** cells divide every 12 hours.
- **Hair** grows faster in the summertime than in the winter.
- **Hair** shed by the average person 60 years old tops 4 million hairs.
- **Hair** loss can be caused by more than 300 drugs.
- **Hair** twisted into a rope could pull a weight of 15 tons.
- **Hair** grows 0.039 mm at our temples and 0.044 mm at the vertex in a 24-hour period.
- **Hair** absorbs moisture then stretches and elongates, allowing it to vary in length by up to 2%.
- **Hair** loss is considered to be a genuine form of disease by the FDA.
- **Hair** is the thickest at age 20 and continues to shrink; by age 70, hair is as fine as baby's hair.
- **Hair** on top of the head usually grows in a clockwise whorl pattern.
- **Hair** follicles secrete sebum, which is composed of fat, cholesterol, proteins, and salts.
- **Hair** length regulations were relaxed by the US Army during the turbulent 1970s: $3^1/_2$ inches was permitted
- **Hairs** on the sea otter count up to 700,000 per $in^2$, the densest of any animal.
- **Hair composition**: 50% carbon, 20% oxygen, 17% nitrogen, 6% hydrogen, 5% sulfur, 2% other
- **Hair** follicles begin to shrink in size around age 40
- **Hair** follicles sensitive to DHT will not regrow hairs and are not suitable for hair transplantation.

- **Hair** loss due to age, not genetics is called 'senescent 'or 'involutional alopecia'.
- **Hair** follicles at the female hairline contain six times more aromatase as those in the male hairline.
- **Hair** count per scalp by hair color: blonde – 140,000; brown – 110,000; black – 108,000; red – 90,000.
- **Hair** loss occurs in more than 50% of men in the United States.
- **Hair** loss occurs in 30 million US women.
- **Hair** loss in women is visible in 40% by age 40.
- **Hair** loss is due to androgenetic alopecia in more than 90% of cases.
- **Hair** growth is controlled by more than 150 genes.
- **Hair** loss is not visually apparent until 50% is lost.
- **Hair** loss genetics: autosomal dominant or polygenic, inherited from either or both parents.
- **Hair** loss incidence in men: 16% by age 18–29, 53% by age 40–49.

## Indications for Hair Transplantation

Hair transplantation, while most frequently performed in larger sessions, is very useful for patients presenting with:

- Denuded hair-bearing areas resulting from face- or brow-lift scars.
- Loss of body hair in such places as pubic, beard, moustache and chest areas.
- Scars on hair-bearing areas acquired from injuries or accidents.
- Scars or denuded areas from birth due to use of forceps or fetal monitors.
- Hair loss due to radiation treatment to scalp area.
- Eyebrow or eyelash loss or scarring.
- Transsexual or gender reassignment.
- Hypopigmented areas damaged from relaxers or traction alopecia.

## Body Hair Transplantation

The follicular unit extraction technique involves extraction of scalp or body hair grafts using a small punch, 1 mm or less. Donor hair can be taken from the chest or back and transplanted to the head.

## Influence of Recipient Sites

A study undertaken in Korea by Dr Jung-Chul Kim examined the influence the recipient site extended to transplanted grafts. Hair was transplanted from the occipital area to the lower leg. After 3 years, hair was transplanted from the leg and re-transplanted to the nape of the neck. Results suggested that the recipient site affects some characteristics of transplanted grafts, such as growth and survival rates. In other words, the transplanted hair attempts to take on the characteristics of the new site.

## Ethnic Considerations

Black, Hispanic, and Asian hair presents its own set of circumstances to be considered when performing hair transplantation:

- Darker skin allows for need of fewer grafts due to less contrast between the skin and the hair.
- Darker skin can lead to keloid formation, hypopigmentation and hypertrophic scars if not carefully assessed pre-transplantation.
- Owing to the curly nature of the follicle, pseudofolliculitis barbae or 'razor bumps' may occur from improperly placed or angled hair follicles. If abscesses form, follicular morbidity is possible.
- Cobblestoning may occur if grafts are placed too high or too low on the scalp and may cause an irregular skin surface that is raised, hardened, and bumpy. Grafts look less attractive.
- Donor site may be less dense; hair can be harvested from fringe areas above the ears.
- 'Halo effect.' A round, unpigmented area of tissue surrounding the edge of the placed graft may occur if grafts are too large.
- The diameter of Asian hair is 80 µm.
- The diameter of Caucasian hair is 70 µm
- The diameter of Black hair is 60 µm.

## Women and Hair Loss

In the USA, 30 million women are affected by some type of hair loss. Many are excellent candidates for hair transplantation and since female hair loss is usually diffuse, the frontal hairline is maintained 85% of the time. Facts about hair loss are listed in Box 24.1.

## Psychology of Hair Loss

- 28% of the men surveyed complained about diffuse hair loss and 48% about baldness; this is

**Facts about female pattern hair loss (FPHL)**

- Affects 65–75% of females presenting with alopecia
- Affects nearly 25% of women aged 35–40
- Affects nearly 50% of women beyond the age of 40
- 20% presenting have a family history of androgenetic alopecia

**Box 24.1** Main reasons for female pattern hair loss (FPHL)

reversed in women: 68% complain about diffuse hair loss and 8% about baldness.

- Men receive information on baldness 68% of the time, and women only receive information on baldness 58% of the time.
- Women are more often given vitamins and shampoos, and given twice the amount of psychological advice as men.
- Seldom are either referred to a psychologist or a psychiatrist, although 50% were diagnosed with psychological problems.
- Androgenetic alopecia is a stressful experience for both sexes, but it is substantially more distressing for women.
- Women are almost twice as likely as men to feel very to extremely upset with negative effects of hair loss.
- The psychological impact of androgenetic alopecia is more severe for women than for men.
- Men tend to receive more teasing and social comments about their loss than women.

## Whorl Pattern and Handedness

Hair grows in a clockwise whorl pattern at the crown in the majority of the population. However, Dr AJ Klar published an article in *Genetics*, August 2004 that the whorl corresponds to 'human handedness.' Specifically, most of the public is right handed and hair grows clockwise; the scalp hair-whorl rotation is counterclockwise in only 8.4% of individuals. Nonright-handers (NRHs) show a random mixture of clockwise and counterclockwise swirling patterns.

## Three Shapes: Determined by Ethnicity (see also Fig. 24.1)

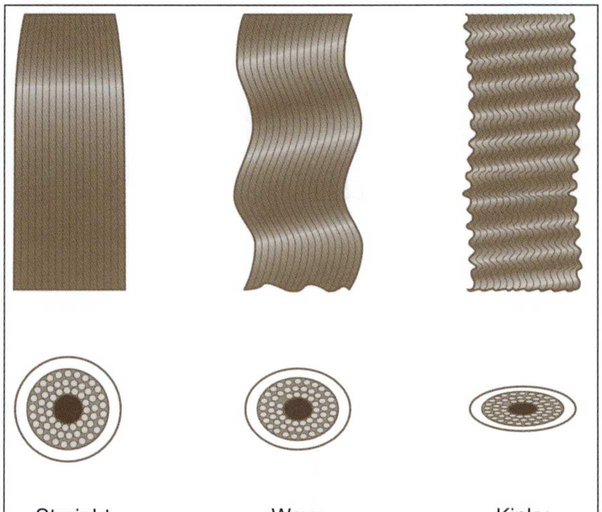


**Fig. 24.1** Depiction of the three hair follicle shapes by ethnicity, left to right; Leiotrichous or straight shaft (Asian); Cynotrichous or wavy shaft (Caucasion); Heliotrichosis or kinky shaft (Black)

- **Leiotrichous:** the thick, round hair shaft causes hair to be straight. Usually seen in Asians, who have a lesser incidence of baldness than Caucasians.
- **Cynotrichous:** a slender, elliptical, and often curved shaft with medium thickness. Most often seen in Caucasian hair
- **Heliotrichous:** ribbon-like, slightly flattened, medium thick, wavy, curly or kinky shaft. Most often seen in the hair shaft of Blacks.

## Further Reading

Cash T, Price V, Savin R 1993 Psychological effects of androgenetic alopecia on women: Comparisons with balding men and with female control subjects. Journal of the American Academy of Dermatology 29(4):568–575

DeKoning EG, Passchier J, Dekker FW 1990 Psychological problems with hair loss in general practice and the treatment policies of general practitioners. Psychological Reports 67:775–778

Hwang S, Kim J-C et al 2002 Does the recipient site influence the hair growth characteristics in hair transplantation? Journal of American Society for Dermatologic Surgery 28(9):795–799

Klar AJ 2003 Human handedness and scalp hair – whorl direction develops from a common genetic mechanism. Genetics 165:269–276

Leavitt ML 2004 Hair loss and women: A physician's perspective. Beautiful Media Publishing, Atlanta, Georgia

Price V 1988 Androgenetic alopecia and hair growth promotion: State-of-the-art present and future. Clinics in Dermatology 6:218–227

Severn W 1971 The long and short of it: Five thousand years of fun and fury over hair. McKay Publishing, New York, p 136

# 25 Core Curriculum in Hair Transplantation Surgery

*Carlos J. Puig*

## Introduction

In 1993, the International Society of Hair Restoration Surgery (ISHRS) was formed to enhance the communication between hair transplantation physicians around the world. The open and honest communications that resulted from this organization's leadership accelerated the development of technologies. This society has promoted the development of a 'core curriculum' for educational purposes.

## Core Curriculum

The Core Curriculum in Hair Restoration Surgery (CCHRS) defines basic science, didactic information, surgical techniques, and pharmacology that are essential to physician competence. In addition, the correct diagnosis and treatment of hair loss are consistent with patient safety and sound esthetic results. The ISHRS hopes that all existing surgical and dermatology training programs that teach hair transplantation surgery procedures will find the CCHRS useful in developing their curriculum relative to the field. This will facilitate the development of a new standard of training within the profession.

The CCHRS is reviewed annually by the ISHRS and contains only those topics and techniques that are evidence based or have proven beneficial to patients through the test of time in application. The CCHRS is designed to be flexible so that it can be expanded or contracted in detail to the level required by the user. A more detailed outline is available on the ISHRS website at: www.ISHRS.org.

Carlos J. Puig DO is the Principle author for The Core Curriculum in Hair Restoration Surgery:

1. Basic science
1.1. Basic science of hair
1.1.1. Scalp anatomy and physiology
1.1.2. Cyclic activity of hair
1.1.3. Androgen-dependent hair
1.1.4. Pathophysiology of androgenic alopecia
1.1.5. Alopecia: classification and incidence
1.1.6. Types of hair
1.1.7. Racial and individual variations
1.1.8. Hair loss etiologies
1.1.9. Excess hair growth
1.1.10. Dermatological scalp conditions
1.2. Epidemiology and demographics of hair loss
1.2.1. Age and androgenetic alopecia (AGA) in men
1.2.2. Female androgenetic alopecia (AGA)
1.2.3. Ethnic variation in the characteristics of skin, scalp, and hair
1.3. Wound healing
1.3.1. Basic science
1.3.2. Factors that influence wound healing
1.3.3. Anatomic and skin type considerations
1.3.4. Microbiology
1.3.5. Biomechanics and histology of normal skin and scars
1.3.6. Wound healing
2. Clinical science
2.1. General surgical principles
2.1.1. Sterile technique
2.1.2. Instrumentation
2.1.3. Instrument preparation
2.1.4. Closure materials
2.1.5. Wound care
2.2. Patient consultation, evaluation, and preparation
2.2.1. Psychology of hair
2.2.2. Patient evaluation
2.2.3. Selection
2.2.4. Standardized photography for hair transplantation
2.2.5. Medicolegal issues in hair replacement

2.2.6. Hair transplantation
2.2.7. Hairline design details
2.2.8. The donor site
2.2.9. Graft preparation techniques
2.2.10. Graft insertion techniques
2.2.11. Postoperative care
2.2.12. Scalp reductions and scalp lifting
2.2.13. Pedicle rotation flaps in the surgical treatment of alopecia
2.3. Development of treatment plan
2.3.1. Patient expectations
2.3.2. Surgical feasibility
2.3.3. Assessments of risks/benefits of treatment plan
2.3.4. Informed consent to include alternative therapies
2.4. Anesthesia
2.4.1. Acetylsalicylic acid (ASA) risk classification
2.4.2. Topical anesthesia
2.4.3. Local anesthesia
2.4.4. Regional anesthesia
2.4.5. Nerve block anesthesia of the scalp
2.4.6. Special considerations
2.4.7. Complications
2.4.8. Pain control and management of the postoperative period
2.5. Emergency preparedness
2.5.1. Management of surgical emergencies
2.5.2. Basic and advanced cardiac life support (ACLS curriculum)
2.5.3. Emergency situations in hair transplantation
2.6. Reconstruction
2.6.1. Surgical techniques
2.6.2. Surgical options
2.7. Complications
2.7.1. General theory, management, and prevention of complications:
2.7.2. Complications of hair transplantation
2.7.3. Complications of flaps in the treatment of baldness
2.7.4. Scar revision
2.8. Strategies in updating old techniques and correcting suboptimal results
2.9. Interdisciplinary care of patient
2.9.1. Interdisciplinary care for complicated cases
2.9.2. Interaction with other medical and surgical specialists to provide optimal care
2.9.3. Education of other medical, surgical, and lay specialists in hair restoration surgery
2.9.4. Nonsurgical hair replacement
2.10. Medical therapy
2.10.1. Current understanding of androgenetic alopecia (AGA) and testosterone
2.10.2. Minoxidil
2.10.3. Finasteride
2.10.4. Dutasteride
2.10.5. Over-the-counter (OTC) treatments and hoaxes
2.11. Special considerations
2.11.1. Hair transplantation in Blacks
2.11.2. Hair transplantation in Asians
2.11.3. Hair transplantation in females
2.11.4. Hair transplantation of the eyebrows
2.11.5. Hair transplantation of the eyelashes
2.11.6. Reconstruction of the temporal points area
2.11.7. Moustache transplantation
2.11.8. Hair transplantation in skin grafts, thin recipient skin, and radiation-induced alopecia
2.11.9. Treatment of the genetically male transsexual
2.11.10. The treatment of female pattern alopecia
2.11.11. Synthetic hair
2.11.12. Automation techniques in hair restoration surgery
2.11.13. Scalp reconstruction techniques
2.11.14. Ethics, marketing and patient consent
3. Professional/regulatory topics
3.1. Medicolegal issues
3.1.1. Risk assessment in the surgical patient
3.1.2. Medical record documentation
3.1.3. Quality assurance (QA) and continuous quality improvement (CQI)
3.1.4. Informed consent
3.1.5. Photographic reproduction
3.2. Regulatory issues
3.2.1. Occupational safety and health administration (OSHA)
3.2.2. Blood-borne pathogens (BBPs)
3.3. Professional ethics
3.3.1. Professional ethical standards
3.3.2. Selection of the most cost-effective treatment plan given patient goals
3.3.3. Realistic expectations
3.3.4. Professional marketing

Reprinted from Dermatologic Surgery 30: 2005; with permission.

# 26 Photographic Results in Hair Transplantation

## Introduction

This chapter presents before and after pictures for patients with a variety of hair loss problems treated by the authors of the chapters in this book. Each set of images demonstrates the type of high-quality work available in the world today.

### Case 1: Male pattern hair loss
### Surgeon: Dowling B. Stough, MD

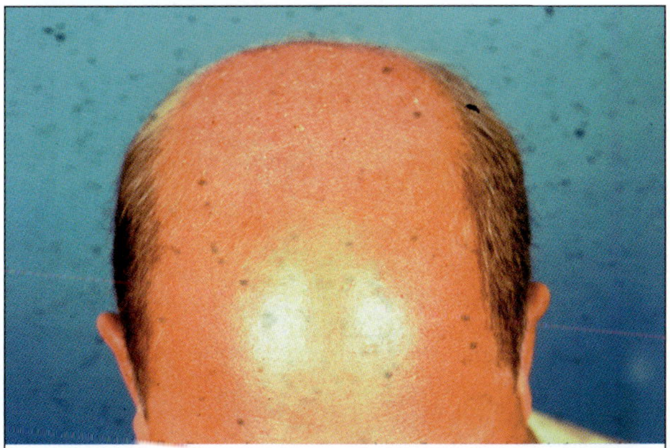

Before

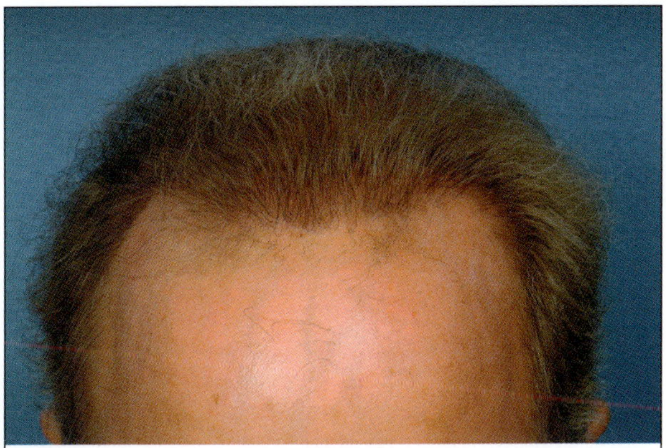

After

### Case 2: Male pattern hair loss
### Surgeon: Robert S. Haber, MD

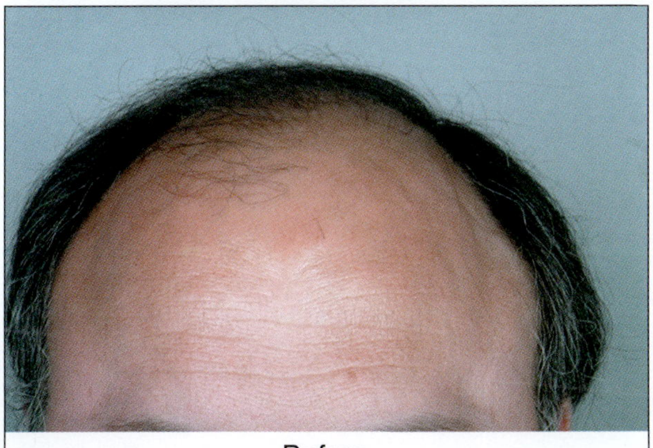

Before

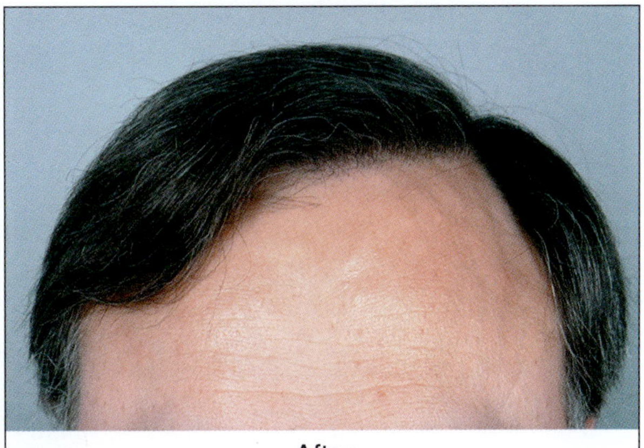

After

**Case 3: Correction of visible plugs**
**Surgeon: Bobby Limmer, MD**

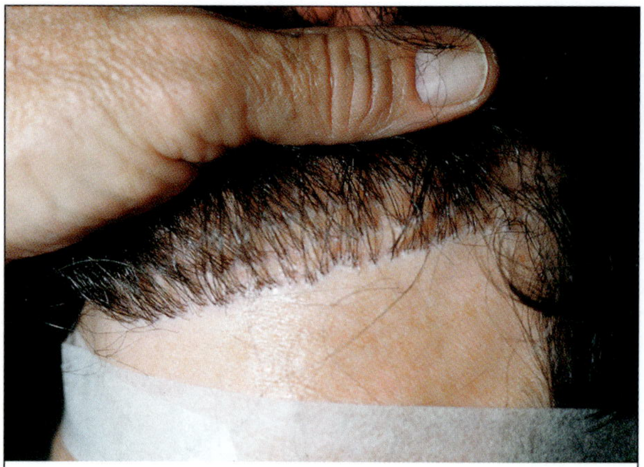

Before

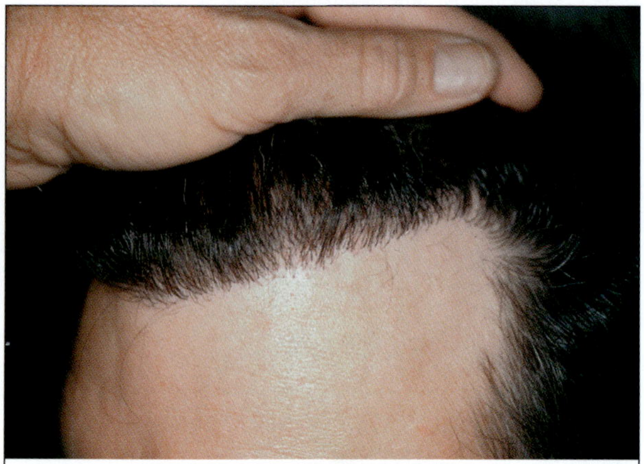

After

**Case 4: Eyebrow reconstruction**
**Surgeon: Michael Beehner, MD**

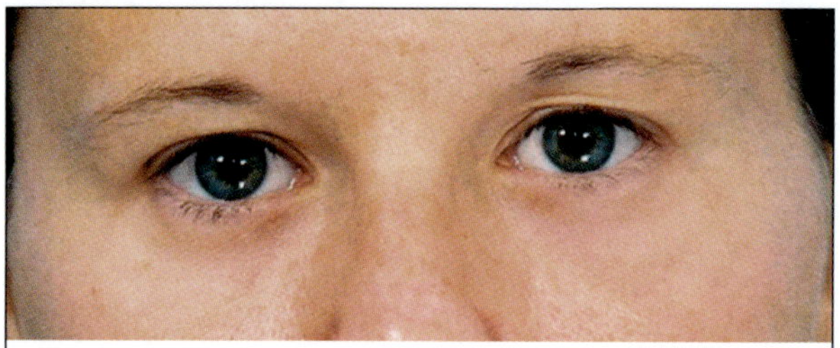

Before

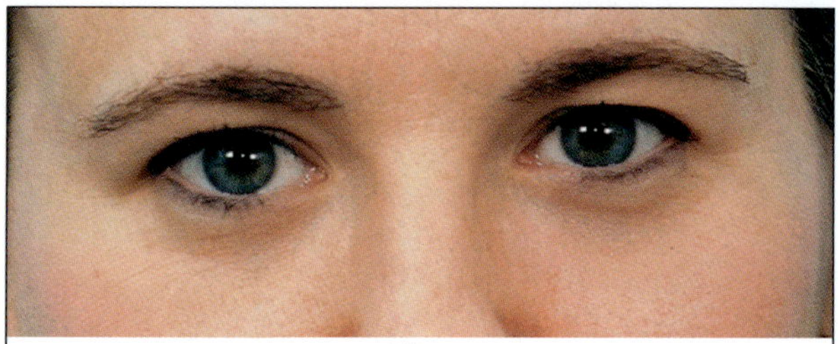

After

**Case 5: Male pattern hair loss**
**Surgeon: Damkerng Pathomvanich, MD**

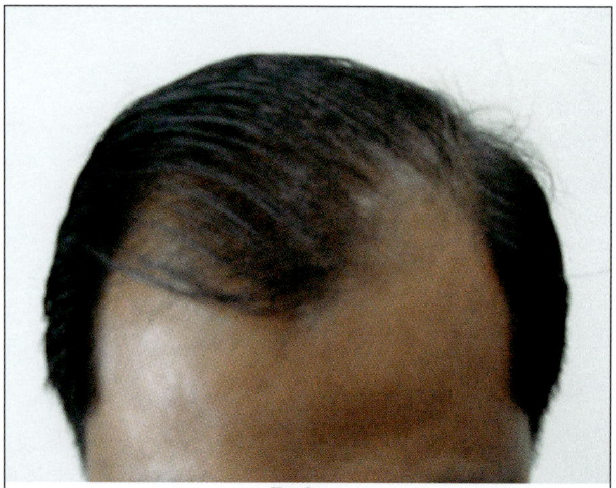

Before

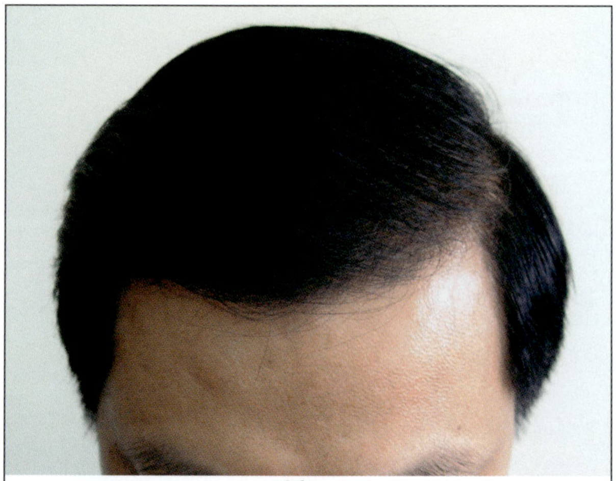

After

**Case 6: Correction of visible plugs**
**Surgeon: James E. Vogel, MD**

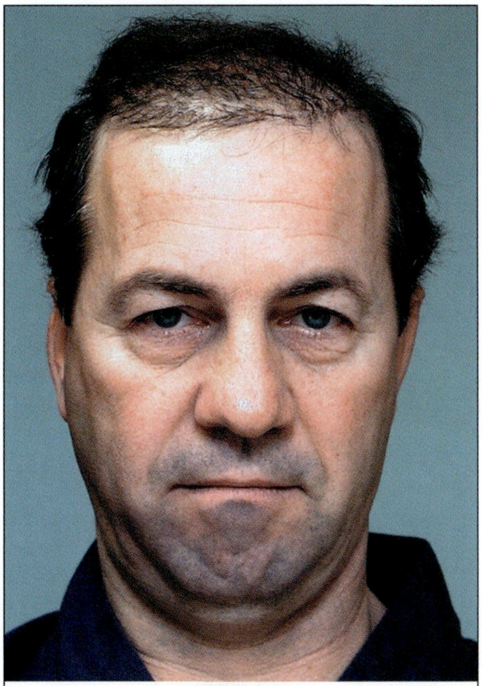
Before

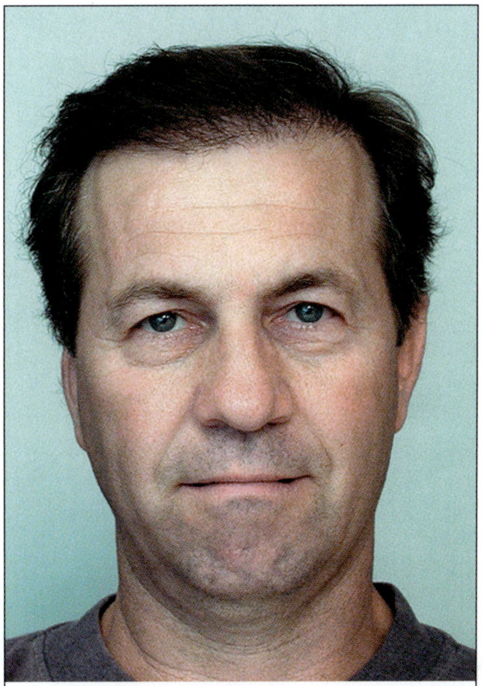
After

**Case 7: Male pattern hair loss**
**Surgeon: Victor Hasson, MD**

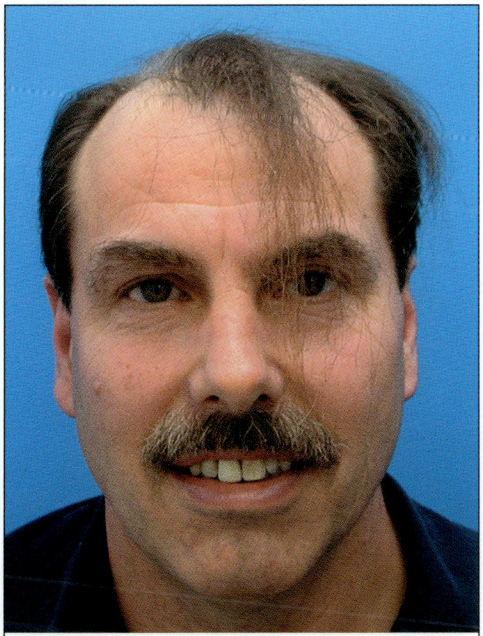
Before

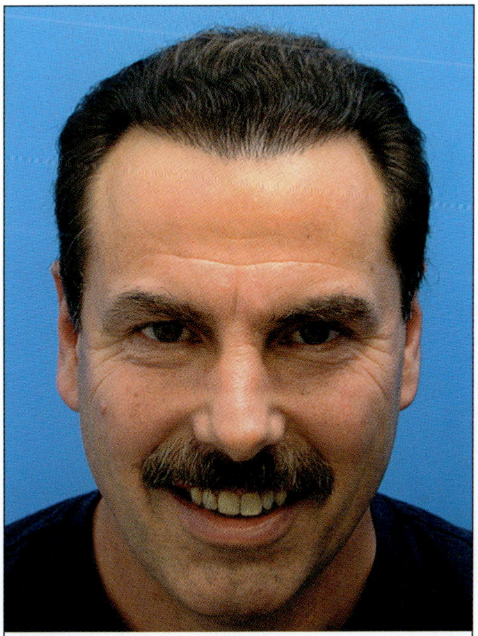
After

## Case 8: Male pattern hair loss
## Surgeon: Jerry E. Cooley, MD

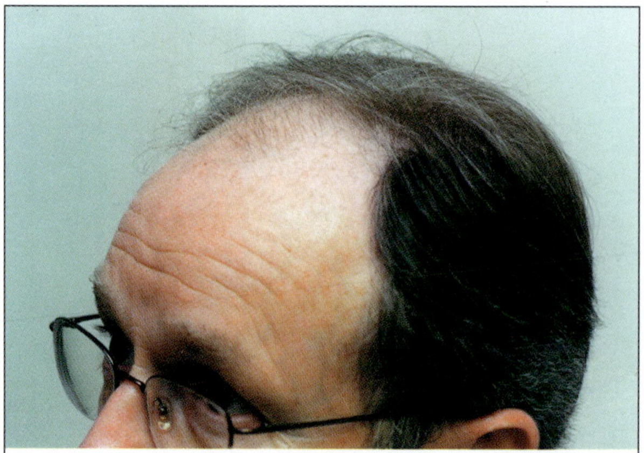
Before

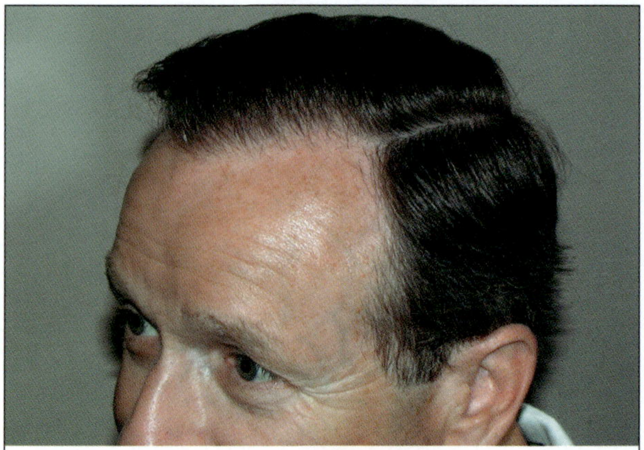
After

## Case 9: Male pattern hair loss
## Surgeon: James A. Harris, MD

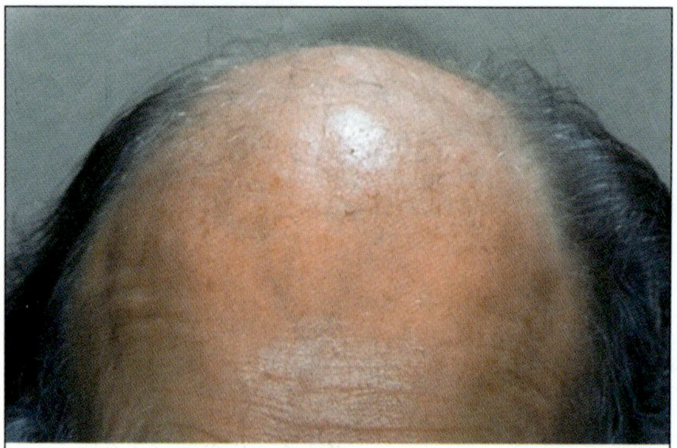
Before

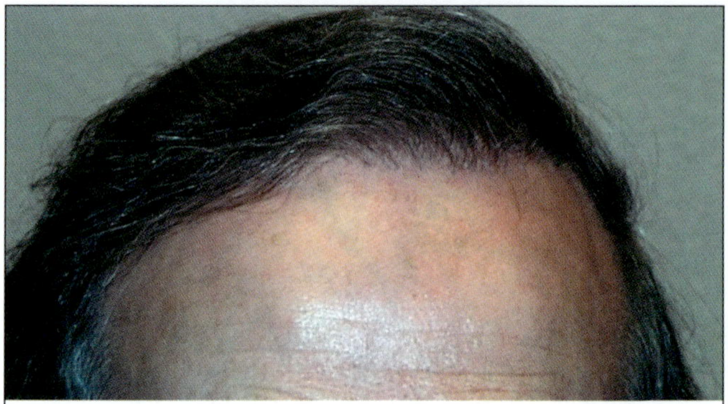
After

## Case 10: Female pattern hair loss
## Surgeon: Francisco Jimenez, MD

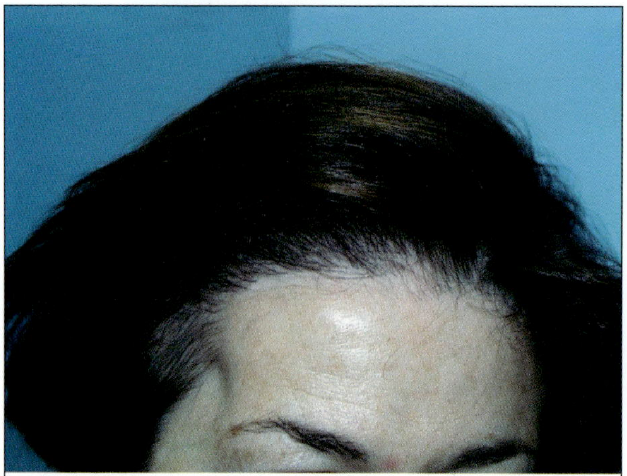
Before

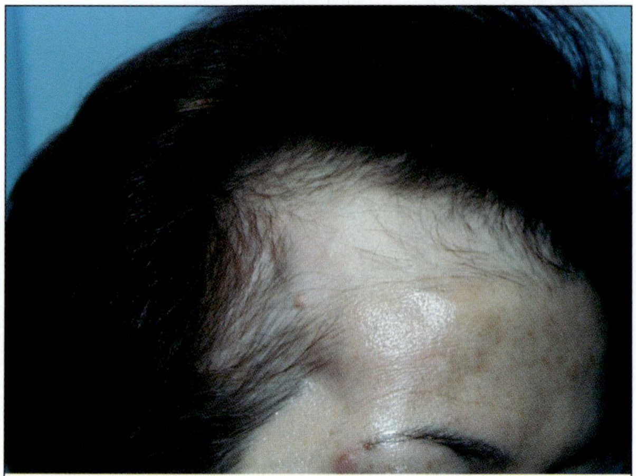
After

## Case 11: Male pattern hair loss
## Surgeon: Robert M. Bernstein, MD

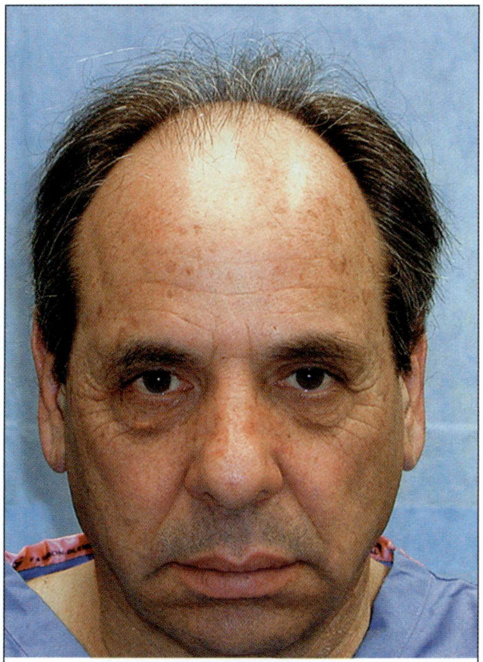
Before

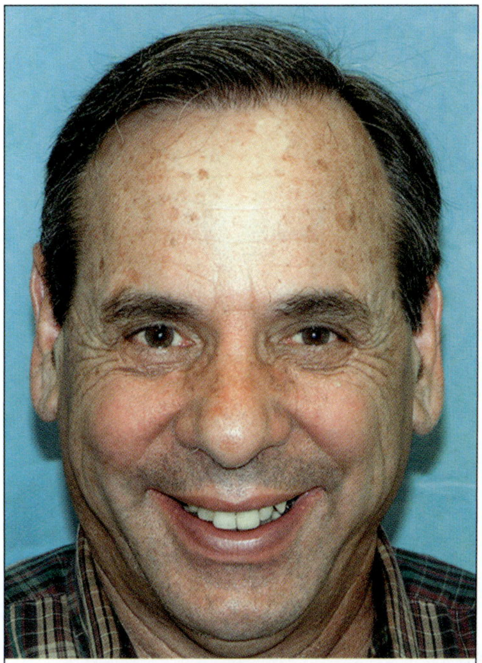
After

## Case 12: Male transgender transplantation
## Surgeon: Bernard Cohen, MD

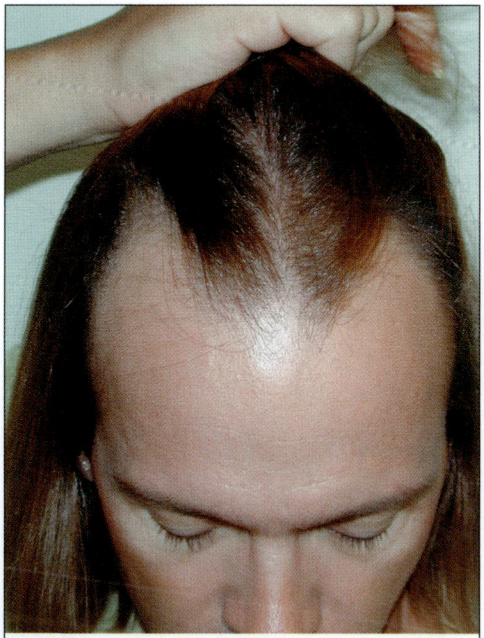
Before

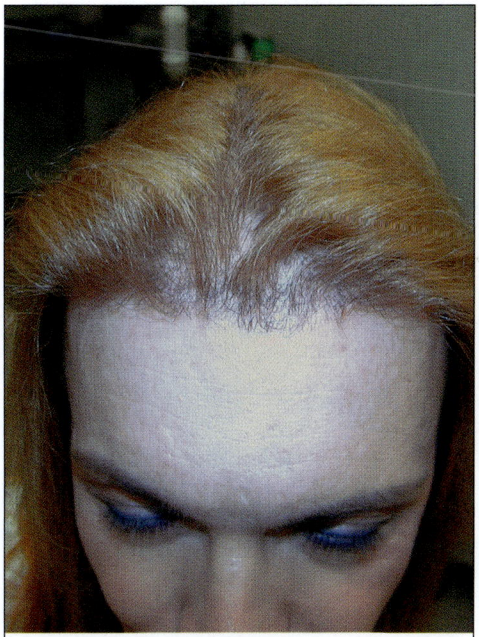
After

**Case 13: Male pattern hair loss**
**Surgeon: Russell Knudsen, MD**

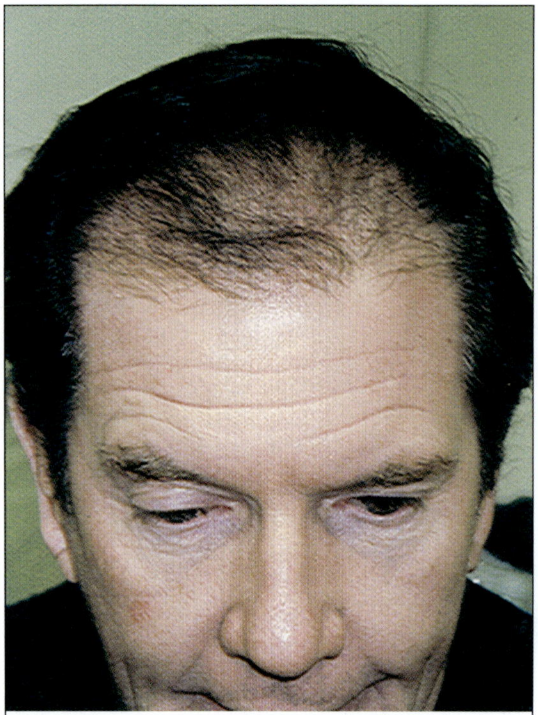
Before

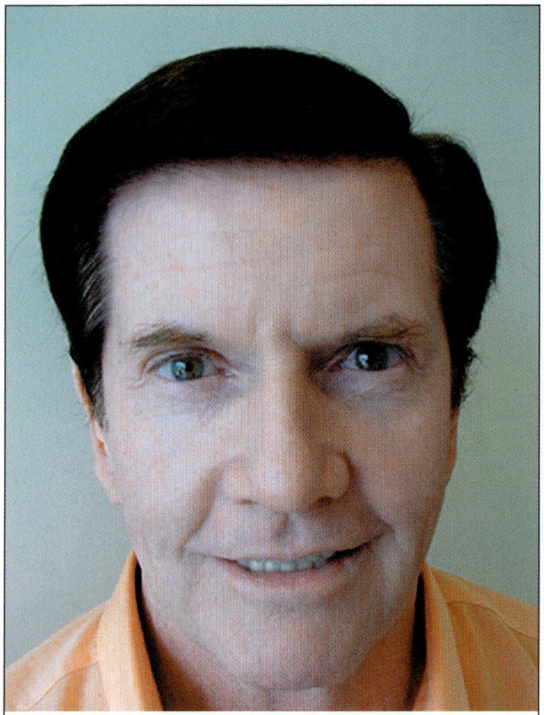
After

**Case 14: Female pattern hair loss**
**Surgeon: Matt L. Leavitt, DO**

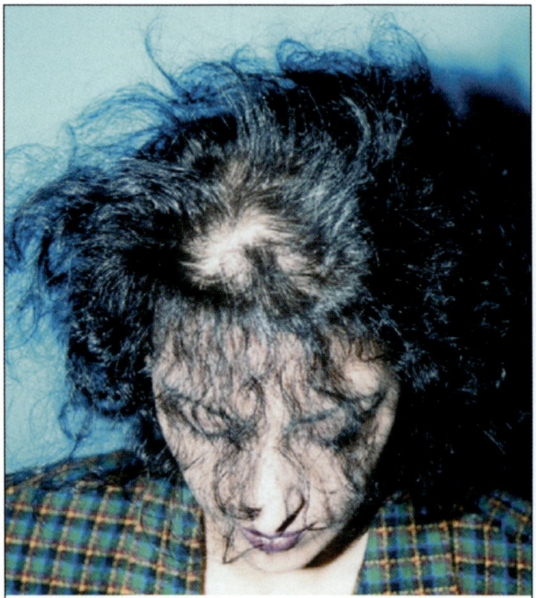
Before

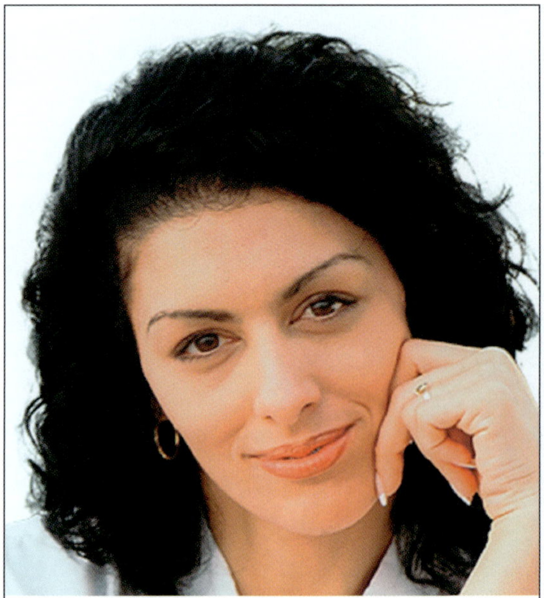
After

## Case 15: Male sideburn scar correction
## Surgeon: Bradley Limmer, MD

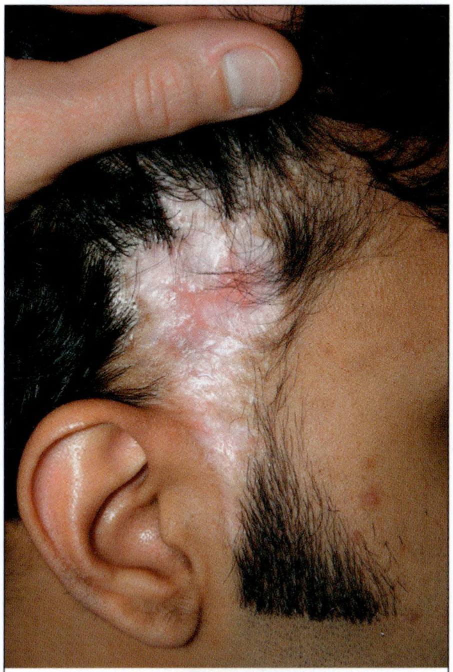

Before

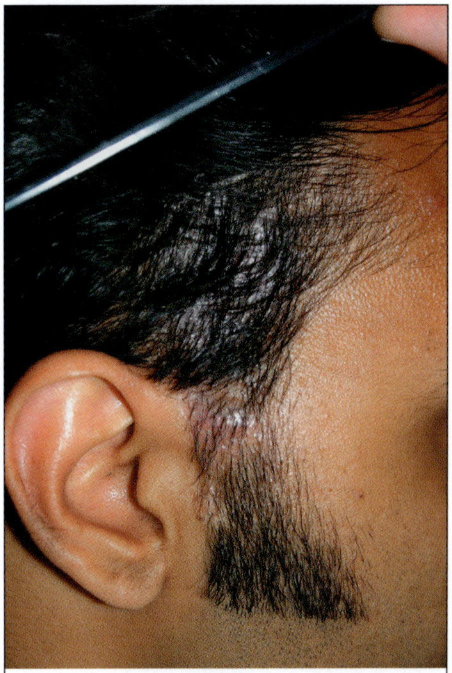

After

## Case 16: Male pattern hair loss
## Surgeon: Mario Marzole, MD

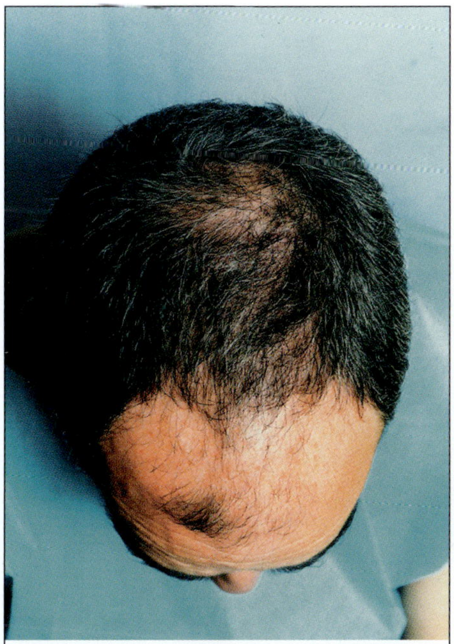

Before

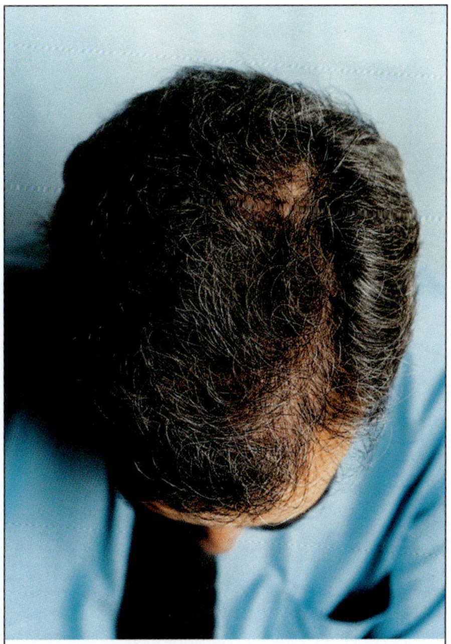

After

## Case 17: Male pattern hair loss
## Surgeon: William M. Parsley, MD

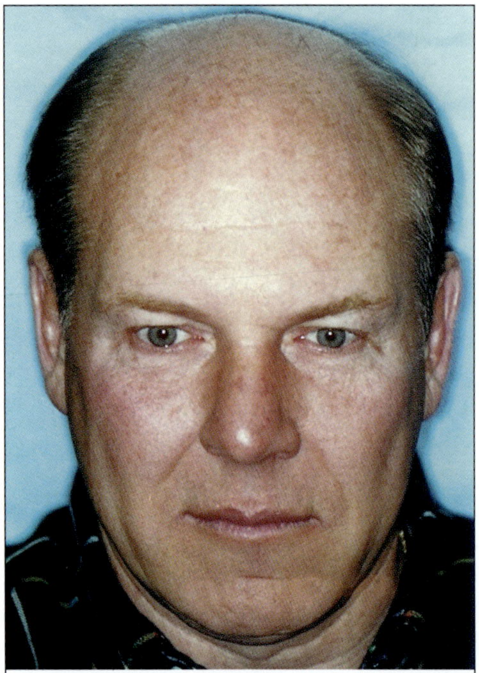

Before

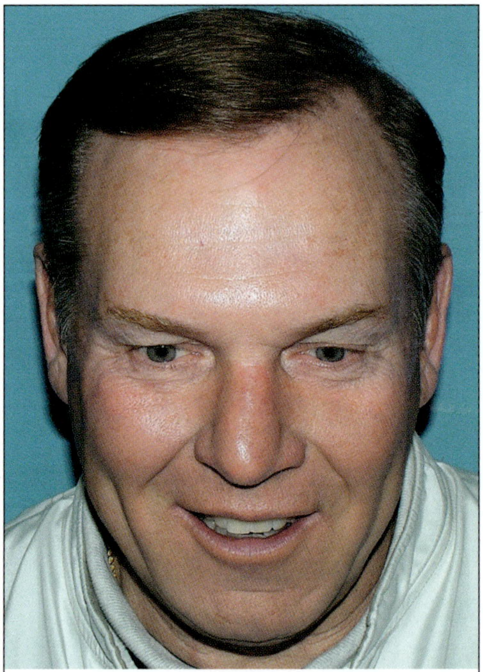

After

## Case 18: Male pattern hair loss
## Surgeon: William Rassman, MD

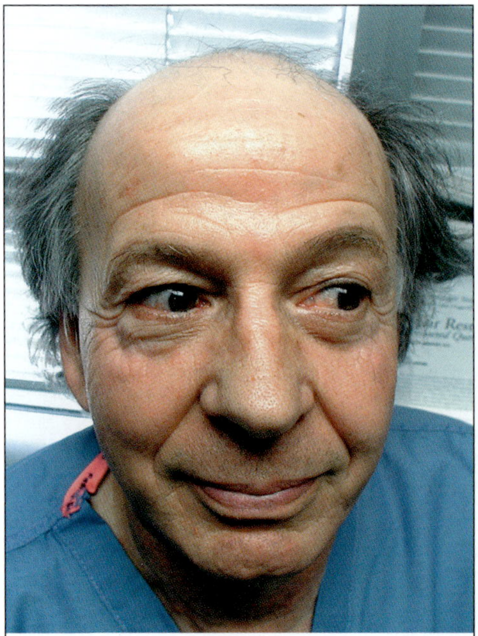

Before

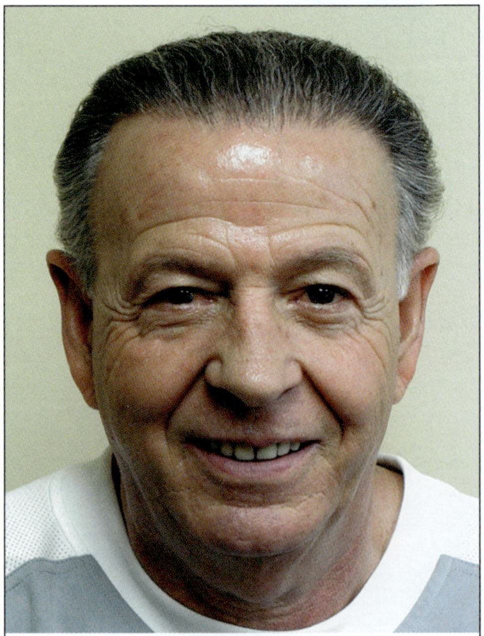

After

## Case 19: Male pattern hair loss
## Surgeon: Paul T. Rose, MD

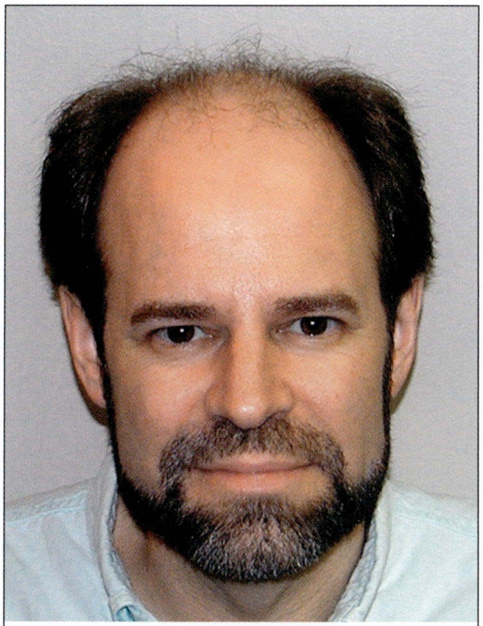
Before

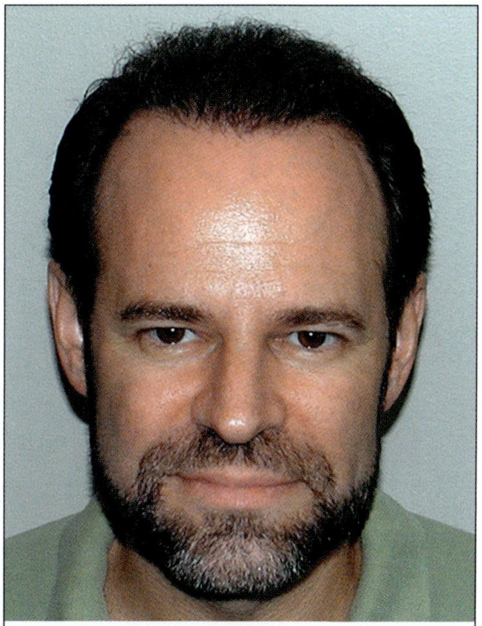
After

## Case 20: Male pattern hair loss
## Surgeon: Marc R. Avram, MD

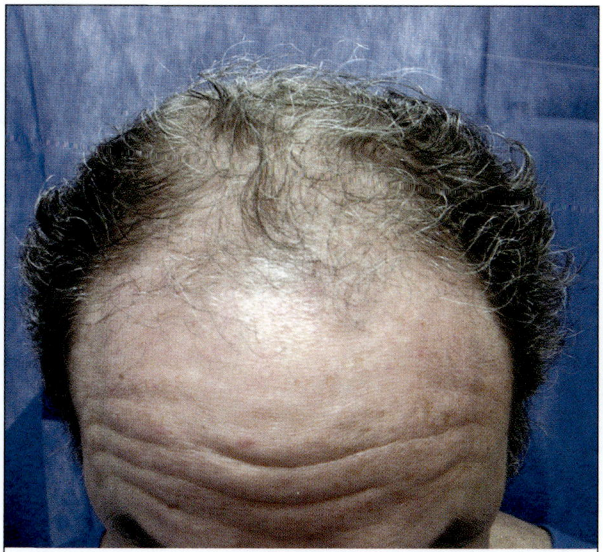
Before

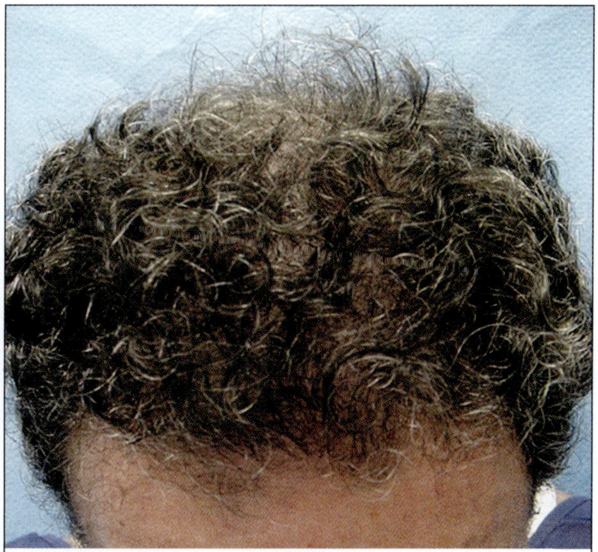
After

## Case 21: Male pattern hair loss
## Surgeon: David Seager, MD

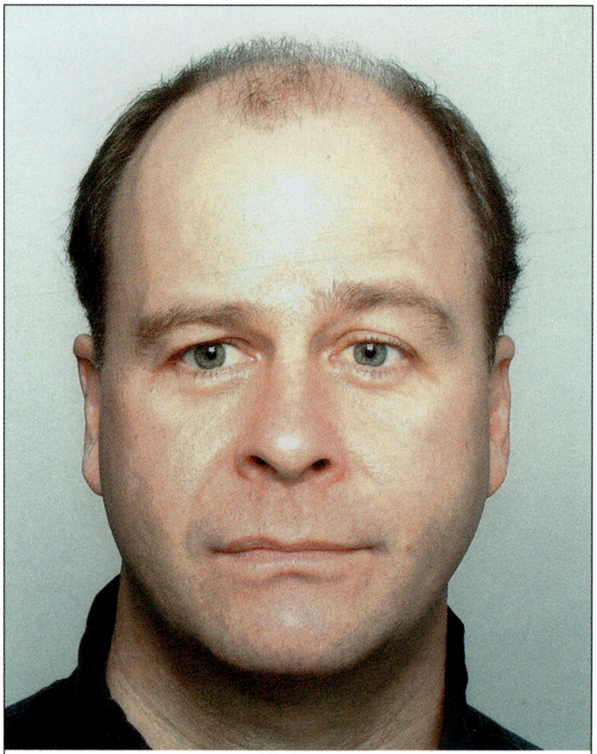

Before

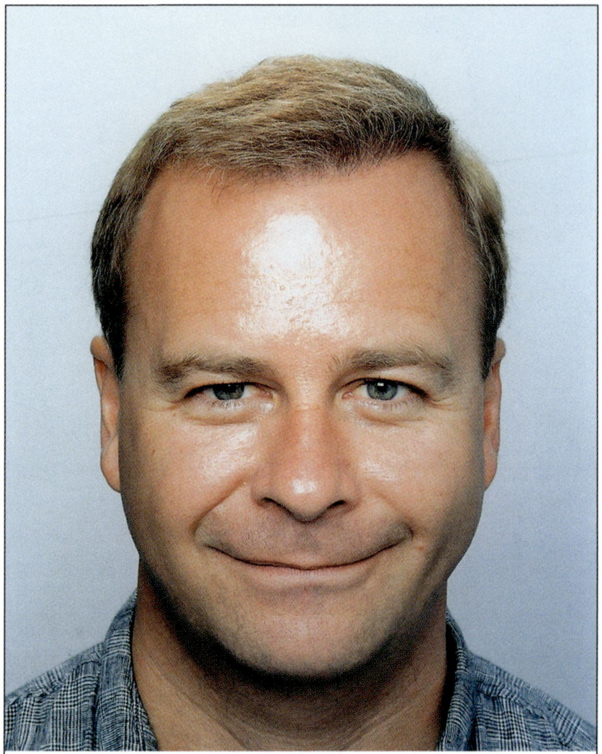

After

# Index

**Notes:** Page numbers in *italics* refer to figures while those in **bold** refer to tables/boxed material.
**Abbreviations:** abbreviations used as subentries include: FPHL, female pattern hair loss and MPHL, male pattern hair loss.

## C



## D

## E



## F

## R



## S

## ELSEVIER DVD-ROM LICENSE AGREEMENT

PLEASE READ THE FOLLOWING AGREEMENT CAREFULLY BEFORE USING THIS DVD-ROM PRODUCT. THIS DVD-ROM PRODUCT IS LICENSED UNDER THE TERMS CONTAINED IN THIS DVD-ROM LICENSE AGREEMENT ("Agreement"). BY USING THIS DVD-ROM PRODUCT, YOU, AN INDIVIDUAL OR ENTITY INCLUDING EMPLOYEES, AGENTS AND REPRESENTATIVES ("You" or "Your"), ACKNOWLEDGE THAT YOU HAVE READ THIS AGREEMENT, THAT YOU UNDERSTAND IT, AND THAT YOU AGREE TO BE BOUND BY THE TERMS AND CONDITIONS OF THIS AGREEMENT. ELSEVIER INC. ("Elsevier") EXPRESSLY DOES NOT AGREE TO LICENSE THIS DVD-ROM PRODUCT TO YOU UNLESS YOU ASSENT TO THIS AGREEMENT. IF YOU DO NOT AGREE WITH ANY OF THE FOLLOWING TERMS, YOU MAY, WITHIN THIRTY (30) DAYS AFTER YOUR RECEIPT OF THIS DVD-ROM PRODUCT RETURN THE UNUSED, PIN NUMBER PROTECTED, DVD-ROM PRODUCT, AND ALL ACCOMPANYING DOCUMENTATION TO ELSEVIER FOR A FULL REFUND.

**DEFINITIONS** As used in this Agreement, these terms shall have the following meanings:

"Proprietary Material" means the valuable and proprietary information content of this DVD-ROM Product including all indexes and graphic materials and software used to access, index, search and retrieve the information content from this DVD-ROM Product developed or licensed by Elsevier and/or its affiliates, suppliers and licensors.

"DVD-ROM Product" means the copy of the Proprietary Material and any other material delivered on DVD-ROM and any other human-readable or machine-readable materials enclosed with this Agreement, including without limitation documentation relating to the same.

**OWNERSHIP** This DVD-ROM Product has been supplied by and is proprietary to Elsevier and/or its affiliates, suppliers and licensors. The copyright in the DVD-ROM Product belongs to Elsevier and/or its affiliates, suppliers and licensors and is protected by the national and state copyright, trademark, trade secret and other intellectual property laws of the United States and international treaty provisions, including without limitation the Universal Copyright Convention and the Berne Copyright Convention. You have no ownership rights in this DVD-ROM Product. Except as expressly set forth herein, no part of this DVD-ROM Product, including without limitation the Proprietary Material, may be modified, copied or distributed in hardcopy or machine-readable form without prior written consent from Elsevier. All rights not expressly granted to You herein are expressly reserved. Any other use of this DVD-ROM Product by any person or entity is strictly prohibited and a violation of this Agreement.

**SCOPE OF RIGHTS LICENSED (PERMITTED USES)** Elsevier is granting to You a limited, non-exclusive, non-transferable license to use this DVD-ROM Product in accordance with the terms of this Agreement. You may use or provide access to this DVD-ROM Product on a single computer or terminal physically located at Your premises and in a secure network or move this DVD-ROM Product to and use it on another single computer or terminal at the same location for personal use only, but under no circumstances may You use or provide access to any part or parts of this DVD-ROM Product on more than one computer or terminal simultaneously.

You shall not (a) copy, download, or otherwise reproduce the DVD-ROM Product in any medium, including, without limitation, online transmissions, local area networks, wide area networks, intranets, extranets and the Internet, or in any way, in whole or in part, except for printing out or downloading nonsubstantial portions of the text and images in the DVD-ROM Product for Your own personal use; (b) alter, modify, or adapt the DVD-ROM Product, including but not limited to decompiling, disassembling, reverse engineering, or creating derivative works, without the prior written approval of Elsevier; (c) sell, license or otherwise distribute to third parties the DVD-ROM Product or any part or parts thereof; or (d) alter, remove, obscure or obstruct the display of any copyright, trademark or other proprietary notice on or in the DVD-ROM Product or on any printout or download of portions of the Proprietary Materials.

**RESTRICTIONS ON TRANSFER** This License is personal to You, and neither Your rights hereunder nor the tangible embodiments of this DVD-ROM Product, including without limitation the Proprietary Material, may be sold, assigned, transferred or sublicensed to any other person, including without limitation by operation of law, without the prior written consent of Elsevier. Any purported sale, assignment, transfer or sublicense without the prior written consent of Elsevier will be void and will automatically terminate the License granted hereunder.

**TERM** This Agreement will remain in effect until terminated pursuant to the terms of this Agreement. You may terminate this Agreement at any time by removing from Your system and destroying the DVD-ROM Product. Unauthorized copying of the DVD-ROM Product, including without limitation, the Proprietary Material and documentation, or otherwise failing to comply with the terms and conditions of this Agreement shall result in automatic termination of this license and will make available to Elsevier legal remedies. Upon termination of this Agreement, the license granted herein will terminate and You must immediately destroy the DVD-ROM Product and accompanying documentation. All provisions relating to proprietary rights shall survive termination of this Agreement.

**LIMITED WARRANTY AND LIMITATION OF LIABILITY** NEITHER ELSEVIER NOR ITS LICENSORS REPRESENT OR WARRANT THAT THE DVD-ROM PRODUCT WILL MEET YOUR REQUIREMENTS OR THAT ITS OPERATION WILL BE UNINTERRUPTED OR ERROR-FREE. WE EXCLUDE AND EXPRESSLY DISCLAIM ALL EXPRESS AND IMPLIED WARRANTIES NOT STATED HEREIN, INCLUDING THE IMPLIED WARRANTIES OF MERCHANTABILITY AND FITNESS FOR A PARTICULAR PURPOSE. IN ADDITION, NEITHER ELSEVIER NOR ITS LICENSORS MAKE ANY REPRESENTATIONS OR WARRANTIES, EITHER EXPRESS OR IMPLIED, REGARDING THE PERFORMANCE OF YOUR NETWORK OR COMPUTER SYSTEM WHEN USED IN CONJUNCTION WITH THE DVD-ROM PRODUCT. WE SHALL NOT BE LIABLE FOR ANY DAMAGE OR LOSS OF ANY KIND ARISING OUT OF OR RESULTING FROM YOUR POSSESSION OR USE OF THE SOFTWARE PRODUCT CAUSED BY ERRORS OR OMISSIONS, DATA LOSS OR CORRUPTION, ERRORS OR OMISSIONS IN THE PROPRIETARY MATERIAL, REGARDLESS OF WHETHER SUCH LIABILITY IS BASED IN TORT, CONTRACT OR OTHERWISE AND INCLUDING, BUT NOT LIMITED TO, ACTUAL, SPECIAL, INDIRECT, INCIDENTAL OR CONSEQUENTIAL DAMAGES. IF THE FOREGOING LIMITATION IS HELD TO BE UNENFORCEABLE, OUR MAXIMUM LIABILITY TO YOU SHALL NOT EXCEED THE AMOUNT OF THE LICENSE FEE PAID BY YOU FOR THE SOFTWARE PRODUCT. THE REMEDIES AVAILABLE TO YOU AGAINST US AND THE LICENSORS OF MATERIALS INCLUDED IN THE SOFTWARE PRODUCT ARE EXCLUSIVE.

If this DVD-ROM Product is defective, Elsevier will replace it at no charge if the defective DVD-ROM Product is returned to Elsevier within sixty (60) days (or the greatest period allowable by applicable law) from the date of shipment.

Elsevier warrants that the software embodied in this DVD-ROM Product will perform in substantial compliance with the documentation supplied in this DVD-ROM Product. If You report a significant defect in performance in writing to Elsevier, and Elsevier is not able to correct same within sixty (60) days after its receipt of Your notification, You may return this DVD-ROM Product, including all copies and documentation, to Elsevier and Elsevier will refund Your money.

YOU UNDERSTAND THAT, EXCEPT FOR THE 60-DAY LIMITED WARRANTY RECITED ABOVE, ELSEVIER, ITS AFFILIATES, LICENSORS, SUPPLIERS AND AGENTS, MAKE NO WARRANTIES, EXPRESSED OR IMPLIED, WITH RESPECT TO THE DVD-ROM PRODUCT, INCLUDING, WITHOUT LIMITATION THE PROPRIETARY MATERIAL, AND SPECIFICALLY DISCLAIM ANY WARRANTY OF MERCHANTABILITY OR FITNESS FOR A PARTICULAR PURPOSE.

If the information provided on this DVD-ROM Product contains medical or health sciences information, it is intended for professional use within the medical field. Information about medical treatment or drug dosages is intended strictly for professional use, and because of rapid advances in the medical sciences, independent verification of diagnosis and drug dosages should be made.

IN NO EVENT WILL ELSEVIER, ITS AFFILIATES, LICENSORS, SUPPLIERS OR AGENTS, BE LIABLE TO YOU FOR ANY DAMAGES, INCLUDING, WITHOUT LIMITATION, ANY LOST PROFITS, LOST SAVINGS OR OTHER INCIDENTAL OR CONSEQUENTIAL DAMAGES, ARISING OUT OF YOUR USE OR INABILITY TO USE THE DVD-ROM PRODUCT REGARDLESS OF WHETHER SUCH DAMAGES ARE FORESEEABLE OR WHETHER SUCH DAMAGES ARE DEEMED TO RESULT FROM THE FAILURE OR INADEQUACY OF ANY EXCLUSIVE OR OTHER REMEDY.

**U.S. GOVERNMENT RESTRICTED RIGHTS** The DVD-ROM Product and documentation are provided with restricted rights. Use, duplication or disclosure by the U.S. Government is subject to restrictions as set forth in subparagraphs (a) through (d) of the Commercial Computer Restricted Rights clause at FAR 52.22719 or in subparagraph (c)(1)(ii) of the Rights in Technical Data and Computer Software clause at DFARS 252.2277013, or at 252.2117015, as applicable. Contractor/Manufacturer is Elsevier Inc., 360 Park Avenue South, New York, NY 10010 USA.

**GOVERNING LAW** This Agreement shall be governed by the laws of the State of New York, USA. In any dispute arising out of this Agreement, You and Elsevier each consent to the exclusive personal jurisdiction and venue in the state and federal courts within New York County, New York, USA.